AF688823

A Clinician's Guide to Joint Replacement

A Clinician's Guide to Joint Replacement

Editor: Finley Heron

AMERICAN
MEDICAL PUBLISHERS
www.americanmedicalpublishers.com

AMERICAN
MEDICAL PUBLISHERS
www.americanmedicalpublishers.com

Cataloging-in-Publication Data

A clinician's guide to joint replacement / edited by Finley Heron.
p. cm.
Includes bibliographical references and index.
ISBN 978-1-63927-846-6
1. Arthroplasty. 2. Total hip replacement. 3. Artificial joints. 4. Joints--Surgery.
5. Hip joint--Diseases--Treatment. 6. Orthopedics--Diagnosis. 7. Orthopedics--Treatment.
I. Heron, Finley.
RD686 .C55 2023
617.472 059 7--dc23

© American Medical Publishers, 2023

American Medical Publishers,
41 Flatbush Avenue,
1st Floor, New York,
NY 11217, USA

ISBN 978-1-63927-846-6 (Hardback)

This book contains information obtained from authentic and highly regarded sources. Copyright for all individual chapters remain with the respective authors as indicated. All chapters are published with permission under the Creative Commons Attribution License or equivalent. A wide variety of references are listed. Permission and sources are indicated; for detailed attributions, please refer to the permissions page and list of contributors. Reasonable efforts have been made to publish reliable data and information, but the authors, editors and publisher cannot assume any responsibility for the validity of all materials or the consequences of their use.

Trademark Notice: Registered trademark of products or corporate names are used only for explanation and identification without intent to infringe.

Contents

Preface

Joint replacement is a surgical procedure concerned with the replacement of a damaged joint with an artificial joint. The artificial joints used in orthopedic surgeries are composed of metals, ceramics or plastics. There are various types of joint replacement surgeries, namely, hip replacement, shoulder replacement and knee replacement. Electrocardiogram, chest-X rays, CT scan and MRI are some commonly used pre-operative evaluation tests. A joint replacement surgery helps to relieve the symptoms like joint pain, joint stiffness and inflammation. There are some risks and complications associated with joint replacement, including heart attack, stroke, urinary tract infection, venous thromboembolism and pneumonia. This book includes some of the vital pieces of work being conducted across the world, on various topics related to joint replacement. It strives to provide a fair idea about this medical procedure and to help develop a better understanding of the latest advances related to this medical procedure.

This book is a comprehensive compilation of works of different researchers from varied parts of the world. It includes valuable experiences of the researchers with the sole objective of providing the readers (learners) with a proper knowledge of the concerned field. This book will be beneficial in evoking inspiration and enhancing the knowledge of the interested readers.

In the end, I would like to extend my heartiest thanks to the authors who worked with great determination on their chapters. I also appreciate the publisher's support in the course of the book. I would also like to deeply acknowledge my family who stood by me as a source of inspiration during the project.

Editor

1

Institutionally Adopted Perioperative Blood Management Program Significantly Decreased the Transfusion Rate of Patients Having Primary Total Hip Replacement Surgery

Hargita Dömötör,[1] Ádám L. Varga,[1] Róbert Sződy,[2] Ferenc Tóth,[2] and Gábor Nardai[1]

[1]*Department of Anesthesiology and Intensive Care, Péterfy Hospital and National Institute of Trauma, Budapest, Hungary*
[2]*Department of Traumatology, Péterfy Hospital and National Institute of Trauma, 1081, Fiumei út 17, Budapest, Hungary*

Correspondence should be addressed to Gábor Nardai; nardai@hotmail.com

Perioperative transfusion in patients undergoing orthopedic surgery increases the number of postoperative complications. Thus, we have introduced an institution-tailored perioperative blood management program (PBM) to decrease the amount of blood transfused in patients going through primary total hip replacement (THR) surgery. We have conducted a before-after observational cohort study in two predetermined observational periods. Demographic and clinical data, ASA scores, laboratory parameters, features of surgical procedure, and anesthesia were registered. Parameters of perioperative fluid administration, transfusion rate, and postoperative complications were also assessed. One hundred patients in the first and 108 patients in the second observational period were enrolled. Eventhough the ratio of posttraumatic THR procedures increased (9% vs. 17%), the PBM protocol has been utilized effectively and a significant decrease in perioperative blood transfusion rate has been observed (61% vs. 21%). The abolishment of routine preoperative LMWH prophylaxis (90% vs. 16%), intraoperative use of tranexamic acid (10% vs. 84%), and the encouraged exploitation of our postoperative observational facility (5% vs. 39%) were abided by our colleagues. Patients still requiring transfusion had lower preoperative hemoglobin levels (129 vs. 147 g/l), scored higher in ASA (ASA III: 46% vs. 19%), and more often presented postoperative hypotension (40% vs. 7%), oliguria (23% vs. 5%), and infections (9% vs. 2%). We conclude that the individualized perioperative blood management protocol was successfully implemented and yielded a lower transfusion rate and better outcomes. Our study suggests that a partial, institution-tailored PBM program may be suitable and beneficial in countries where the modalities of perioperative blood management are limited.

1. Introduction

Total hip replacement surgery is one of the most common orthopedic procedures with a considerable risk of bleeding. We have high-quality evidence that excessive transfusion, besides depleting the national blood reserve, increases the number of postoperative complications, hospital length-of-stay [1], and costs [2]; thus, every healthcare provider has a responsibility to take measures to reduce blood transfusion rates. In our institution, a preliminary audit has shown that among patients undergoing THR, the transfusion rate is above 50% (local audit 2012, data not shown). This result validated the creation of a program aiming to reduce blood use in perioperative care. The program incorporated the elements of the internationally approved perioperative blood management (PBM) concept: preoperative anemia screening and management, reduction of perioperative blood loss, postoperative anemia tolerance, and individualized transfusion therapy [3]. However, whether partial implementation of the program results in transfusion benefit is yet to be clarified. A local clinical advisory board was set up to determine which of the possible measures could both be feasible and have merit in our institution's setting.

2. Methods

2.1. Development of the Institution-Tailored Protocol (Table 1). Clinical advisory board (senior anesthesiologist—leader, consultant orthopedic surgeons, and critical care specialists) assembled the interventions integrated into the local PBM program, and the following elements were introduced by institutional guidelines and staff education: (a) careful preoperative screening program for anemia (Hgb < 120 g/l). The preoperative anesthesia visits for patients undergoing THR have been scheduled at least 3 weeks prior to surgery whenever possible. Anemic patients were referred for anemia management, and surgeries were delayed if necessary. (b) Individualized vs. routine administration of preoperative LMWH, based on the patient's risk of thromboembolism. (c) Routine administration of 15 mg/kg intravenous bolus tranexamic acid on incision has been incorporated in our THR protocol as it is shown that tranexamic acid can significantly reduce intraoperative blood loss, and if the presence of contraindications is carefully evaluated, complications are rare [4]. (d) Leaving wound drains after major joint replacement surgery is a controversial topic among orthopedic surgeons. Due to the complexity and controversy of the topic, the omission of wound drain use has not been made mandatory, but only encouraged and ultimately entrusted to the surgeon's judgment. (e) Viscoelastometry-based point-of-care, goal-directed hemostasis treatment using rotational thromboelastometry (ROTEM) has been introduced in the management of major/massive surgical bleeding. (f) The practice of restrictive transfusion is one that requires both extensive training of personnel and the development of facilities that allow continuous monitoring of the patients in the early postoperative period. We have extended the postoperative high-dependency unit with the capacity to observe patients undergoing major joint replacement with moderate-to-high cardiovascular or bleeding risk for the critical first 24 hours led by an anesthetist. (g) We have also conducted institution-wide education among doctors and nurses working in surgical wards on the principles and practice of restrictive transfusion policy. Single unit transfusion and clinical reassessment applicable has also become a recommended, although not obligatory, policy. These measures ensure patient safety while allowing practitioners to determine the patient's individual physiologic tolerance of anemia, thus providing a wider range of tolerable hemoglobin levels. (h) To ratify this novel policy, we have established an administrative control on transfusion that requires practitioners to specify the indication (hemodynamic instability, chest pain, dyspnea, and active bleeding) of transfusion on the request form if the patient's hemoglobin level is above 80 g/l.

Perioperative erythropoietin treatment as a modality of anemia management has not been implemented due to its unavailability in Hungary.

The routine use of cell salvage devices has not been incorporated in our policy either. Eventhough they are proven to be efficient in reducing the transfusion ratio, this concerns mostly procedures with the anticipated blood loss of more than 1000 ml [3]; whereas, in our institution, the average intraoperative blood loss during THR is 300–800 ml (local audit 2012, data not shown); thus, we deemed the cost-benefit ratio unfavourable.

The summary of the measures implemented compared to general PBM elements is given in Table 1.

2.2. Data Collection. A periinterventional, single-center, before-after study with prospective data collection was approved by local clinical directory board. Patients: adult patients having primary THR surgery in a three-month period of 2013 and 2016. Data were collected from electronic charts of the hospital informatics system, blood bank, and paper-based charts of anesthesia, surgery, and postoperative care until discharge. TXA dose has been predetermined as 15 mg/kg single bolus infusion at the incision. Oliguria and anuria (urine output < 0,5 ml/kg/h) have been recorded in the 6th, 12th, and 24th hours postoperatively. Perioperative hypotension was defined as systolic blood pressure under 100 Hg mm measured intraoperatively and in the first 24 hours postoperatively. Comparisons were made between the 2013 and 2016 groups regarding demographics, clinical data, type of anesthesia, basic features, and indication of surgical procedure. We have also examined the utilization ratio of PBM measures, the corresponding change in transfusion rate, complications, and hospital length-of-stay. Long term follow-up (3 months) of infection-related complications (surgical and systemic) has only been performed in the after period (2016) using the data of the electronic hospital chart.

2.3. Statistical Analysis. Data are given as mean with 95% confidence interval or as a percentage of the total and the amount of blood transfused as a ratio with the number of patients that received transfusion in the denominator. The significance of differences between groups was analyzed by Mann–Whitney, chi-square, and Fischer tests as applicable. A p value < 0.05 was considered statistically significant.

3. Results

3.1. Comparison of the Population of 2013 and 2016. Demographic and clinical data of the population are given in Table 2.

There were no significant differences between demographic data, preexisting clinical features, modality of anesthesia, length, and technique of surgery between 2013 and 2016 as given in Table 2. Eventhough it did not achieve statistical significance, the increase of posttraumatic surgeries (vs. osteoarthritis) is notable.

There has been a significant increase in the utilization of all institutionally approved PBM measures (Table 3). The use of tranexamic acid has become part of the routine unless contraindications are present. Admission ratio to postoperative high-dependency units increased significantly, granting greater safety to patients with higher anesthetic risk. A restrictive hemoglobin trigger has been kept unless an indication of keeping a higher hemoglobin level was present.

Table 1: Elements of the general PBM program as integrated into our institutional protocol.

Anemia screening/correction	Preoperative screening	Yes	Surgery, if Hgb > 120 g/l
	Anemia correction, iron supplements	Yes	
	Anemia correction, EPO treatment	No	Off label in Hungary
Minimizing blood loss	Less invasive surgical technique	No	Not changed during study period
	Tranexamic acid administration	Yes	Liberal use
	Autologous blood donation	No	Not supported by national blood service
	Hemostasis optimization, preoperative	Yes	Preoperative LMWH only if high risk
	Hemostasis optimization, intra/postoperative	Yes	Viscoelastometry-guided protocol
	Cell salvage techniques	No	Not beneficial
	Normothermia	Yes	
Increasing anemia tolerance	Advanced postoperative care	Yes	Postop HDU introduced
Rational hemotherapy	Restrictive transfusion threshold	Yes	Transfusion, if Hgb < 80 g/l

Table 2: Demographic and clinical data of the population. Data are shown as mean (CI 95%) and percentage of the total.

	2013 ($n = 100$)	2016 ($n = 108$)	
Age (years)	68 (65–70)	68 (66–69)	ns
Female (%)	70	64	ns
ASA III. (%)	22	21	ns
BMI (kg/m^2)	28.1 (27.8–28.9)	28 (27.7–29.0)	ns
Preoperative Hgb level (g/l)	138 (135–141)	126 (123–129)	ns
Antiplatelet therapy (%)	16	10	ns
Indication: hip fracture (%)	9	16,6	ns
Neuraxial anesthesia (%)	80	84	ns
Length of surgery (min)	90 (84.9–95.1)	100 (95–105)	ns
Cemented THR (%)	73	74	ns

Table 3: Implementation ratio of the elements of the local PBM program.

	2013 ($n = 100$)	2016 ($n = 108$)	
Preoperative LMWH (%)	90	16	$P< 0.05$
Tranexamic acid (i.v.) (%)	10	84	$P < 0.05$
Wound drainage (%)	100	89	$P < 0.05$
Postoperative HDU admission (%)	5	39	$P < 0.05$
Transfusion trigger < 80 g/l (%)	5	86	$P < 0.05$

A significant difference has been observed in the transfusion ratio of the before and after groups (61% vs. 21%), eventhough there was no significant disparity in fluid administration, postoperative hemoglobin levels, and hospital length-of-stay. In the after group, patients suffered from postoperative hypotension significantly less frequently (12% vs. 35%), but there was no significant difference in the incidence of oligoanuria. The amount of blood received by patients transfused has shown minimal change (Table 4).

3.2. Assessment of Clinical Features and Transfusion Requirements in 2016. Clinical data and complications between transfused and not transfused patients in 2016 are given in Table 5.

Between the transfused and not transfused groups, there was no significant difference in age, surgical, and anesthetic technique. Patients that received transfusion had a significantly higher anesthetic risk (ASA III, 20% vs. 50%), and their preoperative hemoglobin levels were significantly lower. They received tranexamic acid significantly less often (64% vs. 91%) and presented hypotension (7% vs. 40%) and oliguria (5% vs. 23%) in the first 24 hours at a significantly higher rate. Infection rates were significantly higher among patients who needed to receive a blood transfusion (Table 5).

4. Discussion

Based on the results above, we can declare that our institution-tailored perioperative blood management protocol was successfully implemented and had a significant impact on postoperative transfusion rates and complications. This supports the assumption that it is not required to execute every element of the PBM program to beneficially influence perioperative transfusion needs.

Improving hemostasis in the entire perioperative period and upgrading postoperative care are the most important pillars of success in our opinion. Research data are conflicted regarding preoperative or postoperative administration of prophylactic LMWH concerning perioperative blood loss. Robust studies found no difference in the effectiveness regarding prevention of thromboembolic events between those whose LMWH prophylaxis were initialized preoperatively and those who were started postoperatively if no indication other than the surgery itself was present [5]. Recent studies focusing on the effect of timing of LMWH

Table 4: Fluid management, transfusion rate, and complications. Data are shown as mean (CI 95%) and percentage of the total.

	2013 ($n = 100$)	2016 ($n = 108$)	
Crystalloids administered, intraoperative (ml)	3421 (3280–3560)	2872 (2720–3030)	ns
Crystalloids administered, postoperative (ml)	1319 (1160–1480)	2113 (1940–2280)	ns
Min. Hgb. level in postoperative 24 hours (g/l)	101 (98.5–104)	104 (101–107)	ns
Transfusion ratio (%)	61	21	$P < 0.05$
Units transfused RBC/number of transfused patients	3	2,8	ns
Postoperative hypotension/24 hours (%)	35	12	$P < 0.05$
Postoperative oligoanuria/24 hours (%)	5	8	ns
Hospital length-of-stay (days)	12	11	ns

Table 5: Clinical data and complications between transfused and not transfused patients in 2016. Data are shown as mean (CI 95%) and percentage of the total.

	Transfusion ($n = 85$)	Transfusion+ ($n = 22$)	
Age (years)	68	73	ns
ASA III (%)	20	50	$P < 0.05$
Length of surgery (min)	98 (93–103)	104 (84–119)	ns
Cemented THR (%)	72	84	ns
Indication: hip fracture (%)	14	27	ns
Preoperative Hgb level (g/l)	143 (140–146)	126 (129–133)	$P < 0.05$
Tranexamic acid i.v. (%)	91	64	$P < 0.05$
Neuraxial anesthesia (%)	86	77	ns
Postoperative hypotension/24 hours (%)	7	40	$P < 0.05$
Postoperative oligoanuria/24 hours (%)	5	23	$P < 0.05$
Infection rate* (%)/<3 months	2	9	$P < 0.001$

*Surgical and systemic infections.

prophylaxis on bleeding risk were not conclusive [6, 7]. In patients with the indication of hip fracture, immobilization as a major risk factor is present; thus, this portion of patients received preoperative prophylactic LMWH.

Between 2013 and 2016, the listed contraindications of tranexamic acid administration had become more permissive due to novel clinical data on its safety, thus further augmenting its liberal use.

In 2013, viscoelastometry has not been available in our institution. A ROTEM device was introduced in 2014, and from that point, it has become part of the everyday routine as part of the hemostatic diagnostics and management of trauma and surgical patients. The insights and experience gained using viscoelastometry are in themselves great tools in hemostatic management, and whenever the need arises, viscoelastometric measurements are readily available ensuring patient safety as it is proven invaluable across all surgical fields frequently encountering massive blood loss and consequential multiple forms of coagulopathy [8, 9]. As part of our PBM program using ROTEM-guided hemostatic management has become institutionally recommended with the indication of substantial intraoperative bleeding.

We have observed a major decrease in the incidence of postoperative hypotension. We consider this a consequence of better hemostatic practice and not the more appropriate hemodynamic management. The fact that the amount of crystalloid infusions used remained unchanged and vasopressor use was also similar (data not shown) supports this assumption. There was no detectable difference in the incidence of oliguria in the first 24 hours. There has also been a drastic increase in the number of patients spending the postoperative first 24 hours in a high-dependency unit where their fluid balance was carefully evaluated, thus again increasing the reported incidence. Taking this into consideration together with the substantial drop in the incidence of hypotension and the relatively unchanged amount of administered intravenous fluids, we postulate that the data from 2013 underestimates the incidence of oliguria.

Surgical technique was unchanged between 2013 and 2016, and all our institution's surgeons used the anterolateral surgical approach (Watson-Jones). One has to consider that the improvement of the manual skills of our surgical staff and more vigilant surgical hemostasis may have a role in the reduction of our transfusion rates. Whether this is significant is beyond the scope of our study. Postoperative wound drainage insertion is a conflicting issue. The amount of data is vast, and the results are conflicting regarding both long- and short-term complications [10], the effects on wound healing and infection rate. Concerning the topic of postoperative transfusion rates and hospital length-of-stay, evidence suggests that leaving a wound drain can be detrimental [11]. Based on this evidence, we concluded to encourage but not recommend to omit wound drainage. The introduction of this new practice was detectable in results.

The study shows that yet there are no ultimate predictors regarding the need for perioperative transfusion, there are several shared characteristics among patients deemed necessary to be given blood, and the early recognition and evaluation of these characteristics play a crucial part in adequate fluid and blood management. Among these, the most self-explanatory is lower preoperative hemoglobin levels. Eventhough, before elective surgery, anemia is usually successfully managed, it is obvious that patients at the lower end of the normal range concerning the hemoglobin level are at higher risk for postoperative symptomatic anemia. Of course, it also can be taken into consideration that THR surgery is usually performed at a relatively advanced age and at that the age group with a lower preoperative hemoglobin level may frequently be associated with underlying disease or frailty.

It is shown that patients that needed blood transfusion perioperatively received tranexamic acid at a lower ratio. This could have been a consequence of a lapse in the implementation of this modality, and some of the most common diseases such as anamnestic thromboembolic events and/or medical anticoagulation are among the contraindications of the administration of tranexamic acid.

It is a long-standing and widely accepted fact that postoperative hypotension and oliguria are good, easily assessable markers of hypovolemia and can be predictors of adverse outcome [12]. It is important to note the fact that hypotension and oliguria are not always the result of hypovolemia and/or anemia but can also be caused by the many conditions associated with surgical and other iatrogenic insults that result in the impairment of cardiac output such as decompensation due to fluid overload, vasoplegia, and acute kidney injury. Understandably, patients with the worse clinical conditions are more susceptible to such effects. The fact is that in the transfusion group, the incidence of these in the first 24 hours postoperatively is congruent with our earlier observation that these patients were overall in a worse clinical condition.

It is shown that the transfusion group had an elevated postoperative infection rate. That is in accordance with the aforementioned difference in the overall clinical condition of these patients as well. There are compelling data including many surgical fields that perioperative transfusion is a risk factor of postoperative infection [1, 13–15]. It is up to debate whether there is causality established by the immunosuppressive effects of transfusion [16] or it is merely a statistical correlation deriving from the same premise that those requiring transfusion are either in a worse preoperative clinical condition and/or underwent greater surgical stress.

We acknowledge the limitations of this study; this is a single-center study, and as such, it cannot give information regarding the applicability of the process in different institutes. Pillars and parts of the PBM program would be differentially important in other systems. As a before-after study that incorporated multiple interventions, we cannot determine the ratio of the overall efficiency that could be attributed to a single measure. Regarding the overall efficiency, as mentioned above, we cannot determine to which extent the success can be attributed to the PBM measures and to what extent are the changing surgical techniques and skills responsible.

5. Conclusion

We conclude that our institution-tailored PBM program was successful and the consequential results have deemed it a worthy endeavor. We have greatly decreased our perioperative transfusion ratio, thus both reducing the risk of transfusion-associated complications and lifting the burden from our National Blood Reserve. We have also conducted a successful training program resulting in a more professional approach to precision medicine. As a result, short-term postoperative complications were significantly decreased. Our results encourage other hospitals to attempt implementing their own institution-tailored PBM protocols even if application in full is not feasible.

References

[1] V. A. Ferraris, D. L. Davenport, S. P. Saha, P. C. Austin, and J. B. Zwischenberger, "Surgical outcomes and transfusion of minimal amounts of blood in the operating room," *Archives of Surgery*, vol. 147, no. 1, pp. 49–55, 2012.

[2] A. Kleinerüschkamp, P. Meybohm, N. Straub, K. Zacharowski, and S. Choorapoikayil, "A model-based cost-effectiveness analysis of Patient Blood Management," *Blood Transfus*, vol. 17, pp. 16–26, 2019.

[3] N. Desai, N. Schofield, and T. Richards, "Perioperative patient blood management to improve outcomes," *Anesthesia & Analgesia*, vol. 127, no. 5, pp. 1211–1220, 2018.

[4] M. Goldstein, C. Feldmann, H. Wulf, and T. Wiesmann, "Tranexamic acid prophylaxis in hip and knee joint replacement," *Deutsches Aerzteblatt Online*, vol. 114, pp. 824–830, 2017.

[5] N. Strebel, M. Prins, G. Agnelli, and H. R. Büller, "Preoperative or postoperative start of prophylaxis for venous thromboembolism with low-molecular-weight heparin in elective hip surgery?" *Archives of Internal Medicine*, vol. 162, no. 13, pp. 1451–1456, 2002.

[6] P. O. Borgen, O. E. Dahl, and O. Reikeras, "Preoperative versus postoperative initiation of dalteparin thromboprophylaxis in THA," *HIP International*, vol. 20, no. 3, pp. 301–307, 2010.

[7] P. O. Borgen, O. E. Dahl, and O. Reikerås, "Blood loss in cemented THA is not reduced with postoperative versus preoperative start of thromboprophylaxis," *Clinical Orthopaedics and Related Research*, vol. 470, no. 9, pp. 2591–2598, 2012.

[8] K. Görlinger, A. Pérez-Ferrer, D. Dirkmann et al., "The role of evidence-based algorithms for rotational thromboelastometry-guided bleeding management," *Korean Journal of Anesthesiology*, vol. 72, no. 4, pp. 297–322, 2019.

[9] L. Spiezia, F. Vasques, A. Behr et al., "Perioperative coagulation assessment of patients undergoing major elective orthopedic surgery," *Internal and Emergency Medicine*, vol. 11, no. 6, pp. 793–801, 2016.

[10] M. Nanni, F. Perna, C. Calamelli et al., "Wound drainages in total hip arthroplasty: to use or not to use? Review of the literature on current practice," *Musculoskeletal Surgery*, vol. 97, no. 2, pp. 101–107, 2013.

[11] H. Xu, J. Xie, Y. Lei, Q. Huang, Z. Huang, and F. Pei, "Closed suction drainage following routine primary total joint arthroplasty is associated with a higher transfusion rate and longer postoperative length of stay: a retrospective cohort study," *Journal of Orthopaedic Surgery and Research*, vol. 14, no. 1, p. 163, 2019.

[12] J. Lesko and J. R. Johnston, "Oliguria," *AACN Clinical Issues: Advanced Practice in Acute and Critical Care*, vol. 8, no. 3, pp. 459–468, 1997.

[13] K. A. Horvath, M. A. Acker, H. Chang et al., "Blood transfusion and infection after cardiac surgery," *The Annals of Thoracic Surgery*, vol. 95, no. 6, pp. 2194–2201, 2013.
[14] C. Rhee, L. Lethbridge, G. Richardson, and M. Dunbar, "Risk factors for infection, revision, death, blood transfusion and longer hospital stay 3 months and 1 year after primary total hip or knee arthroplasty," *Canadian Journal of Surgery*, vol. 61, no. 3, pp. 165–176, 2018.
[15] Y.-K. He, H.-Z. Li, and H.-D. Lu, "Is blood transfusion associated with an increased risk of infection among spine surgery patients?: A meta-analysis," *Medicine (Baltimore)*, vol. 98, no. 28, Article ID e16287, 2019.
[16] M. A. Blajchman, "Immunomodulation and blood transfusion," *American Journal of Therapeutics*, vol. 9, no. 5, pp. 389–395, 2002.

2

Thumb Interphalangeal Joint Replacement as an Alternative to Joint Fusion

Laurence Grüber, Georges Kohut, and Théa Voser

Clinique Générale Saint-Anne, Cabinet Kohut. Rue Hans-Geiler 6, Fribourg 1700, Switzerland

Correspondence should be addressed to Laurence Grüber; gruberlaurence@gmail.com

Academic Editor: Benjamin Blondel

Arthrodesis is the generally accepted treatment for symptomatic osteoarthritis of the interphalangeal (IP) joint of the thumb. For 7 thumbs in 5 patients, an IP joint replacement was offered as a pain alleviating and motion conserving treatment option for osteoarthritis. In these cases, an offlabel use of the SR-PIP prosthesis was performed. All patients did well postoperatively with reasonable pain-free range of motion of the interphalangeal joint except one patient who required further surgeries for recurring joint instability. Radiologically, though, an osteolysis around the stems that could lead to loosening of the prosthesis and progressing periarticular ossifications that might cause a blockage of the joint were observed. IP joint arthroplasty represents a viable option on the short term; however, further studies should be conducted to ensure their long-term sustainability.

1. Introduction

Osteoarthritis of the interphalangeal (IP) joint of the thumb is not a rare occurrence [1]. When this condition remains symptomatic after conservative management, arthrodesis is the generally admitted treatment [2]. It provides the patient with a stable, nonmoving, but also, pain-free joint. Lin et al. [3] demonstrated in their three-dimensional analysis of the thumb joints in regular daily activities that the spherical grip for a ball with a diameter of 6.3 cm exhibited the largest IP joint flexion with an average of 49°. Twisting a key only needed 22° of flexion. In the literature, for the IP joint, a functional arc of motion between 2° and 43° is considered necessary, when its normal active range of motion is 73° in flexion and 5° in extension [4]. As a result, it would seem logical to try to keep this joint active to maintain the function of the hand as normal as possible and avoid an overload of the metacarpophalangeal (MCP) and carpometacarpal (CMC) joints. Until this day, however, to the best of our knowledge, there have been no studies comparing the dexterity of the hand with the IP joint blocked or kept freely moving. There also is no proof that blocking the IP joint might speed up the development of arthritis in the MCP and CMC joints. Very few reports about IP joint arthroplasty have been described so far [5, 6]. We offered this alternative technique to patients desiring to keep some motion of the IP joint, assuming that they would benefit from it, by reducing pain and improving dexterity in their activities and potentially avoiding an early onset of arthritis in the more proximal joints of the thumb.

1.1. Cases Presentation. We report a consecutive case series of 7 arthroplasties of the IP joint of the thumb implanted over a four year period on 5 patients (2 bilateral). Patients presented with a painful degenerative osteoarthritis of the IP joint that was resistant to a well-conducted orthopedic treatment, with concomitant arthritis in the CMC and MCP joints. Patients with jobs that required heavy workloads were not given this option. In addition, we excluded patients whose bone stock was insufficient, as well as thumbs with nonfunctioning tendons. All these patients would clearly benefit more from an arthrodesis. We included 5 subjects who were willing to keep some motion at the tip of the thumb. These patients had to understand that they were offered an offlabel procedure and consent to it. We describe our thumb IP arthroplasty technique with the use of the SR-PIP prosthesis (Stryker). This device consists of titanium, cobalt chrome, and ultrahigh molecular weight polyethylene and is indicated for the replacement of the proximal interphalangeal joint of the long fingers.

For this study, we reviewed all the patients we had previously operated for a thumb IP arthroplasty. They all accepted to come in for medical follow-up consultation. During this meeting, patients underwent a series of questions, a clinical examination, followed by photographic pictures of the hands, and a standard AP and lateral radiographs of the thumb.

During surgery, the joint was accessed by a posterior approach. A Y-shaped incomplete tenotomy of the extensor pollicis longus tendon was performed. Part of the extensor tendon was always spared on the edges of the joint. The collateral ligaments were preserved. Osteophytes were resected on the proximal phalanx. Part of the head of the proximal phalanx was resected by an osteotomy. The medullary canal was enlarged with reamers to adjust the contours for a proper fit of the trial components. Part of the base of the distal phalanx was resected with a burr, in order to accommodate for the volume of the trial component. The medullary canal was prepared in the same manner as for the proximal phalanx. Trial reduction was performed. The size of the prosthesis was chosen so as to allow easy flexion passively, complete extension, and minimal lateral play. Definitive components were cemented. The tendon was repaired using a running absorbable suture. Postoperatively, the thumb was immobilized with a splint for three weeks, maintaining the IP in complete extension. Progressive rehabilitation was then followed.

All our subjects were females. The average age at surgery was 65.9 years. The medium follow-up period was 2.6 years, with a minimum of 18 months. In six of the operated hands, concomitant surgeries were performed. Two underwent a distal interphalangeal (DIP) joint arthrodesis of a long finger. One had three DIP arthrodesis of long fingers. One had an osteophyte resection on the DIP of the index finger. Two had a proximal interphalangeal (PIP) joint arthroplasty of a long finger.

For all patients, X-ray controls were obtained before and after surgery (Figure 1), as well as at the last follow-up. Regrettably, strict AP X-rays of the thumb IP joint were not always obtained before surgery.

1.2. Pre- and Postoperative Images. At the last follow-up visit, one patient reported pain exclusively during physical activities. No patient presented pain at rest. No pain was reproduced by direct palpation or mobilization of the joint. The average visual analogue scale (VAS from 0 to 10) of our cohort after the surgery approximates was 0.3, even with activities. It cannot be compared to the preoperative score, as pain level using the VAS has not been asked before surgery.

Medium active range of motion in the IP joint before surgery was 40.8 degrees (information only in 6 cases), while it was 58.1 degrees at the latest follow-up (Table 1). One of the patients showed nearly no mobility. One other presented an impressive range of motion (ROM) of 110°. The global overall mobility of the thumb was good, with an average Kapandji score of 8.9. Postoperatively, the thumb-index (key) pinch strength was at an average of 5.7 kg on the operated thumbs. The same strength was measured on the nonoperated thumbs. It must be emphasized that only 3 measures could be done on thumbs that had not been through a surgery, as 2 patients underwent the surgery on both sides. In comparison, the key pinch of healthy female has been found to be about 7.8 kg on the dominant hand and 8.2 kg on the nondominant hand [7].

One patient needed reoperation. She presented with recurrent dislocation of the joint. It was believed to result from the undersizing of the prosthesis, as it did not recur after replacing it by a larger size at revision. It is important to note that it did not diminish the thumbs overall functioning afterwards. Otherwise, no severe perioperative complications were observed, such as intraoperative fractures, deep infection, or wound contracture.

At the last follow-up, one patient presented with a very limited range of motion in the IP joint. This occurrence was associated with the finding of massive ossifications around the prosthesis. The recognition of growing osteophytes, and ossification, in the substance of the capsule and collateral ligaments was frequent on follow-up X-rays, but had some clinical relevance only in this one case, with one patient presenting with a reduced range of motion. One other patient presented with a significantly high mobility. This situation was not associated with symptoms of instability. No abnormality was seen on the X-rays.

One other observation on successive imaging is the appearance of a radiolucent line around the metaphyseal region of the proximal phalanx prosthesis in two cases. This line could correspond to a stress shielding of the bone in this cemented prosthesis where the cement coating was confined to the stem region on the radiographs. It was first observed at the last follow-up at about two years after surgery.

Two further cases showed a millimetric radiolucent line, surrounded by a sclerotic rim, around the contours of the prosthesis and cement on both the proximal and the distal phalanx. Again, these were first seen at the last follow-up at 3 and 5 years postop. Since no follow-up X-rays were done between the end of the first year of follow-up and the last examination, this line could have appeared at any moment in this time frame. These patients had no symptoms at rest, but one reported pain during regular daily activities. Even though no definition of wear exists regarding finger prosthesis, this appearance makes us suspect this diagnosis, especially in the presence of pain in one patient. As long as the patient experiences only mild discomfort, no further care is required.

Axial deviation could also be an issue. Lack of preoperative AP X-rays of the thumb IP in some cases limits the information available regarding this topic. One case showed an oblique implantation of the stem of the prosthesis on P1, with a valgus of 20° that stayed stable on the follow-up X-rays. Another case showed a preoperative valgus of 18° that was partly corrected with surgery, with 10° persisting postoperatively. One last case presented a 15° valgus deviation that persisted on the postoperative X-rays.

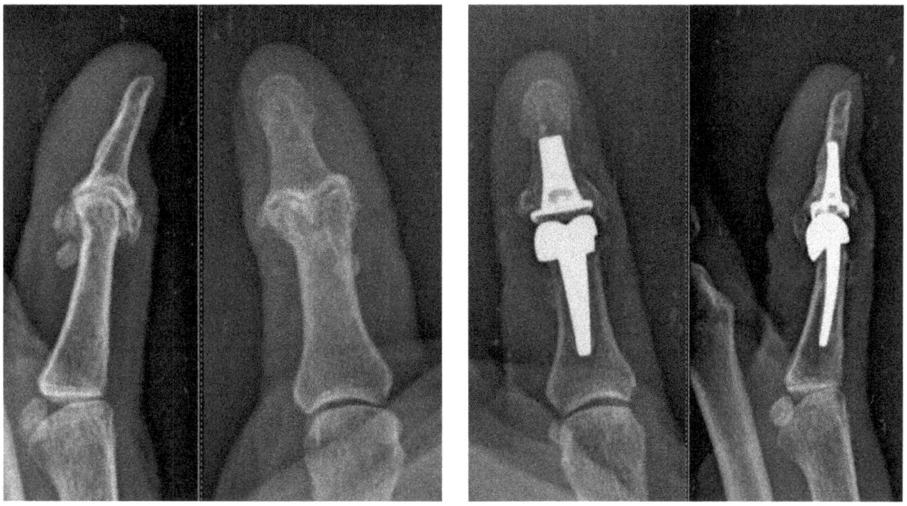

(a) (b)

FIGURE 1: Pre- and postoperative X-rays.

TABLE 1: Pre- and postoperative assessments.

Patient	Age (yo) at surgery	Time from surgery (yo)	VAS	ROM IP (°) Preop	ROM IP (°) postop	ROM MCP (°) postop	Kapandji	Pinch arthropl (kg)	Pinch opp (kg)	Reoperation
1	70.4	5	0	30	56	34	9	7.5	5.5	0
2	69.3	2.9	2	55	80	46	9	6	6	0
3	62	2	0	70	110	44	9	3.5	—	0
4	61.7	2.3	0	?	60	38	9	5	—	0
5	73.1	2.5	0	50	10	45	8	6	5.5	0
6	61.8	2.4	0	25	40	64	9	6	—	0
7	62.8	1.5	0	15	51	66	9	6	—	3
Tot	65.9	2.6	0.3	40.8	58.1	48, 1	8.9	5.7	5.7	0.4

None of our patients complained of instabilities of the replaced IP joint. We did notice, however, in 5 of 7 cases, a tendency for radial angulation of the joint while applying moderate force. The observed angulation was between 2° and 15°. In 4 cases, the joint had a valgus deviation at rest, while in 1 case, the joint had a varus deviation. In 2 cases, a radiolucent line was seen on the X-ray. None of the patients showed ulnar angulation during testing.

Lastly, three of five patients complained of cosmetic discomfort of the thumb. Admittedly, it was often thicker, and in some cases, it presented with a slight valgus deviation. But at present time, all patients would choose to go through the procedure again.

2. Discussion

This new technique, described in this article is interesting and seductive. Till this day, only two papers have reported on this subject, both of which were published in April 2019. Schindele et al. [5] reported their results of thumb IP arthroplasty in a 53-year-old patient, presenting with bilateral thumb IP osteoarthritis. She benefited from a silicone arthroplasty on the first side and a surface gliding implant arthroplasty on the second side. Follow-up was for 6 and 4 years, respectively. The patient was satisfied with the outcome. She presented no pain. Active motion on the first side was 35°/0/0° and 25°/0/40° on the second side.

She presented a 20° radial deviation of the IP joint of the thumb with the silicone arthroplasty, and the patient noticed some instability. She was, however, happy with the overall outcome.

McKee et al. [6] reported a 15-year-old trauma patient, who presented with an intra-articular fracture and adjacent laceration at the distal portion of the proximal phalanx of the thumb resulting in near complete loss of the interphalangeal joint after a table saw accident. This patient had a surface gliding implant arthroplasty and a tendon repair. Follow-up was for 22 months. The range of motion of the IP joint was 40°, which can be considered good in this badly injured joint. The patient reported no pain. The DASH score was 6.82.

In our experience though, the implantation of the prosthesis in this location is not a simple procedure, due to the tightness of the soft tissue in this approach. However, in their case report, Schindele et al. [5] did free the radial collateral ligament. This management could simplify the procedure. Consequences on joint stability should be further assessed.

Overall, patients presented a very high satisfaction rate after arthroplasty of the IP joint. They did not report any limitations in everyday activities. It must be emphasized, however, that the reported results of the arthrodesis are evenly good. In the study by Ameline et al., including thumb interphalangeal and finger distal interphalangeal joints arthrodesis, patients presented a VAS of 0.46 [8]. The current literature does not provide any control study comparing the surgical procedure on the IP joint of the thumb, to the orthopedic treatment, not even with the arthrodesis. [9].

Nevertheless, we think that low-demanding activities of daily living, such as small precision tasks, would appear more difficult to patients with arthrodesis and require compensation by the MP and CMC joint. As a result, this might lead to fast evolving arthritis of the CMC joint, especially in people with an MP joint with a limited range of motion. This remains an assumption, however, since as stated earlier, no comparative study has studied the surgical treatment of IP joint arthroplasty yet.

We believe IP arthroplasty has a role in the treatment of arthritis of this joint as it could help patients maintain some motion, and at the same time, it could help with some precision tasks. We understand that the retrospective design of the study, the limited number of cases, as well as a medium follow-up of 2.6 years represent important drawbacks to our study. It remains, though, by far, the largest series reported to date.

The suspected instability observed remains of unknown significance. These symptoms did not in absolute correlate clinically and radiologically. A bigger case load would probably answer our questions. The significance of the radiolucent lines observed on our X-rays also has to be further assessed, as they could mean an evolution towards implant loosening. We had no such severe evolution in our cohort yet. If failure of an implant happened in our patients, an implant removal and secondary arthrodesis should be performed. In this condition, arthrodesis would most probably require a bone graft to compensate with the bone stock loss. Further studies must be carried out, comparing conservative treatment, arthrodesis, and arthroplasty of the IP joint to better assess the outcome and determine the best treatment option in each situation.

References

[1] D. J. Hunter, Y. Zhang, M. C. Nevitt et al., "Chopstick arthropathy: the Beijing osteoarthritis study," *Arthritis & Rheumatism*, vol. 50, no. 5, pp. 1495–1500, 2004.

[2] A. J. Berger and R. A. Meals, "Management of osteoarthrosis of the thumb joints," *The Journal of Hand Surgery*, vol. 40, no. 4, pp. 843–850, 2015.

[3] H.-T. Lin, L.-C. Kuo, H.-Y. Liu, W.-L. Wu, and F.-C. Su, "The three-dimensional analysis of three thumb joints coordination in activities of daily living," *Clinical Biomechanics*, vol. 26, no. 4, pp. 371–376, 2011.

[4] M. C. Hume, H. Gellman, H. McKellop, and R. H. Brumfield, "Functional range of motion of the joints of the hand," *The Journal of Hand Surgery*, vol. 15, no. 2, pp. 240–243, 1990.

[5] S. Schindele, M. Marks, and D. B. Herren, "Thumb interphalangeal joint replacements with silicone and surface gliding implants. A case report," *Journal of Hand Surgery (European Volume)*, vol. 44, no. 6, pp. 649–651, 2019.

[6] D. McKee and E. L. Domingo-Johnson, "Novel use of joint replacement in a thumb interphalangeal joint," *Case Reports in Orthopedics*, vol. 15, Article ID 2603098, 2019.

[7] U. Puh, "Age-related and sex-related differences in hand and pinch grip strength in adults," *International Journal of Rehabilitation Research*, vol. 33, no. 1, pp. 4–11, 2010.

[8] T. Ameline, V. Bégot, L. Ardouin, C. Hulet, and N. Hanouz, "Arthrodesis of thumb interphalangeal and finger distal interphalangeal joints using the intramedullary X-Fuse implant: retrospective analysis of 38 cases," *Chirurgie de la main*, vol. 34, no. 2, pp. 67–72, 2015.

[9] C. K. Spies, M. Langer, P. Hahn, L. P. Müller, and F. Unglaub, "The treatment of primary arthritis of the finger and thumb joint," *Deutsches Ärzteblatt International*, vol. 115, pp. 269–275, 2018.

3

Early Economic Evaluation Demonstrates that Noncomputerized Tomography Robotic-Assisted Surgery is Cost-Effective in Patients Undergoing Unicompartmental Knee Arthroplasty at High-Volume Orthopaedic Centres

Leo M. Nherera,[1] Sanjay Verma,[2] Paul Trueman,[3] and Simon Jennings[4]

[1]*Health Economics and Market Access, Smith & Nephew, 5600 Clearfork Main St, Fort Worth, TX 76107, USA*
[2]*Health Economics and Market Access, Smith & Nephew, 5 Croxley Green Business Park, Hatters Ln, Watford WD18 8YE, Watford, UK*
[3]*Health Economics and Market Access, Smith & Nephew, 101 Hessle Rd, Hull HU3 2BN, UK*
[4]*London North West University Healthcare NHS Trust, Acton Lane Park Royal, London NW10 7NS, UK*

Correspondence should be addressed to Leo M. Nherera; leo.nherera@smith-nephew.com

Academic Editor: Benjamin Blondel

Background. For over fifty years, unicompartmental knee arthroplasty (UKA) has been used to treat single-compartment osteoarthritis of the knee and is considered a safe alternative to total knee arthroplasty (TKA). The development and use of robotic-assisted surgery (r-UKA) have made the execution of the procedure more precise, and various studies have reported improved radiographic outcomes and implant survival rates; however, its cost-effectiveness is unknown. This study aimed at assessing the cost-effectiveness of noncomputerized tomography (non-CT) r-UKA compared to the traditional unicompartmental knee arthroplasty (t-UKA) method in patients with unicompartmental knee osteoarthritis from the UK payer's perspective. *Methods.* We developed a 5-year four-state Markov model to evaluate the expected costs and outcomes of the two strategies in patients aged 65 years. Failure rates for t-UKA were taken from the British National Joint Registry while data for non-CT r-UKA were obtained from a 2-year observational study. Cost was obtained from the NHS reference cost valued at 2018/19 GBP£, and a discount rate of 3.5% was applied to both costs and benefits. *Results.* For a high-volume orthopaedic centre that performs 100 UKA operations per year, non-CT r-UKA was more costly than t-UKA but offered better clinical outcomes, and the estimated cost per QALY was £2,831. The results were more favourable in younger patients aged less than 55 and sensitive to case volumes and follow-up period. *Conclusion.* Non-CT r-UKA is cost-effective compared with t-UKA over a 5-year period. Results are dependent on case volumes and follow-up period and favour younger age groups.

1. Introduction

For over fifty years, unicompartmental knee arthroplasty (UKA) has been used to treat single-compartment osteoarthritis of the knee and is considered a safe alternative to total knee arthroplasty (TKA) [1, 2]. There are a number of documented surgical benefits associated with UKA when compared with TKA which include less perioperative morbidity, reduced blood loss, and shorter postoperative recovery and rehabilitation [3–5]. A recent systematic review and meta-analysis using data from randomised controlled trials, observational studies, and registry studies reported shorter mean length of stay, better functional patient-reported outcome measure scores, and fewer revisions compared to TKA [6].

UKA procedure volumes are low compared to TKA with suggestions that adoption is limited by perceived technical difficulty in performing the procedure and concerns over the variation in outcomes in the published literature [7, 8]. Failures of UKA have been attributed to medial-lateral mismatch, inadequate stability of the components, and improper alignment [7, 9]. The development and use of robotic-assisted surgery (r-UKA) have made the execution of a technically difficult procedure more precise, and various studies have reported improved radiographic outcomes and in particular improved implant alignment [10–14]. It is estimated that approximately 14% of US UKA surgeries were performed with robotic assistance as of 2012 and this rate is expected to increase [11]. Studies have also observed an association between high-volume centres and better outcomes, in particular revision rates [15–17].

The capital costs of robotic assistance mean that a crude comparison of procedural costs of traditional instrumentation versus robotic-assisted UKA would favour the traditional procedure [12]. However, it is important that the incremental costs associated with robotic-assisted surgery consider potential impacts on clinical outcomes. Cost-effectiveness analyses can help to reduce decision uncertainty by allowing a comparative analysis of both the costs and health outcomes (revisions avoided) of traditional unicompartmental knee arthroplasty (t-UKA) versus non-CT r-UKA. Our study, therefore, aimed at evaluating the cost-effectiveness of non-CT r-UKA when compared to that of t-UKA in the UK. Whilst the evidence on non-CT r-UKA remains limited at the current time, early economic modelling allows for the cost-effectiveness to be estimated based on the available evidence and through extrapolation of outcomes. Over time, early models can be validated as further data are made available.

2. Materials and Methods

2.1. Overview and Modelling Framework. A Markov model with four health states was developed in Microsoft® Excel from the perspective of UK National Health Service payer. The four discrete health states following primary UKA surgery were as follows: (1) successful primary UKA, (2) revision UKA, (3) rerevision UKA, and (4) death. Figure 1 shows the diagrammatic representation of the model structure.

The model considers a cohort of 100 patients with a mean age of 65 years who are eligible for primary UKA. This age group was considered to be broadly representative of a typical patient for UKA surgery according to registry data [7, 18].

The model estimates the costs and outcomes of treating 100 patients managed with either non-CT r-UKA (Navio Smith & Nephew, Memphis, TN) compared with t-UKA. Given limitations in the data, the model recognises the difference in surgical approach but makes no attempt to distinguish the effectiveness of particular implant designs. Following primary UKA surgery with or without robotic assistance, patients can enter a successful primary UKA state, but remain at risk of entering a revision surgery state due to UKA failure, i.e., all-cause revision. For patients that transition into the revision surgery state, these patients can enter into a successful postrevision state or are at further risk of transition to a rerevision surgery state. No further surgical options were considered beyond a second revision (rerevision), as we assumed patients will be converted to total knee arthroplasty. Lastly, patients may transition to the death state from any other health state and experience no further transitions. Individuals in the model can transition between the health states each year. The model has a 5-year time horizon. The model estimates the number of individuals in each health state every year, considering the risk of health states worsening (e.g., failure).

2.2. Clinical Data Inputs for Traditional UKA and Robotic-Assisted Surgery. Clinical data on traditional UKA were derived from the 2018 National Joint Registry [18] from England and Wales. The NJR was set up in 2002 to collect information on joint replacement operations and performance of implants and surgeons. The failure rate of all UKA surgeries as defined by revisions at 5 years was reported to be 6.1%. Revision was defined as a reoperation resulting in the modification of the primary UKA or conversion to TKA. Rerevision was defined as a reoperation of a revised UKA [19]. Due to the low incidence of revision surgery, a one-year cycle length was utilized and is in consistent with published studies [19, 20]. The following formula was used to convert the reported 5-year rates to annual probabilities for use in the model [21].

$$p = 1 - e^{-rt}, \quad (1)$$

where p is the probability, r is the rate, and t is the unit of time.

Clinical data on the performance of non-CT r-UKA were obtained from a retrospective multicenter, cohort study on patients who had undergone robotic-assisted surgery with 2.3 years of follow-up [7]. Given the limited follow-up data, it was necessary to extrapolate outcomes to 5 years to allow for comparison with NJR data. We adopted a conservative assumption on the effect of robotic surgery on revision rates. We assumed that any incremental benefit of non-CT r-UKA occurs in the first two years in accordance with the available clinical trial data. After this time, the risk of revision surgery was assumed to be the same as traditional UKA from year 3 to 5.

Overall survivorship of the UKA knee implants was 99.2% (95% confidence interval: 94.6% to 99.9%) [7]. These data were used to derive the hazard rate (HR) of revision surgery with non-CT r-UKA compared to t-UKA. Registry data on t-UKA identified 95,836 UKAs, of which 2863 needed a revision at 2 years [18]. This is compared to 1 revision in 128 knees seen in non-CT r-UKA study. The HR was therefore calculated to be 0.20 (95% CI: 0.17 to 0.24; $p < 0.05$). The HR was applied only for the first two years, after which we assumed the revision rates of non-CT r-UKA to be similar to that of t-UKA.

2.3. Mortality Rates. The all-cause age-specific mortality was obtained from UK Life Tables 2015/17 [22] (Table 1). For the base model, 5-year mortality rates following

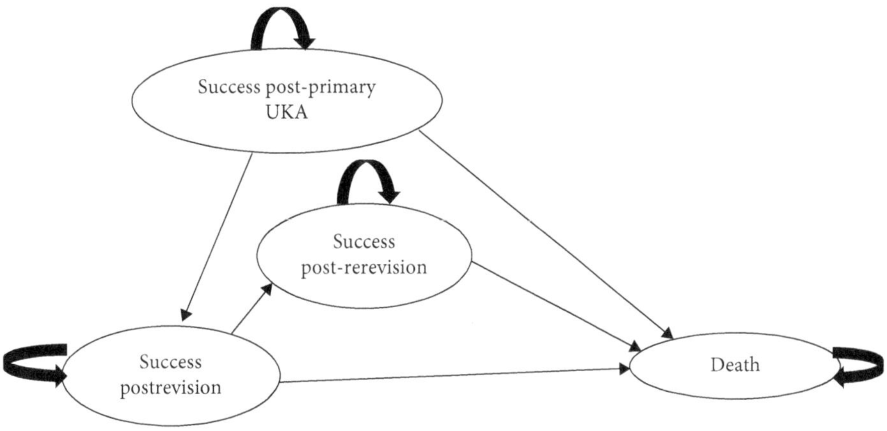

FIGURE 1: Schematic representation of the model structure.

TABLE 1: Model input parameters.

Revision data at 5 years converted to annual probabilities				
Age	Mean	95% LCI	95% UCI	Reference
65	1.19%	1.15%	1.22%	[18]
Rerevision all ages				
All	2.05%	1.89%	2.21%	[18]
Robotic-assisted UKA effectiveness				
	Hazard rate	95% LCI	95% UCI	
Revision	0.2000	0.1700	0.2400	[7]
Mortality following surgical procedure				
Age	Mean	95% LCI	95% UCI	
65	4.44%	4.42%	4.47%	[18]
All-cause mortality				
Age 65	4.9%			[22]
Quality of life weights				
Postsurgery	0.750	0.600	0.938	[19]
Revision	0.565	0.452	0.706	[19]
Rerevision	0.4630	0.370	0.579	[19]
Mortality	0.000	0.000	0.000	[19]
Costs GBP £2018/19				
Revision/rerevision	£10,390	£7,793	£12,988	[23]
Arthroplasty	£6,267	£4,700	£7,833	[23]
Rehabilitation	£289	£217	£361	[23]
Consumables (burr, drape, discs)	£260	£195	£325	Manufacturer
Robotics costs	£358,000	£286,400*	£429,600*	Manufacturer
Annual service contract (year 2–5)	£21,500			Manufacturer

NJR = National Joint Registry of England and Wales; LCI = lower value of the 95% confidence interval; UCI = upper value of the 95% confidence interval; *assumed ±20%.

surgery were used. We assumed that both primary non-CT r-UKA and t-UKA had no impact on mortality; hence, similar mortality rates were experienced in both groups of patients. We made a further assumption that the probability of death after revision surgery due to UKA was the same in both the non-CT r-UKA- and t-UKA-treated patients.

2.4. Health-Related Quality of Life (HRQOL) and Utility Data Used in the Model. Outcomes of the analysis are presented as cost per revision avoided and cost per quality-adjusted life year (QALYs). QALYs are a measurement of quality of life defined on a scale of 0–1. A year of perfect health is equivalent to 1 QALY while a year of less than perfect health is worth less than 1 QALY. This outcome is widely used by health technology assessment bodies (such as NICE) as it generates a common currency which can be used to assess the cost-effectiveness of any health technology. A benchmark of £20,000–£30,000 per QALY is widely considered to represent a cost-effective use of healthcare resources in the NHS. The QALY for each health state is calculated by multiplying the health state utility (revision surgery, healed) by the model life span using the roll-back method. Utility data used were obtained from the published literature [19].

2.5. Case Volume and Healthcare Resource Costs. As robotic surgery requires capital expenditure, the cost per case will be dependent on procedural volumes. A previous study defined a high-volume arthroplasty centre as one which conducts >12 UKA cases per year or >200 TKA cases annually [19]. In the base case model, we considered a high-volume orthopaedic centre which conducts 100 UKA procedures per annum, similar to a previously published study of robotic surgery [19]. A break-even analysis was performed to evaluate the minimum surgical volume required to achieve cost-neutral non-CT r-UKA utilization and this issue was further assessed in sensitivity analyses.

The model adopted a payer perspective—considering only those costs and benefits that are incurred by the health service (the UK National Health Services) or the insurer (Table 1). Both future costs and benefits were discounted by 3.5% annually in accordance with the recommendations of the NICE reference case [24].

Costs included in the model were measured in GBP Pound sterling and were obtained from NHS reference costs [23, 25]. The reference costs include the procedure, implant, theatre, physician, and anaesthetic among other costs. The capital cost of CT-image free robotic system was estimated to be £358,000, which is the list price in the UK. This was adjusted in sensitivity analyses. Using the information on the assumed device life span (5 years) and discount rate (3.5%), we calculated the discounted annual equivalent costs (present value) of £79,290. In addition to the purchase price, the robot requires an annual service contract fee after the first year of ownership reported to be £21,500 per annum by the manufacturer. The annual equivalent costs, the annual service contract costs, and consumables were then summed and divided by the expected case volume of 100 cases per year to determine the cost per case of the robotic equipment. This cost was estimated to be £1,225 per case. Procedure costs were estimated as a weighted average from National Health Service (NHS) reference costs based on the relevant healthcare resource group (HRG) codes presented in Table 1.

2.6. Cost-Effectiveness Analysis and Sensitivity Analysis. The incremental cost-effectiveness ratio (ICER) is the added cost per additional unit of health benefit in this model measured as revisions avoided and QALYs. This is calculated as the difference between the expected costs of non-CT r-UKA and t-UKA divided by the difference between the expected numbers of QALYs between the two strategies over 5 years:

$$\text{ICER} = \frac{\Delta\text{cost}}{\Delta\text{QALYs}}. \tag{2}$$

A one-way and probabilistic sensitivity analysis (SA) was implemented to evaluate the impact of uncertainty around the underlying data on base case model conclusions. One-way SA was implemented by varying some of the model parameters one at a time using lower and upper values reported in the literature and assessing the impact this had on model conclusions. Values were varied ±20% if ranges were not reported in the literature in accordance with other published economic studies. Furthermore, structural sensitivity analyses were conducted to assess the uncertainty of structural assumptions such as age, volume of cases seen, and time horizon which may affect outcomes. As age is a key variable in determining rates of revision surgery, we considered patient cohorts aged <55 years, 65–74 years, and >75 years to estimate the impact on outcomes. Probabilistic sensitivity analysis (PSA) was implemented by assigning statistical distributions to input parameters and vary the inputs simultaneously to assess the impact on model results. Clinical data inputs were assigned the lognormal distribution while the cost and utility data were assigned the gamma and beta distribution, respectively. The results of the PSA are presented on a cost-effectiveness acceptability curve. The curve shows the probability that each intervention is cost-effective at different willingness-to-pay (WTP) values. The WTP value is what the payer is prepared to pay for an additional unit of clinical benefit in this model measured in QALYs.

3. Results

3.1. Base Case Results. We report the results of a high-volume centre that performs 100 UKA procedures per year. Non-CT r-UKA was more costly than t-UKA but offered better clinical outcomes (there were fewer revisions and more QALYs) as shown in Table 2, and the estimated cost per QALY was £2,831.

3.2. Structural and One-Way Sensitivity Analysis. The base results are reported for a 65-year-old cohort of both males and females. In a separate analysis, we considered different age groups and non-CT r-UKA remained cost-effective across all age groups. However, the results were more favourable for the younger age group aged <55 years compared to those aged over 75 years. Gender, however, demonstrated only modest differences between the two cohorts (ICER male: £3,374; ICER female: £2,332/QALY). Extending the follow-up period beyond 5 years improved the cost-effectiveness of non-CT r-UKA, with it becoming cost saving with a follow-up beyond 7 years. One-way sensitivity analysis results suggest non-CT r-UKA is not sensitive to changes in key assumptions of revision probability, non-CT r-UKA effectiveness, and discount rate. Changes in these input parameters showed small changes in the estimated ICER, suggesting the reliability of the initial model assumptions. Sensitivity analysis results are summarised in Table 3.

Table 2: Cost-effectiveness results of non-CT r-UKA compared to t-UKA for 100 treated patients.

Intervention	Costs	Number of revisions avoided	Cumulative QALYs	Incremental costs	Complications avoided	Cost/ complication avoided	Difference in QALYs	Cost/ QALY
Traditional UKA	£853,034	86	431					
Robotic-assisted UKA	£879,852	96	440	£26,8178	11	£2,521	9.47	£2,831

Table 3: Structural and one-way sensitivity analysis.

Parameter	Cost per QALY
Base case	**£2,831**
All age groups	£3,353
Age <55	Non-CT r-UKA dominating
Age 65–74	£6,578
Age >75	£10,283
Males	£3,373
Females	£2,332
2-year follow-up	£33,704
7-year follow-up	Non-CT r-UKA dominating
Revision probability lower value	£3,686
Revision probability upper value	£2,039
Non-CT r-UKA effectiveness lower value	£2,358
Non-CT r-UKA effectiveness upper value	£3,520
Discount rate lower value	£690
Discount rate upper value	£2,831
Cost of robotics/case lower value	£1,157
Cost of robotics/case upper value	£5,676

Non-CT r-UKA: noncomputerized tomography robotic-assisted unicompartmental knee arthroplasty.

The probability that non-CT r-UKA is cost-effective at a willingness-to-pay figure of £20,000/QALY is 100% as shown by the cost-effectiveness acceptability curve in Figure 2.

3.3. Number of Cases and Break-Even Analysis. As the cost per case is dependent on volume, we also varied the number of UKA procedures conducted to determine the impact on the cost-effectiveness ratio. Unsurprisingly, increasing the volume of procedures reduces the cost per case of robotic-assisted surgery and in doing so, improved the cost-effectiveness. Therefore, for high-volume facilities, the cost-effectiveness of non-CT r-UKA is favourable while for low-volume facilities the cost-effectiveness is less favourable. For example, for a centre that sees 20 patients per year, the cost per QALY is estimated to be £43,581, while for those that see more than 138 patients, non-CT r-UKA becomes cost saving compared to traditional UKA (see Figure 3).

4. Discussion

We assessed the cost-effectiveness of non-CT r-UKA compared to t-UKA from a UK health service perspective. Our base case analysis showed that non-CT r-UKA offered better clinical outcomes (fewer revisions) and hence more QALYs at an increased cost. The estimated cost per QALY is £2,831 for a high-volume facility that sees 100 patients per year, which is well within what is considered cost-effective in the NHS. This result is unlikely to be a chance finding as confirmed by the probabilistic sensitivity analysis.

Our study is the first of its kind comparing the cost-effectiveness of non-CT r-UKA with t-UKA based on clinical data from the UK. A previous study of robotic-assisted surgery for UKA based on data from the United States generated a cost-effectiveness ratio of $47,180 per QALY, significantly more than the current analysis. Whilst both studies adopted a cohort of 100 patients and based their analyses on 2-year follow-up data on robotic-assisted UKA, there were some notable differences in the methodologies and data sources. The differences result from a number of variables including higher procedural costs in the United States, differences in the time horizon adopted in the analyses, and differences in the robotic surgical systems considered.

Currently, the uptake of UKA is estimated to be less than 10% of total arthroplasties, yet UKA has been found to offer better clinical outcomes at lower costs when compared to TKA [26–28]. Cost savings have been attributed to reduced length of stay and reduced use of healthcare services, such as fewer outpatient visits in the first 2 years after the index surgery [27]. However, there is also a relationship between procedure volume and outcomes. A systematic review that compared TKA with UKA noted that centres that perform 20% of their arthroplasty practice as UKA achieve lower rates of revision for unexplained pain or failures [6]. It is speculated that one of the reasons low-volume centres observe higher failure rates of UKA is poor patient selection where surgeons are more likely to offer UKA to patients with partial-thickness cartilage loss which is associated with poor outcomes compared to patients with bone-on-bone arthritis [26, 27].

Our study corroborates this finding, indicating that non-CT r-UKA is cost-effective in centres conducting more than 30 non-CT r-UKA procedures per year and this improves dramatically in centres performing over 100 cases per year. Increasing the volume of non-CT r-UKA surgery and the frequency of procedures for individual surgeons ensures that surgeons reduce the learning curve, maintain their knowledge of the procedure, and ultimately, deliver improved outcomes [6, 29].

Robotic-assisted surgery has the potential to reduce variation in practice and promote more consistent outcomes in UKA, thereby enabling a shift in case mix and more widespread use of UKA for appropriate patients. This, in

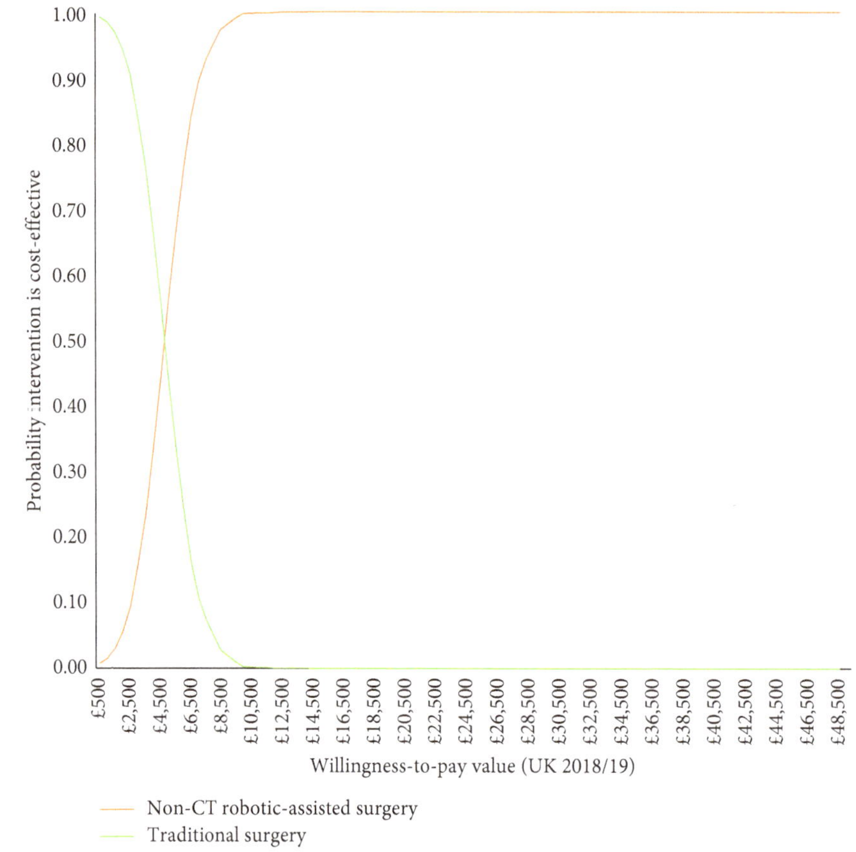

FIGURE 2: Cost-effectiveness acceptability curves.

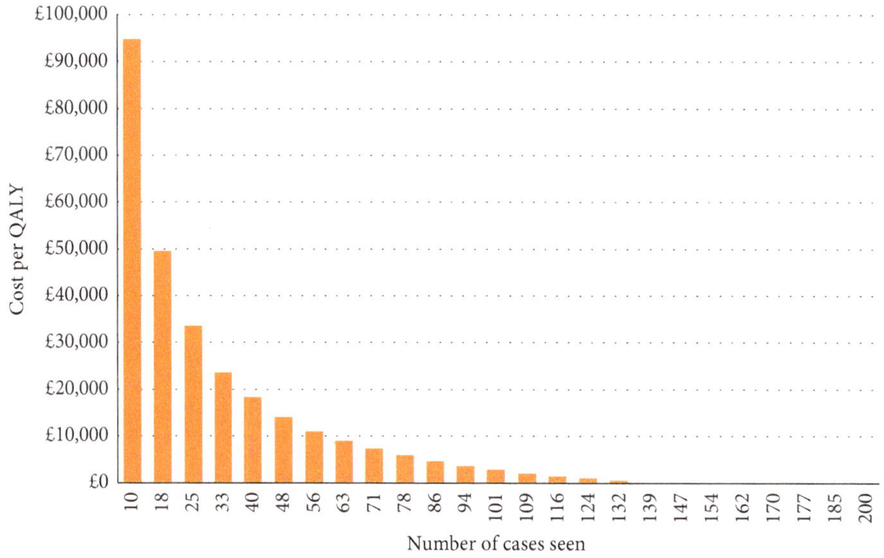

FIGURE 3: Number of procedures and the resultant cost per QALY.

turn, may allow for more rapid recovery than TKA procedures and a shorter hospital stay. However, it is vital that surgeons have access to appropriate training on non-CT r-UKA and increase their procedure volume to maintain familiarity with the approach.

The current analysis should be considered as an "early" economic evaluation of robotic-assisted UKA, acknowledging that there are currently limited data on the effectiveness of this approach, particularly in terms of patient follow-up. In recognition of this, we made a number of conservative assumptions such as limiting the impact of non-CT r-UKA on revisions to 2 years following surgery and assumed that non-CT r-UKA had no impact on rerevisions and quality of life. These assumptions have the potential of underestimating the true benefits of non-CT r-UKA compared to t-UKA. However, we cannot quantify this benefit due to the lack of information in the published studies that were included in the analysis.

We also derived baseline rates of revision for UKA from registry data. Whilst these data are widely used for evaluations of this sort, they provide a mean rate which includes data from high- and low-volume surgeons. Given the complexity of UKA, it seems likely that high-volume surgeons may have better outcomes which would alter the findings of this analysis. We have attempted to address his through sensitivity analyses around the hazard rate although further research is required to generate comparable cohorts of patients and surgeons.

We conducted a number of one-way sensitivity analyses which demonstrated that the model was sensitive to case volume. Centres with higher case volume are bound to benefit more from non-CT r-UKA since the cost per case falls as the capital is deployed across greater numbers of patients. The model was based on an assumed cohort of 100 patients, as is typical in studies of this type. However, we recognise that the throughput of UKA is currently below this in a significant number of facilities. Sensitivity analyses illustrate the importance of volume and emphasise that robotic-assisted surgery will be more cost-effective in facilities that are designed to maximise their use of the capital equipment.

The model is also sensitive to assumptions around follow-up for instance if the model is analysed over 2 years, the estimated cost per QALY increases to £33,704 while if the model is analysed over 7 years, the model becomes cost saving. Ultimately, this issue can only be addressed through further long-term follow-up of robotic-assisted UKA patients to determine whether the short-term outcomes are sustained or even improve relative to traditional UKA.

Economic evaluation should be an iterative process and refined as uncertainty around the model parameters decreases. Our study is supported by robust clinical evidence based on a single multicentre retrospective cohort study with 2.3 years' worth of survivorship data in 128 patients. We appreciate these data are indicative of the potential benefits of non-CT r-UKA and that the analysis would need to be refined as more data become available. "Early" economic models are intended to inform decision making and investments early in the life cycle of promising technologies. Healthcare providers have the option of being risk-averse and delaying investment decisions indefinitely until uncertainty is addressed, or more assertive in their adoption of new technologies. In the case of orthopaedic interventions, where 5- and even 10-year outcomes are considered to be the gold standard of evidence, this is challenging. Delaying a decision on the adoption of a new technology for 10 years may reduce the risk of a bad investment but also deprives patients' access to promising technologies. Furthermore, by the time evidence is available, further technological advances are likely to have occurred. Early economic models, which incorporate sensitivity analyses to identify critical uncertainties, can help decision makers to make more informed choices about if and when they adopt promising innovative technologies.

5. Conclusion

According to our economic analysis, the use of non-CT robotics-assisted UKA may be more cost-effective when compared to traditional UKA for patients with knee osteoarthritis when performed at high-volume orthopaedic centres with experienced clinicians. These findings remained robust when different assumptions were tested. Future studies with longer time horizons are warranted to elucidate what benefits may persist beyond the reported two years and also to validate these preliminary findings. Clinicians and policy makers should consider adopting robotics as they strive to provide high-quality, value-based healthcare. This will allow the generation of more clinical data necessary to perform a definitive economic analysis in the near future.

References

[1] R. A. Berger, R. M. Meneghini, J. J. Jacobs et al., "Results of unicompartmental knee arthroplasty at a minimum of ten years of follow-up," *The Journal of Bone and Joint Surgery-American Volume*, vol. 87, no. 5, pp. 999–1006, 2005.

[2] N. F. Soohoo, H. Sharifi, G. Kominski, and J. R. Lieberman, "Cost-effectiveness analysis of unicompartmental knee arthroplasty as an alternative to total knee arthroplasty for unicompartmental osteoarthritis," *The Journal of Bone and Joint Surgery-American Volume*, vol. 88, no. 9, pp. 1975–1982, 2006.

[3] L. P. Hunt, Y. Ben-Shlomo, E. M. Clark et al., "45-day mortality after 467 779 knee replacements for osteoarthritis from the National Joint Registry for England and Wales: an observational study," *The Lancet*, vol. 384, no. 9952, pp. 1429–1436, 2014.

[4] A. D. Liddle, A. Judge, H. Pandit, and D. W. Murray, "Adverse outcomes after total and unicompartmental knee replacement in 101 330 matched patients: a study of data from the National Joint Registry for England and Wales," *The Lancet*, vol. 384, no. 9952, pp. 1437–1445, 2014.

[5] C. L. Cool, K. A. Needham, A. Khlopas, and M. A. Mont, "Revision analysis of robotic arm-assisted and manual unicompartmental knee arthroplasty," *The Journal of Arthroplasty*, vol. 34, no. 5, pp. 926–931, 2019.

[6] H. A. Wilson, R. Middleton, S. G. F. Abram et al., "Patient relevant outcomes of unicompartmental versus total knee replacement: systematic review and meta-analysis," *BMJ*, vol. 364, p. l352, 2019.

[7] A. K. Battenberg, N. A. Netravali, and J. H. Lonner, "A novel handheld robotic-assisted system for unicompartmental knee arthroplasty: surgical technique and early survivorship," *Journal of Robotic Surgery*, vol. 14, no. 1, pp. 55–60, 2020.

[8] S. W. Bell, I. Anthony, B. Jones, A. MacLean, P. Rowe, and M. Blyth, "Improved accuracy of component positioning with robotic-assisted unicompartmental knee arthroplasty," *The Journal of Bone and Joint Surgery*, vol. 98, no. 8, pp. 627–635, 2016.

[9] E. K. Song, M. N, S.-H. Lee, B.-R. Na, and J.-K. Seon, "Comparison of outcome and survival after unicompartmental knee arthroplasty between navigation and conventional techniques with an average 9-year follow-up," *The Journal of Arthroplasty*, vol. 31, no. 2, pp. 395–400, 2016.

[10] Y.-W. Moon, C.-W. Ha, K.-H. Do et al., "Comparison of robot-assisted and conventional total knee arthroplasty: a controlled cadaver study using multiparameter quantitative three-dimensional CT assessment of alignment," *Computer Aided Surgery*, vol. 17, no. 2, pp. 86–95, 2012.
[11] J. H. Lonner, J. R. Smith, F. Picard, B. Hamlin, P. J. Rowe, and P. E. Riches, "High degree of accuracy of a novel image-free handheld robot for unicondylar knee arthroplasty in a cadaveric study," *Clinical Orthopaedics and Related Research*, vol. 473, no. 1, pp. 206–212, 2015.
[12] D. J. Jacofsky and M. Allen, "Robotics in arthroplasty: a comprehensive review," *The Journal of Arthroplasty*, vol. 31, no. 10, pp. 2353–2363, 2016.
[13] A. Gilmour, A. D. MacLean, P. J. Rowe et al., "Robotic-arm-assisted vs conventional unicompartmental knee arthroplasty. The 2-year clinical outcomes of a randomized controlled trial," *The Journal of Arthroplasty*, vol. 33, no. 7, pp. S109–S115, 2018.
[14] J. F. Plate, A. Mofidi, S. Mannava et al., "Achieving accurate ligament balancing using robotic-assisted unicompartmental knee arthroplasty," *Advances in Orthopedics*, vol. 2013, 6 pages, 2013.
[15] T. W. Hamilton, J. M. Rizkalla, L. Kontochristos et al., "The interaction of caseload and usage in determining outcomes of unicompartmental knee arthroplasty: a meta-analysis," *The Journal of Arthroplasty*, vol. 32, no. 10, pp. 3228–3237, 2017.
[16] M. Badawy, A. M. Fenstad, C. A. Bartz-Johannessen et al., "Hospital volume and the risk of revision in Oxford unicompartmental knee arthroplasty in the Nordic countries -an observational study of 14,496 cases," *BMC Musculoskelet Disord*, vol. 18, p. 388, 2016.
[17] A. D. Liddle, H. Pandit, A. Judge, D. W. Murray et al., "Effect of surgical caseload on revision rate following total and unicompartmental knee replacement," *The Journal of Bone and Joint Surgery*, vol. 98, no. 1, 8 pages, 2016.
[18] National Joint Registry for England and N. I. Wales, "15th annual report 2018," 2017.
[19] W. E. Moschetti, J. F. Konopka, H. E. Rubash, and J. W. Genuario, "Can robot-assisted unicompartmental knee arthroplasty Be cost-effective? A Markov decision analysis," *The Journal of Arthroplasty*, vol. 31, no. 4, pp. 759–765, 2016.
[20] F. A. Sonnenberg and J. R. Beck, "Markov models in medical decision making," *Medical Decision Making*, vol. 13, no. 4, pp. 322–338, 1993.
[21] R. L. Fleurence and C. S. Hollenbeak, "Rates and probabilities in economic modelling," *Pharmacoeconomics*, vol. 25, no. 1, 6 pages, 2007.
[22] Office of National Statistics, *National Life Tables: UK 2015–17*, Office of National Statistics, London UK, 2019, https://www.ons.gov.uk/peoplepopulationandcommunity/birthsdeathsandmarriages/lifeexpectancies/datasets/nationallifetablesunitedkingdomreferencetables.
[23] National Health Service, *NHS Reference Costs 2017/18*, National Health Service, England UK, 2019, https://improvement.nhs.uk/resources/reference-costs/.
[24] National Institute for Health and Care Excellence, "Guide to the methods of technology appraisal," National Institute for Health and Care Excellence, London UK, 2019, http://www.nice.org.uk/media/D45/1E/GuideToMethodsTechnologyAppraisal2013.pdf.
[25] C. Lesley and A. Burns, *Unit Costs of Health and Social Care*, Personal Social Services Research Unit, University of Kent, England UK, 2017.
[26] E. Burn, A. D. Liddle, T. W. Hamilton et al., "Cost-effectiveness of unicompartmental compared with total knee replacement: a population-based study using data from the National Joint Registry for England and Wales," *BMJ Open*, vol. 8, no. 4, 2018.
[27] D. J. Beard, L. J. Davies, J. A. Cook et al., "The clinical and cost-effectiveness of total versus partial knee replacement in patients with medial compartment osteoarthritis (TOPKAT): 5-year outcomes of a randomised controlled trial," *The Lancet*, vol. 394, no. 10200, pp. 746–756, 2019.
[28] G. Peersman, W. Jak, T. Vandenlangenbergh, C. Jans, P. Cartier, and P. Fennema, "Cost-effectiveness of unicondylar versus total knee arthroplasty: a Markov model analysis," *The Knee*, vol. 21, pp. S37–S42, 2014.
[29] K. J. Palmer, G. J. Lowe, G. D. Coughlin, N. Patil, and V. R. Patel, "Launching a successful robotic surgery program," *Journal of Endourology*, vol. 22, no. 4, pp. 819–824, 2008.

4

Robotic Assistance in Unicompartmental Knee Arthroplasty Results in Superior Early Functional Recovery and is More Likely to Meet Patient Expectations

Meredith P. Crizer, Amer Haffar, Andrew Battenberg, Mikayla McGrath, Ryan Sutton, and Jess H. Lonner

Rothman Orthopaedic Institute at Thomas Jefferson University, Philadelphia, PA, USA

Correspondence should be addressed to Jess H. Lonner; jess.lonner@rothmanortho.com

Academic Editor: Allen L. Carl

Robotic technology has reduced the errors of implant alignment in unicompartmental knee arthroplasty (UKA), but its impact on functional recovery after UKA is poorly defined. The purpose of this study was to compare early functional recovery, pain levels, and satisfaction in UKA performed with either robotic assistance or conventional methods. A retrospective analysis was performed on 89 matched consecutive patients who underwent outpatient UKA by a single physician using either conventional instruments ($n = 39$) or robotic methods ($n = 50$), with otherwise identical perioperative protocols. Outcomes studied included Lower Extremity Functional Score (LEFS), new Knee Society Score (KSS), Knee Injury and Osteoarthritis Outcome Score for Joint Replacement (KOOS-JR.), VR/SF-12, Visual Analog Scale (VAS) pain scores, and perioperative opioid consumption. Patients in the robotic cohort had superior early functional outcomes, with greater LEFS (conventional = 23; robotic = 31) at 1 week post-op ($p = 0.015$) and KOOS-JR (conventional = 74; robotic = 81) at up to 6 months post-op ($p = 0.037$); these two values remained statistically significant after mixed-model regression analysis ($p = 0.010$; $p = 0.023$), respectively. At 1 year post-op, expectations were more likely to be met in those who received robotic assistance ($p = 0.06$). No differences were reported with respect to postoperative opioid usage ($p = 0.320$), reoperations ($p = 1.00$), and complications ($p = 0.628$). Robotic-assisted UKA resulted in more rapid recovery and less early postoperative pain and were more likely to meet expectations than conventional UKA, although functional differences equilibrated by 1 year postoperatively. Further follow-up is necessary to determine if implant durability is impacted by robotics.

1. Introduction

Unicompartmental knee arthroplasty (UKA) is an effective alternative to total knee arthroplasty (TKA) in patients with osteoarthritis (OA) localized to a single tibiofemoral compartment of the knee [1–3]. UKA has several potential advantages over TKA including faster recovery times, superior postoperative function, more physiological gait, shorter hospital stay, lower blood loss, decreased postoperative morbidity, reduced postoperative opioid consumption, and lower perioperative costs [4–6].

Despite these benefits and the remarkable mid- and long-term success and durability of UKA performed by high-volume UKA surgeons [7–11], UKA failures, and the need for revision related to component malposition, may occur more frequently compared to TKA, particularly in the hands of lower volume surgeons [3, 12–17]. Nationwide insurance statistics and international joint arthroplasty registries have demonstrated that UKA's fail and require revision at a substantially greater rate than TKA at all time points [3, 18, 19]. In a multicenter analysis of 418 failed UKAs, it was reported that 12% of aseptic failures of UKA were attributed to faulty implantation and malpositioning of components and that 49% of these failures occurred within 5 years postoperatively [20]. Other studies have shown that excessive tibial slope and small errors of 2° or 3° in the coronal plane increase the risk of mechanical failure after UKA [14–17]. Conventional methodology for UKA has been shown to result in outliers of greater than 2° in as many as 40–60% of procedures [12, 21].

Robotic assistance was introduced to improve the accuracy of implantation in UKA, and indeed, a number of studies have shown that to be the case [22–28]. Studies have shown reduction in surgical error with robotic assistance compared to manual methods of surface preparation [23, 24, 26]. It has been posited that optimizing component alignment and positioning, as well as quantifying soft tissue balance, would lead to improvement in patient outcomes. Nonetheless, it is unknown whether the improved precision and reduced error with robotics impact clinical function and implant survivorship in UKA [29–33]. The purpose of this study is to compare early recovery, pain levels, short-term functional outcomes, and implant durability in patients undergoing UKA using either conventional manual instrumentation or a robotic sculpting tool.

2. Materials and Methods

After obtaining institutional review board approval, a retrospective cohort study (level III) of matched consecutive UKA cases operated on by a single surgeon at two facilities was conducted. UKA was performed with conventional instrumentation ($n = 39$) or robotic technology ($n = 50$) depending on the geographic location of the procedure and access to robotic technology at one center or another. Surgeries were performed consecutively from August 2015 to April 2018. In the conventional cohort, ZUK implants (Smith and Nephew, Memphis, TN) were used while Stride implants (Smith and Nephew, Memphis, TN) were used in the robotic cohort. The primary investigator's criteria for UKA include the presence of medial unicompartmental arthritis, as well as minimum flexion arc of 90°, flexion contracture of less than 5°, varus deformity of less than 10°, a competent anterior cruciate ligament, and absence of pain or exposed bone in the patellofemoral and lateral compartments. Patients were included in the analysis if they underwent outpatient unilateral medial UKA, and those who underwent lateral UKA and simultaneous bilateral UKA were excluded. Demographics and comorbidities were similar between groups (Table 1).

In all cases, a fixed-bearing fully cemented UKA was utilized. In the robotic cohort, the Navio handheld robotic sculptor (Smith and Nephew, Memphis, TN) was used. Navio is an image-free semiautonomous robotic system that utilizes optical-based navigation with an imageless system to provide 3D morphed images. The precision of Navio has been shown to result in mean rotational errors within 1.04°–1.88° and 1.48°–1.98° of the femoral and tibial implants, respectively, with mean femoral and tibial transitional errors reported to be within 0.72–1.29 mm and 0.79–1.27 mm, respectively [24]. It relies on intraoperative surface and limb mapping and registration to plan condylar bone resections and quantify soft tissue balancing. The system provides protective control against inadvertent bone removal by modulating the exposure and speed of the motorized bur. In the conventional instrumentation cohort, proximal tibial resection was performed with an extramedullary tibial cutting guide, and a spacer block technique was used for femoral preparation.

Table 1: Summary of cohort demographics.

Dependent variable	Conventional $N = 39$	Robotic $N = 50$	p value
Gender			1.000
Female	17 (43.6%)	21 (42.0%)	
Male	22 (56.4%)	29 (58.0%)	
Age (years)	58 (13)	63 (11)	0.073
BMI	28.3 (4.06)	28.1 (4.45)	0.783
CCI	0.37 (0.63)	0.52 (0.93)	0.367
CCI (age adjusted)	1.76 (1.58)	2.34 (1.64)	0.099

Values are reported in means and standard deviations, with the exception of gender, which is reported in means and percentages relative to the entire cohort. CCI: Charlson Comorbidity Index.

In the robotic system studied, an algorithm is followed to establish the tightness or laxity in the hemicompartment after virtual positioning of the components. After arthrotomy and removal of the medial osteophytes, a valgus stress is applied to the knee (in the case of medial UKA) as it is passively moved from full extension to deep flexion. After surface mapping and 3-dimensional planning of implant sizes, their position and orientation are "virtually" established. A graphic representation of gap spacing through an entire range of motion is created. Adjustments can be made in the virtual positioning of the components—including tibial slope and depth of resection, or femoral component flexion, anteriorization, and distalization—to achieve the desired soft tissue balance across the entire flexion arc. The goal is to adjust the implant positions and orientations such that the gaps in extension and flexion are balanced according to surgeon preferences, with roughly 2 mm of laxity between the components through a full arc of motion, and avoiding overcorrection of alignment into the opposite compartment.

In the conventional technique used in this study, the distal femoral resection was based on the tibial cut, with the goal of leaving 2 mm of laxity between the articulating surfaces of the femoral and tibial trial components, confirmed by a 2 mm spacer device.

Perioperative protocols for anesthesia, surgical incision, periarticular capsular injection, physical therapy, pain management, and overall care were otherwise identical. At our institution, postoperative rehabilitation includes immediate weight bearing as tolerated with a walker, followed by a transition to a cane at the discretion of the physical therapist. Upon restoration of adequate quadriceps strength and balance, patients were allowed to ambulate without assistance. Self-directed exercises began on the day of surgery, and formal physical therapy was initiated within 4 days after surgery, including range of motion and isometrics.

The primary patient-reported outcomes (PROs) studied were Knee Injury and Osteoarthritis Outcome Score for Joint Replacement (KOOS-JR), new Knee Society Score (KSS), Lower Extremity Functional Score (LEFS), Visual

Analog Scale (VAS) pain scores (0–100), and Veterans RAND 12-Item Health Survey (VR-12/SF-12) including both mental and physical health scores. The LEFS, new Knee Society Score, and KOOS-JR surveys are reliable, validated, and responsive measurements of lower body and knee health outcomes while VAS and VR-12/SF-12 are accurate and precise measurements of pain and physical and mental health, respectively [34–37]. PROs were collected 30 days preoperatively, and with the exception of new KSS, at 1 week, 6 weeks, 12 weeks, and 2 years postoperatively for VR-12/SF-12 and KOOS-JR. Postoperatively, the new KSS was assessed only at one year postoperatively. VAS pain scores were collected preoperatively and weekly at 1, 2, 3, 6, and 12 weeks. A linear mixed-effects model was used to assess differential change over time between the two groups. Secondary outcomes studied were postoperative opioid consumption up to 3 months after surgery, reoperations, revisions, and postoperative complications.

Mean age, BMI, KOOS-JR, LEFS, new KSS, VR-12/SF-12, and VAS scores were analyzed with *t*-tests for significance. A *p* value of <0.05 was set as the threshold to establish statistical significance of the results. Means of reported VAS pain scores were adjusted for group baseline differences. A linear mixed-effects model was utilized to assess differential changes among patients in the two cohorts.

Total 1 month preoperative and total 3 month postoperative opioid usage were determined using the Pennsylvania Prescription Drug Monitoring Program (PDMP) and New Jersey Prescription Monitoring Program (NJ PMP). These statewide databases have a reported accuracy of up to 97% and collect all information for filled prescriptions of all controlled substances. Opioid usage was reported in morphine milligram equivalents (MME).

3. Results

KOOS-JR scores increased for both cohorts over time. The robotic cohort had higher preoperative KOOS-JR scores than the conventional cohort ($p = 0.029$), and remained significantly higher at 6 weeks ($p = 0.001$) and 6 months ($p = 0.0037$) following surgery. While the robotic cohort had higher KOOS-JR scores at 2-year follow-up, the difference between the two cohorts was not statistically significant at that timeframe ($p = 0.469$) (Table 2).

Both cohorts experienced an increase in LEFS throughout the duration of the study. LEFS scores were significantly higher in the robotic cohort than in the conventional group at 1 week post-op but were similar at 6 weeks and 12 weeks post-op (Table 2). Mixed-model regressions were run to assess whether the improvement in LEFS and KOOS-JR was attributable to cohort placement. LEFS improved at 6 weeks and 12 weeks post-op ($p < 0.001$ at both time points). Similarly, KOOS-JR increased at 6 weeks, 12 weeks, 6 months, and 1 and 2 years following surgery ($p < 0.001$ at all time points). These regressions showed that the increase in LEFS attributable to robotic assistance is 8.47, 95% CI [2.25; 14.69] ($p = 0.010$); for KOOS-JR, these values were 7.26, 95% CI [1.18; 13.33] ($p = 0.023$).

Table 2: A summary of functional outcomes.

Dependent variable	Conventional	Robotic	*p* value
LEFS 1 week	23 (11)	31 (14)	0.015
LEFS 6 weeks	55 (10)	59 (13)	0.181
LEFS 12 weeks	59 (12)	62 (12)	0.324
Pre-op KOOS-JR[2]	49 (12)	57 (14)	0.029
6-week KOOS-JR	67 (8)	76 (9)	0.001
12-week KOOS-JR	68 (10)	74 (13)	0.131
6-month KOOS-JR	74 (10)	81 (11)	0.037
1-year KOOS-JR	77 (13)	84 (15)	0.100
2-year KOOS-JR	82.9 (20)	86.2 (17)	0.469

Values are reported in means and standard deviations. LEFS: Lower Extremity Functional Scale; KOOS-JR: Knee Injury and Osteoarthritis Outcome Score for Joint Replacement.

Preoperatively, there were no significant differences between groups in baseline total KSS score, or the individual component scores for functional activities, expectations, satisfaction, or symptoms. At 2 years after surgery, there was a significant improvement in all KSS elements compared to preoperative scores, with the patients in the robotic cohort more likely to have had their expectations met ($p = 0.006$). Those who received robotic assistance during UKA had higher satisfaction scores than those who did not and this approached statistical significance ($p = 0.068$). Otherwise, there were no differences between subsets (Table 3).

There was no significant difference in the mean preoperative ROM in the conventional cohort ($113^\circ \pm 8^\circ$) and in the robotic cohort ($116^\circ \pm 8^\circ$) ($p = 0.054$). Likewise, at 2 years after UKA, the ROM in each group was similar (robotic cohort ROM: $131^\circ \pm 11^\circ$; conventional cohort ROM: $131^\circ \pm 8^\circ$) ($p = 0.825$).

The difference in pre-op VAS pain scores was statistically significant ($p = 0.001$) between the two groups, as patients in the robotic-assisted cohort experienced an average VAS score of 44 while patients in the conventional cohort had a VAS pain score of 62. Patients who had robotic UKA experienced less pain at 1 week and 2 weeks post-op, but these findings were not statistically significant ($p = 0.146$ and $p = 0.234$, respectively). At 3 weeks post-op, patients in the robotic cohort had lower VAS pain scores (26) than those in the conventional cohort (39) ($p = 0.018$). These differences equilibrated by 6 weeks post-op (Table 4). No difference was found in 1 month total preoperative narcotic usage nor 3 month total postoperative narcotic usage between the two cohorts ($p = 0.282$ and $p = 0.320$, respectively) (Table 4). VAS scores are reported on a scale of 0–100 while opioid usage is reported in morphine milligram equivalents (MME).

Mixed-model regression analysis was run to control for baseline differences and elucidate whether cohort placement resulted in greater reduction of VAS pain scores over time. VAS scores decreased up until 6 weeks post-op ($p < 0.001$). No difference was found in changes in VAS scores that were attributable to cohort placement (−0.23, 95% CI: −1.37, 0.91, $p = 0.699$).

Patients in both the robotic and conventional cohorts had statistically similar physical (SF-12 PCS) and mental health scores (SF-12 MCS) preoperatively ($p = 0.691$ and $p = 0.760$, respectively). Despite similar baseline measures, at 6 weeks,

TABLE 3: A summary of preoperative, 2 year postoperative new Knee Society Scores, and 2 year postoperative VAS satisfaction scores.

Dependent variable	Conventional	Robotic	p value
Pre-op KSS functional activities (0–100)	47 (18)	48 (18)	0.811
Pre-op KSS patient expectations (0–15)	14 (3)	13 (3)	0.390
Pre-op KSS satisfaction (0–40)	16 (6)	16 (7.5)	0.552
Pre-op KSS symptoms (0–25)	9 (6)	12 (6)	0.148
2-year post-op KSS functional activities (0–100)	74 (19)	82 (17)	0.208
2-year post-op KSS patient expectations (0–15)	8 (2)	11 (3)	0.006
2-year post-op KSS satisfaction (0–40)	28 (10)	34 (9)	0.068
2-year post-op KSS symptoms (0–25)	20 (5)	21 (5)	0.269
2-year post-op VAS satisfaction	86 (20)	92 (18)	0.301

TABLE 4: A summary of VAS scores and opioid usage.

Dependent variable	Conventional	Robotic	p value
Pre-op VAS pain	62 (18)	44 (22)	0.001
1-week post-op VAS pain	60 (18)	53 (18)	0.146
2-week post-op VAS pain	46 (20)	39 (15)	0.234
3-week post-op VAS pain	39 (19)	26 (16)	0.018
6-week post-op VAS pain	23 (16)	18 (16)	0.370
12-week post-op VAS pain	21 (21)	16 (16)	0.552
Pre-op opioid usage (MME)	6 (7)	8(8)	0.282
Post-op opioid usage (MME)	660 (237)	714 (268)	0.320

TABLE 5: Preoperative and postoperative SF-12 PCS and SF-12 MCS values.

Dependent variable	Conventional	Robotic	p value
Pre-op SF-12 PCS	36 (8)	35 (9)	0.691
6-week SF-12 PCS	39 (8)	43 (9)	0.099
12-week SF-12 PCS	45 (8)	48 (7)	0.140
2-year SF-12 PCS	48 (10)	50 (11)	0.601
Pre-op SF-12 MCS	57 (8)	56 (11)	0.760
6-week SF-12 MCS	56 (8)	57 (7)	0.658
12-week SF-12 MCS	58 (5)	57 (9)	0.644
2-year SF-12 MCS	51 (7)	55 (7)	0.017

Values are reported in means and standard deviations.

the robotic cohort had a higher SF-12 PCS score (43 ± 9) than the conventional cohort (39 ± 8), approaching, but not achieving, statistical significance ($p = 0.099$) (Table 5).

SF-12 MCS scores were found to be significantly higher in the robotic cohort (55 ± 7) than in the conventional cohort (51 ± 7), ($p = 0.017$). Differences in SF-12 PCS equilibrated by 12 weeks. Both groups demonstrated statistically comparable improvement in SF-12 MCS at 6 and 12 weeks.

No patients in our cohort experienced a mechanical failure, infection, or revision after surgery. One patient in the robotic-assisted cohort had a reoperation: irrigation and debridement for traumatic wound dehiscence after a fall two weeks following surgery, while no patients in the conventional cohort had any reoperations. Overall, there was no statistical significance with respect to complications and reoperations between the two cohorts ($p = 0.628$ and $p = 1.00$, respectively).

4. Discussion

Experience with robotic technology for UKA has consistently shown improvements in radiographic alignment [27]. Less certain, and less studied, is the impact of robotic precision on clinical outcomes, postoperative pain, patient satisfaction, and implant durability. This study was an attempt to add additional insight regarding whether UKA performed with robotic technology that quantifies both bone resection parameters and soft tissue balance impacts early outcomes and short-term durability any differently than a matched group of patients undergoing UKA with conventional instrumentation.

Our data show that, in our matched cohorts, robotic assistance during UKA does indeed provide patients with greater early functional recovery up to 6 months following surgery, according to the LEFS and KOOS-JR scores. The LEFS, in particular, has been shown to be extremely responsive to subtle differences early in the postoperative period. Any functional differences in our study equilibrated by 1 year. We found no difference in cumulative 3-month postoperative opioid usage. Finally, we found that patients in the robotic cohort were statistically significantly more likely to have their expectations met at 2-year follow-up. Satisfaction was also higher in the robotic cohort, and this approached statistical significance ($p = 0.068$).

A prospective study by Blyth et al. of 139 patients undergoing medial UKA randomized to using either manual conventional cutting instruments or haptic robotic assistance found significant reductions in pain in the initial two months after robotic UKA [29]. The authors found that, from the first postoperative day, up until week 8 after UKA, the median pain scores for the robotic group were 55.4% lower than those observed in the manual surgery group ($p = 0.040$). Similarly, VAS pain scores for both of our cohorts decreased significantly up until 6 weeks post-op. However, unlike the Blyth study, while VAS pain scores in our series were lower for patients in the robotic cohort at three weeks post-op, mixed-model regression analysis showed no difference between these two cohorts with respect to decrease in VAS pain scores at measured time intervals. Furthermore, Blyth and colleagues reported that, at three months postoperatively, the robotic group had significantly better Knee Society Scores (KSS) than the conventional group ($p = 0.04$), although the KSS may not be an optimal measure of early functional outcomes, and the KSS differences were not apparent at one year after UKA. This is similar to what we found with regard to LEFS and KOOS-JR early in the postoperative period, and similarly, we found no differences in 1-year KSS or KOOS-JR scores. In comparison with those who underwent robotic UKA in the Blyth study, patients who underwent UKA with robotic assistance in our study seemed to have higher KOOS-JR scores. At 1 year post-op, the average KOOS-JR in the robotic-assisted cohort was 84. Using the crosswalk of KOOS-JR to Oxford Knee Scores (OKS) [38], this corresponds to an OKS of 44. In contrast, less than half of the robotic patients in the Blyth study failed to achieve an OKS of 43. Although there was no overall statistical difference between groups, the proportion of patients in the Blyth study achieving a Forgotten Joint Score of >80%—a measure of the patient's awareness of their joint—was almost double in those who underwent UKA with robotic assistance compared to conventional methods (15% versus 8%, $p = 0.265$).

At one year postoperatively, a greater proportion of patients receiving robotic-assisted surgery improved their UCLA activity scores (69% versus 52%; $p = 0.06$). Importantly, the authors noted that on subgroup analysis of 35 patients considered to be highly active preoperatively, there was statistically better improvement in function with robotic assistance than with conventional techniques for KSS, Oxford Knee Score, and Forgotten Joint Score ($p = 0.0346$) one year after UKA [29], and these superior results persisted at 2-year clinical follow-up [31]. Our study was not adequately powered to review a subset of highly active patients to determine whether we had comparable benefits of robotics in such a cohort.

Other studies have also shown more rapid clinical recovery after UKA performed with robotic assistance compared to conventional methods. In a retrospective review of 28 lateral UKAs, 11 performed with robotic assistance with the same handheld image-free device used in the present study and 17 performed with conventional instruments, Canetti et al. reported a more rapid return to sports with robotic assistance (mean and standard deviation of 4.2 ± 1.8 months compared with 10.5 ± 6.7 months; $p < 0.01$) [33]. However, as the authors point out, surgical approaches varied between the two groups, recall bias may have existed when retrospectively determining interval to return to sport, and it is unclear whether perioperative protocols differed between the groups in that study [33]. Kayani et al. reported on a prospective consecutive cohort study of 146 patients that underwent medial UKA using either conventional jig-based instrumentation or robotic arm assistance. Robotic arm-assisted UKA was associated with reduced postoperative pain ($p < 0.001$), decreased opiate analgesia requirements ($p < 0.001$), shorter time to straight leg raise ($p < 0.001$), decreased number of physiotherapy sessions ($p < 0.001$), and increased maximum knee flexion at discharge ($p < 0.001$) [39]. While these outcomes are encouraging, it is unclear whether pain levels were similar prior to surgery and thus whether the significant differences in postoperative pain levels were truly clinically significant or an equivalent change between groups compared to preoperative pain levels. Furthermore, it is unclear whether perioperative pain management protocols were similar between groups. If they were similar, the reduced opiate requirements in their study is worth highlighting, particularly given that both our study and the study by Blyth et al. found no differences [29].

We found no difference between groups in cumulative postoperative opioid prescriptions in the three months following surgery. This finding is in agreement with the findings of Blyth et al. [29]. However, one weakness in our methodology is that we utilized a statewide database, the Pennsylvania Prescription Drug Monitoring Program (PDMP), to record opioid usage. While this database has a reported accuracy of up to 97% with respect to quantity prescribed, we were unable to track or study patient opioid usage. Moreover, with narcotics being prescribed to patients in accordance with standard protocols, the quantities that were obtained from the statewide database may not accurately reflect postoperative narcotic use, particularly for those who abstain or are low-level users. Further studies which investigate opioid usage between these two methods of UKA are needed.

At this time, mid- and long-term survivorship studies are lacking in robotic-assisted UKA. Nonetheless, several series comparing revision rates and durability to historical controls, registry and insurance databases, and comparable cohorts have shown encouraging results at short term to midterm [27, 30, 31, 40]. A prospective randomized trial found that at 2-year follow-up while no revisions were necessary in the robotic-assisted group, there were 2 revisions (2.8%) in the manual group and more radiolucencies beneath the components in the conventional group [31]. In a matched case-control study of 160 UKA performed with either Navio or a conventional technique using the identical implant (HLS Uni Evolution, Tornier®), Batailler et al. found that, at a mean follow-up of 19.7 months for the robotic-assisted group and 24.2 months for the control group, 5% ($n = 4/80$) of patients in the robotic-assisted UKA group and 9% ($n = 7/80$) in the conventional UKA group required revision to TKA (n. s. d.) [27]. In the conventional group, 86% of revisions were due to component malposition or limb malalignment, compared to none in the robotic-assisted group [27]. In a clinical study of 128 patients undergoing UKA with NAVIO robotic assistance, Battenberg et al. reported that the overall survivorship of the knee implant among novice users was 99.2% (95% confidence interval: 94.6 to 99.9%) after a mean of follow-up period of 2.3 years, compared to a reference survival rate of 95.7% from the Australian registry and 92.6% from a US Medicare database [3, 18, 30].

Similarly, our matched study of UKA performed with conventional instruments or robotics had a low revision rate in both cohorts, with no difference in failure rates, albeit further follow-up will be necessary to clearly determine if there are longer-term benefits to the improved accuracy of implantation and quantified soft tissue balance with robot assistance.

It is unclear why some of the outcome parameters studied in our series were different between the robotic and conventional groups up until 1-year follow-up, given generally otherwise identical surgical approaches and perioperative protocols. One possible explanation may be that quantifying soft tissue balance may impact early function. Robotic assistance during UKA utilizes optical motion capture technology to provide real-time medial and lateral gap balance measurements under valgus/varus strain to induce ligament tension through the arc of flexion [22]. These parameters allow surgeons to achieve the desired ligamentous tension and limb alignment by fine-tuning implant positioning [22].

As with all retrospective studies, ours has several potential limitations. First, ours was a matched cohort of consecutive cases performed with or without robotic assistance based on geographic location and robotic access according to hospital selection. While a randomized prospective study may have been better to eliminate the potential for selection bias, we feel that we were able to mitigate some of the deficiencies of a retrospective cohort study since demographics, patient socioeconomics, preoperative functional scores, and range of motion were matched, we used fixed-bearing cemented UKA implants of similar design in each group, and perioperative protocols such as physical therapy and pain management were identical. A second potential weakness which could serve as a confounding variable for this study is that the operative surgeon has extensive experience with both conventional and robotic techniques, which may have reduced the differences between the two groups. It is possible that surgery performed by less experienced surgeons, or a multicentered study, may or may not yield different results that favor one method over another, in terms of both clinical outcomes and implant survivorship. For instance, Karia et al. have shown that robotic assistance neutralizes surgeon inexperience and improves alignment measures compared to persistent errors with conventional methods in the hands of inexperienced surgeons [41]. We would encourage a study similar to ours by surgeons with variable operative experience with either conventional or robotic techniques to determine the impact of advanced precision on functional outcomes in UKA in their hands. Third, due to matching of the cohorts, our sample size was limited to 39 in the conventional instrumentation group and 50 in the robotic technology arm, which may have increased the risk of type II error. Fourth, our study did not look at the impact of component alignment on functional outcomes, as we had a relatively high incidence of postoperative short radiographs in both groups which were slightly rotated, thus rendering radiographic measurements of alignment inaccurate. Nonetheless, others have studied implant alignment comparisons between conventional and various robotic systems. Fifth, our follow-up was only one year after surgery. While our results show that patients in both groups experienced similar functional outcomes and implant durability at 1-year follow-up, further follow-up is necessary to elucidate whether either technique suffers increased failures at mid- and longer-term follow-up.

5. Conclusion

Robotic-assisted UKA had superior functional outcomes up until 6 months following surgery, with differences equilibrating between the two cohorts by 1 year post-op. While the robotic cohort had lower VAS pain scores at 3 weeks post-op, mixed-model regression analysis showed this decrease was not attributable to cohort placement. We also noticed no difference in cumulative postoperative opioid prescriptions, although we were unable to determine precise opioid usage. Those who received robotic assistance were more likely to have their expectations met and satisfaction was tending to be higher in the robotic cohort as well. Despite these promising early results, further mid- and long-term studies are needed to better assess whether robotic-assisted UKA provides longer-term benefits on clinical functionality, implant durability, and patient satisfaction. Otherwise, if these outcome metrics are not appreciably impacted by using robotic technology, its broader use will only be considered if robotics can be shown to be cost-effective and time-efficient and eliminate instrument tray burden.

References

[1] G. S. Kazarian, J. H. Lonner, M. G. Maltenfort, H. M. K. Ghomrawi, and A. F. Chen, "Cost-effectiveness of surgical and nonsurgical treatments for unicompartmental knee arthritis," *Journal of Bone and Joint Surgery*, vol. 100, no. 19, pp. 1653–1660, 2018.

[2] D. S. Casper, A. N. Fleischman, P. V. Papas, J. Grossman, G. R. Scuderi, and J. H. Lonner, "Unicompartmental knee arthroplasty provides significantly greater improvement in function than total knee arthroplasty despite equivalent satisfaction for isolated medial compartment osteoarthritis," *The Journal of Arthroplasty*, vol. 34, no. 8, pp. 1611–1616, 2019.

[3] E. N. Hansen, K. L. Ong, E. Lau, S. M. Kurtz, and J. H. Lonner, "Unicondylar knee arthroplasty has fewer complications but higher revision rates than total knee arthroplasty in a study of large United States databases," *The Journal of Arthroplasty*, vol. 34, no. 8, pp. 1617–1625, 2019.

[4] P.-E. Schwab, P. Lavand'homme, J. C. Yombi, and E. Thienpont, "Lower blood loss after unicompartmental than total knee arthroplasty," *Knee Surgery, Sports Traumatology, Arthroscopy*, vol. 23, no. 12, pp. 3494–3500, 2015.

[5] S. Shankar, M. W. Tetreault, B. J. Jegier, G. B. Andersson, and C. J. Della Valle, "A cost comparison of unicompartmental and total knee arthroplasty," *The Knee*, vol. 23, no. 6, pp. 1016–1019, 2016.

[6] I. L. Kalbian, T. L. Tan, A. J. Rondon et al., "Reduced opioid requirements following unicompartmental knee arthroplasty compared with total knee arthroplasty," *The Bone & Joint Journal*, vol. 101-B, no. 7_Supple_C, pp. 22–27, 2019.

[7] M. R. O'Rourke, J. J. Gardner, J. J. Callaghan et al., "Unicompartmental knee replacement: a minimum twenty-one-year followup, end-result study," *Clinical Orthopaedics and Related Research*, vol. 440, pp. 27–37, 2005.

[8] D. W. Pennington, J. J. Swienckowski, W. B. Lutes, and G. N. Drake, "Lateral unicompartmental knee arthroplasty: survivorship and technical considerations at an average follow-up of 12.4 years," *The Journal of Arthroplasty*, vol. 21, no. 1, pp. 13–17, 2006.

[9] R. A. Berger, R. M. Meneghini, J. J. Jacobs, and M. B. Sheinkop, "Results of unicompartmental knee arthroplasty at a minimum of ten years of follow-up," *The Journal of*

Bone and Joint Surgery, vol. 87, no. 5, pp. 999–1006, 2005.

[10] M. Ollivier, C. Jacquet, A. Lucet, S. Parratte, and J. N. Argenson, "Long-term results of medial unicompartmental knee arthroplasty for knee avascular necrosis," *The Journal of Arthroplasty*, vol. 34, no. 3, pp. 465–468, 2019.

[11] H. Pandit, T. W. Hamilton, C. Jenkins, S. J. Mellon, C. A. F. Dodd, and D. W. Murray, "The clinical outcome of minimally invasive phase 3 oxford unicompartmental knee arthroplasty," *The Journal of Bone and Joint Surgery*, vol. 97-B, no. 11, pp. 1493–1500, 2015.

[12] P. Hernigou and G. Deschamps, "Alignment influences wear in the knee after medial unicompartmental arthroplasty," *Clinical Orthopaedics & Related Research*, vol. 423, pp. 161–165, 2004.

[13] A. D. Liddle, H. Pandit, A. Judge, and D. W. Murray, "Effect of surgical caseload on revision rate following total and unicompartmental knee replacement," *The Journal of Bone and Joint Surgery*, vol. 98, no. 1, pp. 1–8, 2016.

[14] J.-A. Epinette, B. Brunschweiler, P. Mertl, D. Mole, and A. Cazenave, "Unicompartmental knee arthroplasty modes of failure: wear is not the main reason for failure: a multicentre study of 418 failed knees," *Orthopaedics & Traumatology: Surgery & Research*, vol. 98, no. 6 Suppl, pp. S124–S130, 2012.

[15] G. S. Dyrhovden, S. H. L. Lygre, M. Badawy, Ø. Gøthesen, and O. Furnes, "Have the causes of revision for total and unicompartmental knee arthroplasties changed during the past two decades?" *Clinical Orthopaedics & Related Research*, vol. 475, no. 7, pp. 1874–1886, 2017.

[16] R. Chatellard, V. Sauleau, M. Colmar, H. Robert, G. Raynaud, and J. Brilhault, "Medial unicompartmental knee arthroplasty: does tibial component position influence clinical outcomes and arthroplasty survival?" *Orthopaedics & Traumatology: Surgery & Research*, vol. 99, no. 4 Suppl, pp. S219–S225, 2013.

[17] W. G. Hamilton, M. B. Collier, E. Tarabee, J. P. McAuley, C. A. Engh, and G. A. Engh, "Incidence and reasons for reoperation after minimally invasive unicompartmental knee arthroplasty," *The Journal of Arthroplasty*, vol. 21, no. 6, pp. 98–107, 2006.

[18] Australian Orthopaedic Association National Joint Replacement Registry, "Hip, knee & shoulder arthroplasty-annual report 2018," AOANJRR, New Orleans, LA, USA, 2018.

[19] National Joint Registry, "National joint registry for England, Wales NI and the I of M 15th annual report 2018," 15th Annual report, National Joint Registry, London, UK, 2018.

[20] J. Cobb, J. Henckel, P. Gomes et al., "Hands-on robotic unicompartmental knee replacement," *The Journal of Bone and Joint Surgery*, vol. 88-B, no. 2, pp. 188–197, 2006.

[21] P. Hernigou and G. Deschamps, "Posterior slope of the tibial implant and the outcome of unicompartmental knee arthroplasty," *The Journal of Bone & Joint Surgery*, vol. 86, no. 3, pp. 506–511, 2004.

[22] J. H. Lonner, *Robotics in Knee and Hip Arthroplasty. Current Concepts, Techniques and Emerging Uses*, Springer, New York city, NY, USA, 2019.

[23] N. J. Dunbar, M. W. Roche, B. H. Park, S. H. Branch, M. A. Conditt, and S. A. Banks, "Accuracy of dynamic tactile-guided unicompartmental knee arthroplasty," *The Journal of Arthroplasty*, vol. 27, no. 5, pp. 803–808, 2012.

[24] J. H. Lonner, J. R. Smith, F. Picard, B. Hamlin, P. J. Rowe, and P. E. Riches, "High degree of accuracy of a novel image-free handheld robot for unicondylar knee arthroplasty in a cadaveric study," *Clinical Orthopaedics & Related Research*, vol. 473, no. 1, pp. 206–212, 2015.

[25] S. W. Bell, I. Anthony, B. Jones, A. MacLean, P. Rowe, and M. Blyth, "Improved accuracy of component positioning with robotic-assisted unicompartmental knee arthroplasty," *Journal of Bone and Joint Surgery*, vol. 98, no. 8, pp. 627–635, 2016.

[26] D. Y. Ponzio and J. H. Lonner, "Robotic technology produces more conservative tibial resection than conventional techniques in UKA," *American Journal of Orthopedics (Belle Mead NJ)*, vol. 45, no. 7, pp. E465–E468, 2016.

[27] C. Batailler, N. White, F. M. Ranaldi, P. Neyret, E. Servien, and S. Lustig, "Improved implant position and lower revision rate with robotic-assisted unicompartmental knee arthroplasty," *Knee Surgery, Sports Traumatology, Arthroscopy*, vol. 27, no. 4, pp. 1232–1240, 2019.

[28] Y. Herry, C. Batailler, T. Lording, E. Servien, P. Neyret, and S. Lustig, "Improved joint-line restitution in unicompartmental knee arthroplasty using a robotic-assisted surgical technique," *International Orthopaedics*, vol. 41, no. 11, pp. 2265–2271, 2017.

[29] M. J. G. Blyth, I. Anthony, P. Rowe, M. S. Banger, A. MacLean, and B. Jones, "Robotic arm-assisted versus conventional unicompartmental knee arthroplasty," *Bone & Joint Research*, vol. 6, no. 11, pp. 631–639, 2017.

[30] A. K. Battenberg, N. A. Netravali, and J. H. Lonner, "A novel handheld robotic-assisted system for unicompartmental knee arthroplasty: surgical technique and early survivorship," *Journal of Robotic Surgery*, vol. 14, no. 1, pp. 55–60, 2020.

[31] A. Gilmour, A. D. MacLean, P. J. Rowe et al., "Robotic-arm-assisted vs conventional unicompartmental knee arthroplasty. The 2-year clinical outcomes of a randomized controlled trial," *The Journal of Arthroplasty*, vol. 33, no. 7, pp. S109–S115, 2018.

[32] J. H. Lonner and M. R. Klement, "Robotic-assisted medial unicompartmental knee arthroplasty," *Journal of the American Academy of Orthopaedic Surgeons*, vol. 27, no. 5, pp. e207–e214, 2019.

[33] R. Canetti, C. Batailler, C. Bankhead, P. Neyret, E. Servien, and S. Lustig, "Faster return to sport after robotic-assisted lateral unicompartmental knee arthroplasty: a comparative study," *Archives of Orthopaedic and Trauma Surgery*, vol. 138, no. 12, pp. 1765–1771, 2018.

[34] G. R. Scuderi, R. B. Bourne, P. C. Noble, J. B. Benjamin, J. H. Lonner, and W. N. Scott, "The new knee society knee scoring system," *Clinical Orthopaedics & Related Research*, vol. 470, no. 1, pp. 3–19, 2012.

[35] S. Lyman, Y.-Y. Lee, P. D. Franklin, W. Li, M. B. Cross, and D. E. Padgett, "Validation of the KOOS, JR: a short-form knee arthroplasty outcomes survey," *Clinical Orthopaedics & Related Research*, vol. 474, no. 6, pp. 1461–1471, 2016.

[36] J. M. Binkley, P. W. Stratford, S. A. Lott, and D. L. Riddle, "The lower extremity functional scale (LEFS): scale development, measurement properties, and clinical application," *Physical Therapy*, vol. 79, no. 4, pp. 371–383, 1999.

[37] J. E. Ware, M. Kosinski, and S. D. Keller, "A 12-item short-form health survey," *Medical Care*, vol. 34, no. 3, pp. 220–233, 1996.

[38] B. A. Polascik, C. Hidaka, M. C. Thompson et al., "Crosswalks between knee and hip arthroplasty short forms," *Journal of Bone and Joint Surgery*, vol. 102, no. 11, pp. 983–990, 2020.

[39] B. Kayani, S. Konan, J. Tahmassebi, F. E. Rowan, and F. S. Haddad, "An assessment of early functional rehabilitation and hospital discharge in conventional versus robotic-

arm assisted unicompartmental knee arthroplasty," *The Bone & Joint Journal*, vol. 101-B, no. 1, pp. 24–33, 2019.
[40] L. J. Kleeblad, T. A. Borus, T. M. Coon, J. Dounchis, J. T. Nguyen, and A. D. Pearle, "Midterm survivorship and patient satisfaction of robotic-arm-assisted medial unicompartmental knee arthroplasty: a multicenter study," *The Journal of Arthroplasty*, vol. 33, no. 6, pp. 1719–1726, 2018.
[41] M. Karia, M. Masjedi, B. Andrews, Z. Jaffry, and J. Cobb, "Robotic assistance enables inexperienced surgeons to perform unicompartmental knee arthroplasties on dry bone models with accuracy superior to conventional methods," *Advances in Orthopedics*, vol. 2013, Article ID 481039, 7 pages, 2013.

5

The Value of Routine Intravenous Tranexamic Acid in Total Hip Arthroplasty

J. Chin, J. Blackett, D. C. Kieser, C. Frampton, and G. Hooper

Department of Orthopaedic Surgery and Musculoskeletal Medicine, University of Otago, Christchurch, New Zealand

Correspondence should be addressed to D. C. Kieser; kieserdavid@gmail.com

Academic Editor: Allen L. Carl

Objective. To determine the effect on the need for transfusion when intravenous tranexamic acid (TXA) is administered intraoperatively in patients undergoing total hip arthroplasty (THA). *Method.* A prospective, double blinded, randomised control trial of 88 patients undergoing THA was randomly allocated to receive 1 g of intravenous TXA or normal saline on induction of anaesthesia. All patients received spinal anaesthesia. The primary outcome measure was transfusion rate, and the secondary outcomes were intraoperative blood loss, haemoglobin levels, length of hospital stay, functional scores, and thromboembolic complications. *Results.* 19.0% of patients given TXA required a blood transfusion, compared with 20.5% given placebo ($p = 0.87$). Secondary outcomes included mean intraoperative blood loss, which was 536.5 ml in the TXA group and 469.8 ml in the placebo group ($p = 0.276$). Day 1 haemoglobin levels were 108.9 g/l in the TXA group versus 104.3 g/l in the placebo group ($p = 0.114$). Day 4 haemoglobin levels were 105.0 g/l and 99.8 g/l, respectively ($p = 0.130$). The mean length of stay in those who received TXA was 4.3days, compared with 4.8days in those given placebo ($p = 0.20$). The Oxford Hip Score showed a mean improvement over a 1-year period of 25.9 points in those who received TXA, compared with 26.7 points in those who received placebo ($p = 0.679$). There were two treatment emergent adverse events: a pulmonary embolism (TXA) and a myocardial infarction (placebo). *Conclusions.* 1 g IV TXA administered on induction did not significantly reduce the need for blood transfusion, postoperative blood loss, functional scores, or the length of stay in patients undergoing THA. This trial is registered with ACTRN12610001065088.

1. Introduction

As our agingpopulation increases and our arthroplasty volumes grow [1, 2], interest in prophylactic measures to optimise the recovery period of these patients has evolved. One area of interest has targeted a reduction in intra-operative blood loss. This is extremely important in the elderly who have a lower physiological reserve and greater medical comorbidities, thus limiting their ability to tolerate anaemia and haemodynamic instability. Furthermore, blood transfusions are not without risk with complications including pyrexia, allergy, transfusion reaction, and infection transmission [3].

The implementation of enhanced recovery after surgery (ERAS) protocols, including intraoperative blood loss control, has been seen to reduce patient morbidity, hastening recovery, and reduce hospital length of stay [4]. One measure which has gained favour in intraoperative blood loss control is tranexamic acid (TXA) [5].

TXA is an antifibrinolytic agent that potentiates the inhibition of fibrinolysis by inhibiting the activation of plasminogen to plasmin. This reduces clot breakdown and therefore blood loss. TXA has been used for more than 30 years in cardiac surgery where it has shown to reduce postoperative blood loss, transfusion requirements, and the frequency of early surgical revisions for bleeding [6]. It has been more recently applied in orthopaedics, where research has suggested that TXA is an efficacious and cost-effective method of blood conservation [5, 7–9].

However, there remains a theoretical concern that the use of this medication may increase the incidence of thromboembolic events, especially venous thromboembolic events (VTE) such as deep vein thrombosis (DVT) or pulmonary embolism (PE). Furthermore, it is unknown how many patients are needed to be treated with TXA to identify a clinically significant reduction in intraoperative blood loss or to prevent a blood transfusion.

The aim of this study was to accurately assess the effect of 1 g intravenous (IV) TXA, given immediately prior to skin incision, on the requirement for blood transfusion in patients undergoing elective total hip arthroplasty (THA) for osteoarthritis (OA) or osteonecrosis. In addition, intraoperative blood loss, preoperative and postoperative functional scores, and the risk of clinically significant VTE were recorded.

2. Methods

We performed a double blind, prospective, randomised control trial (RCT) with patients randomised to receive either 1 g IV TXA or a placebo of IV saline prior to skin incision in patients undergoing elective THA for OA or osteonecrosis.

Patients were recruited by the orthopaedic surgeons of Burwood Hospital, Christchurch, New Zealand.

This RCT only included those patients that received a spinal anaesthetic (+/− general anaesthetic) as part of their procedure. This controls for a confounder in that it is thought a spinal anaesthetic protects against blood loss in total hip arthroplasty by reducing arterial and venous pressure [10].

Patients' consent was attained as was ethical approval from the Central Regional Ethics Committee, Wellington, New Zealand.

Patients were excluded if they had contraindications for TXA (history or risk of thrombosis, active thromboembolic disease, and acquired disturbance of colour vision) or were on clopidogrel, ticagrelor, warfarin, dabigatran, or any other anticoagulant. Patients with renal failure or bleeding disorders were also excluded. Those on aspirin were asked to stop one week prior to surgery. This was recommenced on day 1 postoperation. Those patients that did not receive a single-dose spinal anaesthetic were excluded.

2.1. Randomisation and Intervention Delivery. Patients were randomised based on a computer-generated list in a 1 : 1 ratio to TXA or placebo. After the patient was recruited into the study and was in the theatre complex, the randomisation allocation was identified by the unblinded hospital pharmacist who dispensed TXA or placebo in a covered and blinded syringe to the anaesthetist just prior to skin incision.

All patients received a single-dose spinal anaesthetic, with a supplementary general anaesthetic being administered at the discretion of the anaesthetic team.

2.2. Procedure and Outcome Measures. THA was performed through a standard posterior approach. Intraoperative blood loss was estimated by the volume in the suction drains and by weighing the swabs, with the assumption that 1 gram was equivalent to 1millilitre of blood. At closure, a single large-bore drain was inserted deep into the fascia lata. Postoperative drainage was recorded for the first 24 hours, and the drains were then removed. Haemoglobin (Hb) was checked preoperatively, one day postoperatively, and four days postoperatively. A blood transfusion threshold of Hb < 80 g/dl was instated. However, patients with symptomatic anaemia with Hb in excess of 80 g/dl were also transfused on clinical reasoning. Time to discharge was recorded from the clinical notes, rounded to the nearest half day.

Functional outcome scores were recorded in clinic both preoperatively and one year postoperatively. These scores included Oxford Hip Score, Western Ontario and McMaster Universities Arthritis Index (WOMAC), and the High Activity Arthroplasty Score (HAAS).

Symptomatic thromboembolic events were screened at follow-up clinics performed at six weeks and variably over the first six months. Any patient who presented to a health practitioner outside of the orthopaedic follow-up clinics over this period was also recorded.

The primary outcomes were the intraoperative blood loss and the transfusion rate, and secondary outcomes were time to discharge, functional outcome scores, and thromboembolic complications.

The outcome measures were compared between randomised groups using Mann–Whitney *U*-tests, and the percentage of patients requiring a transfusion was compared using Fisher's exact test.

To achieve adequate power, with alpha 0.05 and beta 0.80, a total of 200 patients were required to detect a decrease in a transfusion rate of 50% from 0.3 units per patient to 0.15 units per patient.

3. Results

In total, 189 patients were approached to be recruited for the study, with 88 patients deemed eligible for inclusion. Most patients were excluded following randomisation and administration of intervention/placebo due to progression to general anaesthetic without a spinal anaesthetic or having incomplete data collection (Figure 1.). The mean BMI was 28.9 (18.8 to 41.7).

The total transfusion rate postoperatively, 8 of 42 (19.0%) patients given TXA required a transfusion, compared with 8 of 39 (20.5%) patients given the placebo ($p = 1.00$). The patients who were randomised to TXA required 0.34 blood units per patient, compared with 0.44 units per patient ($p = 0.70$) in the placebo group (Table 1).

Intraoperative blood loss for patients who received TXA was slightly higher than for those who received placebo (Table 1). Mean total estimated intraoperative blood loss in the TXA group was 536.5 ml and 469.8 ml in placebo ($p = 0.276$). Blood loss in swabs was higher in those who received TXA, with a mean of 173.7 g versus 128.8 g ($p = 0.053$), respectively. Blood loss measured from the suction showed a mean of 362.8 ml in those who received TXA and 341.1 ml in the placebo group ($p = 0.681$). Mean total blood loss recorded in the drain showed blood conservation in those who received TXA compared with placebo, with 560.9 ml and 688.4 ml, respectively ($p = 0.22$).

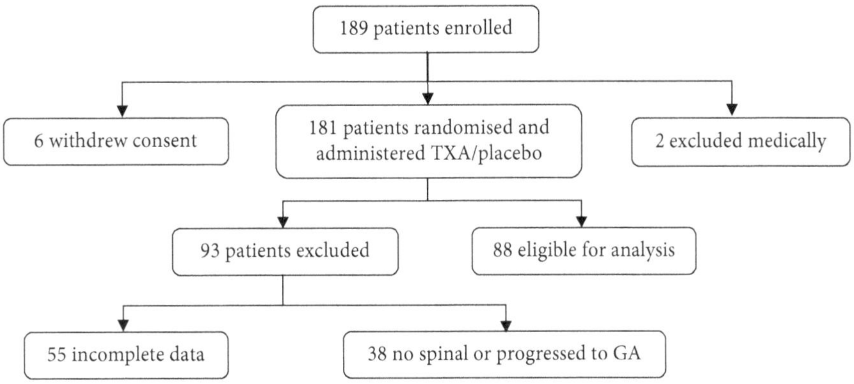

Figure 1: Flowchart of patient inclusion and exclusion.

Table 1: Comparison of intraoperative blood loss and transfusion rates between TXA and placebo.

	TXA	Placebo	p value
Transfusion rate (units/patient)	0.34 (0–3)	0.44 (0–8)	0.70
Number of patients requiring transfusion (n/N, %)	8/42 (19.0%)	8/39 (20.5%)	1.00
Mean perioperative blood loss (mL), mean (range)	536.5 (130–920)	469.8 (57–1359)	0.28
Mean total blood loss in drains (mL), mean (range)	560.9 (0–1860)	688.4 (0–2500)	0.22
Day 1 haemoglobin levels (g/L), mean (range)	108.9 (82–132)	104.3 (80–143)	0.11
Day 4 haemoglobin levels (g/L), mean (range)	105.0 (83–129)	99.8 (75–136)	0.13
Time to discharge (days), mean (range)	4.3 (2.0–7.0)	4.8 (2.0–21.0)	0.20

Day 1 haemoglobin levels were higher in those receiving TXA with mean measurements of 108.9 g/l versus 104.3 g/l ($p = 0.114$). This was supported by day 4 haemoglobin measures with 105.0 g/l in those who received TXA and 99.8 g/l in those who received placebo ($p = 0.130$) (Table 1).

The length of stay did not differ significantly between the two randomised groups (Table 1). The mean length of stay of those who received TXA was 4.3days, compared with 4.8days in those who received placebo ($p = 0.20$).

There was no significant difference between TXA and placebo groups in the improvement of functional scales, comparing the preoperative to the one-year postoperative scores. The Oxford Hip Score showed a mean improvement of 25.9 points in those patients who received TXA, compared with 26.7 points in those who received placebo ($p = 0.679$). The WOMAC scores were improved by 49.9 points in the TXA group, compared with 50.7 points in the placebo group ($p = 0.864$). The mean improvement in the HAAS was 7.5 points in the TXA group, compared with 8.2 points in the placebo group ($p = 0.278$).

There was one patient in the TXA group who had a postoperative pulmonary embolism and one patient in the placebo group who had postoperative myocardial infarction.

4. Discussion

Our results show that a single dose of 1 g IV TXA prior to incision did not significantly reduce the postoperative blood loss following THA. In addition, no significant differences in transfusion rates were noted.

As observed by the American College of Physicians, "although it is tempting to equate statistical significance with clinical importance, critical readers should avoid this temptation. To be clinically important requires a substantial change in an outcome that matters. Statistically significant changes, however, can be observed with trivial outcomes. And because statistical significance is powerfully influenced by the number of observations, statistically significant changes can be observed with trivial (small) changes in important outcomes. Large studies can be significant without being clinically important, and small studies may be important without being significant [11]."

When one considers the financial cost of such treatment, the total drug cost of tranexamic acid (NZ$58) is less than the production cost of a unit of allogenic blood (NZ$158) [12]. However, using the number needed to treat of 67, this study effectively spent $3886 on TXA to save 1 unit of blood. This cost was not retrieved in a significantly shorter duration of stay as shown by the time to discharge.

However, it may be that 1 g IV TXA is not the optimum dose or the method of administration. Studies have shown that higher doses of TXA and additional routes of administration have a significant effect [5, 8, 9, 13]. In an RCT with 150 patients, Yi and colleagues suggested a single-dose IV TXA plus topical TXA reduce blood loss and the need for transfusion, compared with placebo and IV TXA alone.

Another recent RCT by Xie and colleagues compared blood loss in groups receiving 1 g of IV TXA combined with 2 g of topical TXA, 3 g topical TXA, or 1.5 g IV TXA alone [13]. The mean haemoglobin loss in the combined, local, and IV groups was 2.98 ± 0.78, 3.36 ± 0.78, and 3.89 ± 0.72 g/d, respectively.

Poeran and colleagues [5] performed a retrospective cohort study on over 870,000 patients in the United States, which showed that patients who received TXA intraoperatively had lower rates of blood transfusion (7.7% vs

20.1%) and marginally less complications (1.9% vs 2.6%). Those patients who received 2 g or more of TXA had a lower odds ratio of requiring a transfusion compared with those who received 1 g or less (0.31 vs 0.38).

Oremus and colleagues [8] used a randomised controlled study of 98 patients to conclude that patients were less likely to require an autologous blood transfusion if they received 1 g TXA on induction, with a further dose 3hours later. They also found that external blood loss was reduced with the use of TXA.

While there was no significant difference in functional improvement, measurements were taken one year apart. This temporal relationship introduces many variables and may have been more useful if functional scores were recorded in the first week postoperatively.

The rare occurrence of thromboembolic events in the study, compounded with the relatively low background incidence of clinically significant VTE, meant that no statistically significant observations regarding safety were established. Other studies published to date have been able to demonstrate that TXA is safe [14–17]. In particular, a large series of 822 patients assessing the use of TXA in cardiac surgery found no increased risk of thromboembolic events [14].

There were several limitations to this study. Firstly, the sample size was smaller than expected due to incomplete data recordings by theatre staff and progression to general anaesthesia without a spinal anaesthetic. These patients were excluded following randomisation and the procedure. Secondly, when transfusion rate is used as an outcome measure, it introduces some bias due to the variation in clinical triggers for transfusion from clinician to clinician. However, we aimed to assess transfusion rate based on the current management with an intention to treat analysis. Thirdly, we used a standardised dose of 1 g IV TXA, whereas the manufacturer's recommended dose is 15 mg/kg every eight hours over a 24-hour period [17]. Given a mean BMI of our patients of 28.9, we may have underdosed the sample on average, and therefore may have biased our results towards the null hypothesis.

5. Conclusion

The current literature suggests that TXA reduces postoperative blood loss and requirement for transfusion; however, this study did not provide any evidence to support this. Further studies are required to confirm the relationship between TXA and rate of transfusion and blood loss. They also need to establish the duration and dose of TXA appropriate for the type of surgery being performed. Focus is required on measuring outcomes of clinical importance such as cost and time to discharge. The safety of TXA in our general population should be confirmed, including in those who have had previous thromboembolic events.

Acknowledgments

The authors thank Glynny Kieser for her editorial input. This research was supported by New Zealand Orthopaedic Association (grant no. NZOA JB1).

References

[1] S. Kurtz, K. Ong, E. Lau, F. Mowat, and M. Halpern, "Projections of primary and revision hip and knee arthroplasty in the United States from 2005 to 2030," *The Journal of Bone and Joint Surgery-American Volume*, vol. 89, no. 4, pp. 780–785, 2007.

[2] G. Hooper, A. J.-J. Lee, A. Rothwell, and C. Frampton, "Current trends and projections in the utilisation rates of hip and knee replacement in New Zealand from 2001 to 2026," *New Zealand Medical Journal*, vol. 127, no. 1401, pp. 82–93, 2014.

[3] S. G. Sandler, H. Yu, and N. Rassai, "Risks of blood transfusion and their prevention," *Clinical Advances in Hematology&Oncology*, vol. 1, no. 5, pp. 307–313, 2003.

[4] M. Melnyk, R. G. Casey, P. Black, and A. J. Koupparis, "Enhanced recovery after surgery (ERAS) protocols: time to change practice?," *Canadian Urological Association Journal*, vol. 5, no. 5, pp. 342–348, 2011.

[5] J. Poeran, R. Rasul, S. Suzuki et al., "Tranexamic acid use and postoperative outcomes in patients undergoing total hip or knee arthroplasty in the United States: retrospective analysis of effectiveness and safety," *BMJ*, vol. 349, no. 12, p. 7829, 2014.

[6] T. Vaněk and Z. Straka, "Topical use of tranexamic acid in cardiac surgery—a review and meta-analysis of four randomized controlled trials," *Coret Vasa*, vol. 55, no. 2, pp. e184–e189, 2013.

[7] T. C. Kelley, K. K. Tucker, M. J. Adams, and D. F. Dalury, "Use of tranexamic acid results in decreased blood loss and decreased transfusions in patients undergoing staged bilateral total knee arthroplasty," *Transfusion*, vol. 54, no. 1, pp. 26–30, 2014.

[8] K. Oremus, S. Sostaric, V. Trkulja, and M. Haspl, "Influence of tranexamic acid on postoperative autologous blood retransfusionin primary total hip and knee arthroplasty: arandomized controlled trial," *Transfusion*, vol. 54, no. 1, pp. 31–41, 2014.

[9] Z. Yi, S. Bin, Y. Jing, Z. Zongke, K. Pengde, and P. Fuxing, "Tranexamic acid administration in primary total hip arthroplasty: arandomized controlled trial of intravenous combined with topical versus single-dose intravenous administration," *The Journal of Bone and Joint Surgery*, vol. 98, no. 12, pp. 983–991, 2016.

[10] S. Rashiq and B. A. Finegan, "The effect of spinal anesthesia on blood transfusion rate in total joint arthroplasty," *Canadian Journal of Surgery*, vol. 49, no. 6, 2006.

[11] American College of Physicians, "ECP—primer on statistical significance and pvalues," *Effective Clinical Practice*, vol. 4, no. 4, pp. 183-184, 2001.

[12] K. M. Ho and H. Ismail, "Use of intravenous tranexamic acid to reduce allogeneic blood transfusion in total hip and knee arthroplasty: ameta-analysis," *Anaesthetic Intensive Care*, vol. 31, no. 5, pp. 529–537, 2003.

[13] J. Xie, J. Ma, C. Yue, P. Kang, and F. Pei, "Combined use of intravenous and topical tranexamic acid following cementlesstotal hip arthroplasty: arandomised clinical trial," *HIP International*, vol. 26, no. 1, pp. 36–42, 2016.

[14] D. T. Mangano, I. C. Tudor, and C. Dietzel, "The risk associated with aprotinin in cardiac surgery," *The New England Journal of Medicine*, vol. 354, no. 4, pp. 353–365, 2006.

[15] S. Nishihara and M. Hamada, "Does tranexamic acid alter the risk of thromboembolism after total hip arthroplasty in the absence of routine chemical thromboprophylaxis?" *The Bone and Joint Journal*, vol. 97-B, no. 4, pp. 458–462, 2015.

[16] V. Selvaratnam, J. R. Fountain, N. J. Donnachie, T. G. Thomas, and F. A. Carroll, "Does pre-operative tranexamic acid increase the incidence of thromboembolism in primary lower limb arthroplasty?" *Open Journal of Orthopedics*, vol. 3, no. 6, pp. 249–252, 2013.
[17] Pfizer, "Data sheet tranexamic acid," 2013, http://www.medsafe.govt.nz/profs/datasheet/c/Cyklokaprontabinj.pdf.

6

Limb Lengthening after Primary Total Knee Arthroplasty: Customized Patient-Specific Instrumentation Does Not Affect Expected Limb Lengthening

Christopher Fang,[1] Kenneth McAlpine,[2] Michael Gustin,[2] Ruijia Niu,[2] David Freccero,[2] Matthew Gordon,[3] and Eric L. Smith[1]

[1]*Department of Orthopedic Surgery, New England Baptist Hospital, 125 Parker Hill Ave, Boston, MA 02120, USA*
[2]*Department of Orthopedic Surgery, Boston Medical Center, One Boston Medical Center Pl, Boston, MA 02118, USA*
[3]*Department of Orthopedic Surgery, Tufts Medical Center, 800 Washington St, Boston, MA 02111, USA*

Correspondence should be addressed to Eric L. Smith; esmith@nebh.org

Academic Editor: Francesco Liuzza

Introduction. Expectations for limb length differences after TKA are important for patient perception and outcomes. Limb length discrepancies may occur due to postoperative leg length increases, which can lead to decreased patient functionality and satisfaction and even possible litigation. The purpose of this study is to examine the frequency and extent of limb lengthening among various preoperative deformities and between two different implant systems. *Methods.* Preoperative and postoperative full-length standing radiographs were obtained between August 2018 and August 2019 to measure mechanical axis and limb length of operative limbs. Demographic information such as age, sex, and BMI was also collected. Patients were grouped into categories for pre- and postoperative subgroup analysis: valgus, varus, customized implant, and conventional implant. Regression analysis was performed to evaluate significant relationships. *Results.* Of the 121 primary TKAs analyzed, 62% of the knees showed an increase in limb length after TKA, with an average lengthening of 5.32 mm. Preoperative varus alignment was associated with a mean lengthening of 3.14 mm, while preoperative valgus alignment was associated with a mean lengthening of 16.2 mm. Overall, there were no statistically significant differences in limb lengths pre- and postoperatively ($p = 0.23$) and no significant changes in limb length for any subgroup. Further, no variables were associated with limb length changes ($p = 0.49$), including the use of customized implants ($p = 0.2$). *Conclusions.* Limb lengthening after TKA is common and, on average, occurs more significantly in valgus knees. No significant difference in limb lengthening could be demonstrated using customized over conventional implants. Preoperative counseling is important to manage patient expectations.

1. Introduction

The effect of total hip arthroplasty (THA) on leg length changes has been extensively studied in the literature [1]. Despite reports of limb length changes following total knee arthroplasty (TKA) [2], minimal attention has been paid to changes in limb length that can be expected following TKA. The considerable effect of limb length discrepancy (LLD) on patient satisfaction, litigation, and outcomes following TKA warrants further study [3–5]. Given the high rate of success of TKA, patients undergoing the procedure expect excellent results and accurate expectations. However, limb length changes after TKA are not well characterized in the literature.

Changes in postoperative limb length have been shown to increase back pack, sciatica, gait disorders, and patient dissatisfaction [6]. This can occur after TKA due to limb lengthening of the operative leg [2, 6, 7]. Studies from 2012 and 2015 have shown that limb lengthening occurs frequently after TKA, though the extent of the lengthening is unclear [2, 8]. Additionally, recent advances in total joint technology may permit greater control over limb lengthening to allow for more precise outcomes. It has been proposed that patient-specific instrumentation (PSI) in TKA potentially permits a more accurate alignment, with comparable results for alignment restoration and component positioning [9, 10], augmented by three-dimensional computerized CT-scan planned custom implants for preoperative planning. This could potentially affect limb lengthening to a differing extent than conventional alignment techniques.

The purpose of this study is to examine limb lengthening and alignment after TKA in various conditions evaluating conventional and customized TKA implants. Our hypothesis is that overall, there will be an increase in limb length following TKA, and that customized TKAs will not have a different effect on limb lengthening than conventional implants.

2. Methods

2.1. Study Design. After Institutional Review Board approval was obtained, patients undergoing primary TKA were identified through a retrospective review of the database of a single fellowship-trained total joint surgeon from August 2018 through August 2019. Patients were included if they had pre- and postoperative full-length standing radiographs taken with an appropriate reference for image calibration. There were no cutoffs for patient age or BMI for this study. Exclusion criteria included lack of pre- or postoperative imaging, insufficient imaging (i.e., incomplete visualization of the entire limb), lack of magnification reference, flexion contractures >15 degrees, previous lower extremity fracture, or revision surgery. Due to ordering errors, lack of follow-up, or absence of a reference for image calibration, 5% of patients were excluded from the study. Films were sufficient for the remaining patients undergoing TKA.

All operations were performed by a single fellowship-trained surgeon using a medial parapatellar approach with standard flexion and extension gap balancing. Patients received either PFC Sigma (DePuy Orthopaedics, Inc., Warsaw, IN) cruciate retaining implants or customized, CT-based patient-matched implant with patient-specific instrumentation (PSI) (Conformis Inc., Burlington, MA). Indications for customized implants were patient preference, a functioning PCL (all CR), and anatomy that could exceed the limits of a conventional total knee system. Demographic information included age, sex, BMI, days from preoperative date to surgery date, days from postoperative date to surgery date, type of implant, and laterality.

Standing anteroposterior (AP) full-length digital images of the lower extremities were obtained before and after (6 months) the procedure according to institutional policies. Limb measurements were performed by a single researcher using TraumaCad online digital software suite (Brainlab AG, Germany) to determine the limb length and mechanical axis of the operative limb by taking the mean value of two measurements as the final data. Institutional protocol for the inclusion of a metal magnification ball (MB) for image calibration was followed in the majority of cases, and images were calibrated to this 25.3 mm ball. Cases in which MB imaging was absent were excluded.

Measurement tools available on TraumaCAD were used to improve the accuracy and consistency of measurements. A "Circle" tool was utilized to establish the center of the femoral head, and a "Line" tool was used to determine the center of the femoral intercondylar notch, tibial plateau, and plafond, with an "Angle" tool establishing the mechanical axis. Limb length was determined using the "Limb Length" function, which calculated total length using a point at the center of the femoral head to the tip of the medial tibial plafond.

All TKAs were grouped three times discretely for analysis: grouping one consisted of varus and valgus groups, grouping two consisted of "customized" and "conventional" groups, and grouping three consisted of "severe varus," "severe valgus," and "moderate malalignment" groups. Values greater than 10° in either varus or valgus qualified into "severe varus" or "severe valgus," respectively, with the third group of "moderate malalignment" to capture the remaining knees in accordance with previously published studies [2, 8]. The mean limb lengthening and frequency of limb lengthening overall as well as the mean preoperative and postoperative alignment in each group were determined.

2.2. Statistical Analysis. Student's t-tests and Fisher's exact tests were appropriately used to compare demographic information between varus and valgus groups. Student's t-tests were performed to compare the difference in average limb lengthening within varus, valgus, customized, conventional, severe varus, severe valgus, moderate malalignment, and overall groups. Regression analysis was performed on leg length to control for variables including preoperative deformity, implant type, BMI, age, and sex. All statistical analyses were performed using Stata 12.0 software. Significance was defined as $p < 0.05$.

3. Results

We analyzed 121 primary TKAs (111 patients) during the study period. 101 TKAs were divided into the varus group, and 20 TKAs into the valgus group. Patient demographic features are presented in Table 1, which showed no significant differences between the groups (Table 1).

Overall, 62% of the 121 knees demonstrated increased limb length following TKA (Table 2). Average lengthening was 5.32 mm (SD: 4.42 mm; range: −6.2 to 51 mm) (Table 2). Mean preoperative alignment was 6.36° (SD, 0.82°), and postoperative alignment was 2.54° (SD, 0.33°) (Table 2). Mean change in alignment was 3.83° (SD, 0.74°) (Table 2).

60 (59.4%) of the 101 varus knees and 15 (75%) of the 20 valgus knees showed increased limb length after TKA (Table 2). Average lengthening of the varus group was 3.14 mm (SD: 4.92 mm; range: −6.2 to 17 mm), and it was 16.2 mm (SD: 9.79 mm; range: −4.1 to 51 mm) for the valgus group (Table 2). Average mechanical alignment for the varus group was 9.36° (SD, 0.59°) and 2.94° (SD, 0.34°)

Table 1: Patient demographics.

Variable	Whole sample	Valgus (<0)	Varus (>0)	p
# pts	121	20	101	
Age (y)	66.1 (0.7)	66.1 (2.2)	66.1 (0.8)	0.99
BMI (kg/m^2)	33.2 (0.5)	32.5 (0.9)	33.3 (0.5)	0.49
Female	88 (72.7%)	16 (80.0%)	72 (71.3%)	0.42
Days preop	107.0 (9.6)	115.4 (25.8)	105.3 (10.4)	0.70
Days postop	46.9 (3.3)	47.9 (4.5)	46.7 (3.8)	0.89
Sigma	106 (87.6%)	19 (95%)	87 (86.1%)	0.27
Left	57 (47.1%)	12 (60%)	45 (44.6%)	0.21

Table 2: Measurement results.

Parameter	Varus ($n = 101$)	Valgus ($n = 20$)	Customized ($n = 15$)	Conventional ($n = 106$)	Overall ($N = 121$)
Preop alignment*	9.36 (0.59)	8.75 (1.5)	6.2 (1.26)	6.39 (0.93)	6.36 (0.82)
Postop alignment*	2.94 (0.34)	0.5 (0.79)	0.67 (0.69)	2.8 (0.35)	2.54 (0.33)
Change in alignment*	6.42 (5.40)	9.25 (6.97)	5.53 (1.19)	3.58 (0.82)	3.83 (0.74)
Lengthening (mm)*	3.14 (4.92)	16.2 (9.79)	10.73 (10.22)	7.61 (4.81)	5.32 (4.42)
$P^{\dagger}$	0.52	0.11	0.31	0.12	0.23
Percentage lengthening	59.4%	75%	60%	62.3%	62.0%

*Values are expressed as mean (SD). †Comparison of preoperative and postoperative limb length within each subgroup. Alignments are expressed in degrees. Lengthening is expressed in mm.

preoperatively and postoperatively, respectively, with a mean change in alignment of 6.42° (SD, 5.40°) (Table 2). Average mechanical alignment for the valgus group was 8.75° (SD, 1.5°) and 0.5° (SD, 0.79°) preoperatively and postoperatively, respectively, with a mean change in alignment of 9.25° (SD, 6.97°) (Table 2).

After discretely regrouping the 121 TKAs by type of implant, 66 (62.3%) of the 106 conventional knees and 9 (60%) of the 15 customized knees showed increased limb length after TKA (Table 2). The demographics between the two groups were similar with no significant differences. Average lengthening of the conventional group was 7.61 mm (SD, 4.81 mm), and it was 10.73 mm (SD, 10.22 mm) for the customized group (Table 2). Average mechanical alignment for the conventional group was 6.39° (SD, 0.93°) and 2.8° (SD, 0.35°) preoperatively and postoperatively, respectively, with a mean change in alignment of 3.58° (SD, 0.82°) (Table 2). Average mechanical alignment for the customized group was 6.2° (SD, 1.26°) and 0.67° (SD, 0.69°) preoperatively and postoperatively, respectively, with a mean change in alignment of 5.53° (SD, 1.19°) (Table 2). No significant changes in lengthening were found within each subgroup (Table 2).

The 121 TKAs were regrouped in a separate analysis, forming "severe varus," "severe valgus," and "moderate malalignment" groups. 38 (31.4%%) were found to have a severe varus deformity (Table 3). In the severe varus group, 71.1% of patients demonstrated increased limb length following TKA with an average lengthening of 13.9 mm (SD, 56.2 mm) (Table 3). Mean preoperative alignment was 15.34° (SD, 0.7°) compared to 4.68° (0.57°) postoperatively, with a mean change in alignment of 10.66° (SD, 0.78°) (Table 3).

Further, 43 (56.6%) were found to have a severe valgus deformity (Table 3). In the severe valgus group, 71.4% of patients demonstrated increased limb length following TKA with an average lengthening of 29 mm (SD, 44.4 mm) (Table 3). Mean preoperative alignment was 16.28° (SD, 1.71°) compared to 0.14° (SD, 1.22°) postoperatively, with a mean change in alignment of 16.43° (SD, 1.63°) (Table 3).

In the malalignment group, 76 (62.8%) demonstrated increased limb length following TKA with an average lengthening of 1.2 mm (SD, 43.5 mm) (Table 3). Mean postoperative alignment was 1.7° (SD, 3.1°) compared to 4.0° (SD, 5.1°) (Table 3). No significant changes in lengthening were found within each severe deformity subgroup (Table 3).

Regression analysis showed that the average limb lengthening in the valgus group was 11.57 mm ($p = 0.337$) greater than that in the varus group after adjusting for age, sex, BMI, and type of implant (Table 4). Limb lengthening had no relationship with age ($p = 0.79$), sex ($p = 0.67$), BMI ($p = 0.73$), or implant type ($p = 0.2$) (Table 4).

4. Discussion

In THA, limb lengthening effects can be minimized with preoperative planning in order to avoid potential complications [11]. In TKA however, the main operative goals of correcting the preoperative deformity and balancing ligaments may lower control and accuracy of leg length, often increasing operative limb length [2, 7]. Therefore, we sought to investigate the frequency and nature of limb length changes in TKA. We further established that an increase in limb length is routine after TKA. In agreement with past studies [2, 8], our overall values fell within the range of the established literature. Lang et al. and Tipton et al., in studies of 102 and 132 knees, found that 83.3% and 59.1% (compared to our 62%) demonstrated lengthening following TKA with an average increase of 6.3 mm and 4.38 mm (compared to our 5.32 mm) and mean postoperative alignment of 1.0° and 2.76° (compared to our 2.54°), respectively [2, 8].

Table 3: Measurement results stratified by degree of deformity.

Parameter	Moderate malalignment ($n = 76$)	Severe valgus ($n = 7$)	Severe varus ($n = 38$)
Preop alignment*	4.0 (5.1)	16.28 (1.71)	15.34 (0.7)
Postop alignment*	1.7 (3.1)	0.14 (1.22)	4.68 (0.57)
Change in alignment*	2.3 (5.3)	16.43 (1.63)	10.66 (0.78)
Lengthening*	1.2 (43.5)	29 (44.4)	13.9 (56.2)
$P^{\dagger}$	0.80	0.13	0.14
Percentage lengthened	56.6%	71.4%	71.1%

*Values are expressed as mean (SD). †Comparison of preoperative and postoperative limb length within each subgroup. Alignments are expressed in degrees. Lengthening is expressed in mm.

Table 4: Regression analysis on leg length (R-square = 0.04, $p = 0.49$).

	Coefficient	95% confidence interval	p value
Preoperative deformity status			
Valgus	11.57	−12.19–35.31	0.337
Varus	Reference		
Implant type			
Sigma	17.89	−9.6–45.49	0.2
Customized	Reference		
Body mass index	−0.23	−1.53–1.07	0.73
Age	−0.09	−0.73–0.55	0.79
Sex			
Male	4.3	−15.36–23.96	0.67
Female	Reference		

Contradictory to Lang et al., none of our statistical tests were significant, showing no difference in pre- and post-operative limb changes for any subgroup [2], consistent with results found by Tipton et al. [8]. There were large mean magnitudes of leg length increase for the operative limb, but standard deviations contributed to nonstatistically significant results. The difference in operative leg length after surgery was not significantly different from the operative leg length before surgery. Though these authors [2] state that LLD is significant, it may not be clinically important if patients do not appreciate a difference in their limb length. Moreover, a study states that patients only perceive a leg length change of 2 cm or more [12], suggesting that the majority of patients in our study would not perceive a difference in their limb length after surgery. Our findings suggest that limb lengthening occurs frequently after TKA, but not to a statistically significant extent. As the temporal trend may indicate, there is potential that LLD may be decreasing over time as techniques and experience allow more control over leg length after surgery [2, 8]. As differences in leg length changes after TKA are reduced, it is likely that most patients will not perceive any leg length differences outside those with severe valgus knees.

The phenomenon of limb lengthening after valgus knees has been observed by several other authors [2, 8, 13]. The mechanism for these changes is unknown. Perhaps the lengthening could be due to less bone being resected during TKA in a valgus deformity knee. Further, the average change in alignment for valgus knees was also more profound, which could contribute to the overall increased length. This could potentially be avoided with CT-scan preoperative planning and awareness for valgus knee deformities [14]. Further research is needed on the exact mechanism and solutions to significant limb length changes for these patients.

Preoperative counseling is very important for managing expectations, especially in the stiff, severe valgus patient. It is logical that while patients might not perceive a leg length change of 2 cm or less, they might still feel small insignificant changes in their daily lives, despite the lack of functional deficits. While most patients are satisfied with the results of their operation relieving their debilitating pain and restoring function, there are still some patients that may be unhappy with their corrected, longer, and straighter leg. Therefore, it is of value to educate patients at increased risk for significant lengthening, such as those with a severe valgus deformity, to prevent unexpected outcomes.

Consistent with past studies, there was no association of any of the variables on leg length change [2, 8]. Our study furthers this evidence by showing that customized knees do not demonstrate significant leg length changes after surgery and have no relationship with limb lengthening. In other words, customized knees do not differ in postoperative LLD compared to conventional knee implants, further illustrating comparable outcomes for customized implants [10].

Chinnappa et al. found that perceived LLD was associated with decreased satisfaction and poorer functional scores but was not associated with radiographic LLD [13]. Hinarejos et al. found postoperative LLD as described by ≥10 mm to have significant worse functional outcome in KSS [15]. Kim et al. found that >15 mm LLD computer-assisted TKA showed lower functional outcome scores, although the authors state that the correlation was low [16]. Further, they found that results of the perception of LLD questionnaire for those with LLD >15 mm was significantly different from those with LLD <15 mm (23% vs 6%); however, results of the satisfaction questionnaires were similar between groups [16]. Regarding customized single use instruments, Romeo et al. found them to have economical and organizational benefits of reducing costs but noted a lack of difference from conventional instrumentation in terms of clinical outcomes such as radiographic parameters or knee scores [17]. Our study adds to the body of literature regarding LLD and expectations for patients after TKA, with customized implants showing no significant differences in limb lengthening over conventional implants.

The current study has several limitations, including its retrospective nature and relatively small sample size. The current study also relied on standing AP full-length radiography using commercially available software applied onto the radiographs to determine limb lengths and the degree of deformity in the coronal plane only. We did not evaluate changes in the sagittal plane, leaving any deformity that may have only been present in the coronal plane go unrecognized. Standing AP radiographs have been validated as accurate and reliable for use in determining LLD when compared to scanograms [18]. The measurement of leg length was shown to decrease as the degree of limb malalignment increased [18]. Flexion contracture preoperatively may affect limb length measurement, but a study has shown that the measurement is not affected by a contracture less than 15° [19]. Measurements were performed by a single researcher using an online digital software suite, potentiating influence by observer subjectivity. However, to reduce this influence, measurements were repeated a second time and the final data were the mean value of these numbers. The subset of the population that underwent primary TKA with PSI was lower than the other subsets, which could give a false sense of equal proportions across groups and increase the possibility of a type II error. Lastly, clinical significance of LLD after TKA is unclear [20]. Still, our study addresses an outcome variable that needs consideration and further research as subtle differences in pre- and postoperative limb lengths can be important for patient outcomes. Future research implementing prospective and meta-analysis studies are needed to fully understand the effect of subtle limb length differences.

5. Conclusions

In conclusion, our data further supports that limb lengthening is common after TKA. Though not statistically significant, it is reasonable that this increase in leg length for the operative limb represented a restoration of the normal joint space height and alignment of the native knee. This increase in leg length may not be clinically significant nor even perceived by the patient, which may allay negative outcomes seen with LLD. Customized PSI and implants do not affect LLD after TKA as compared to conventional implants.

References

[1] J. Y. Lazennec, D. Folinais, C. Florequin, and A. E. Pour, "Does patients' perception of leg length after total hip arthroplasty correlate with anatomical leg length?" *The Journal of Arthroplasty*, vol. 33, no. 5, pp. 1562–1566, 2018.

[2] J. E. Lang, R. D. Scott, J. H. Lonner, J. V. Bono, D. J. Hunter, and L. Li, "Magnitude of limb lengthening after primary total knee arthroplasty," *The Journal of Arthroplasty*, vol. 27, no. 3, pp. 341–346, 2012.

[3] S. D. Ulrich, A. Bhave, D. R. Marker, T. M. Seyler, and M. A. Mont, "Focused rehabilitation treatment of poorly functioning total knee arthroplasties," *Clinical Orthopaedics and Related Research*, vol. 464, pp. 138–145, 2007.

[4] A. Upadhyay, S. York, W. Macaulay, B. McGrory, J. Robbennolt, and B. S. Bal, "Medical malpractice in hip and knee arthroplasty," *Journal of Arthroplasty*, vol. 22, 2007.

[5] L. T. Samuel, A. A. Sultan, J. M. Rabin et al., "Medical malpractice litigation following primary total joint arthroplasty: a comprehensive, nationwide analysis of the past decade," *The Journal of Arthroplasty*, vol. 34, no. 7, pp. S102–S107, 2019.

[6] J. R. Perttunen, E. Anttila, J. Sodergard, J. Merikanto, and P. Komi, "Gait asymmetry in patients with limb length discrepancy," *Scandinavian Journal of Medicine & Science in Sports*, vol. 14, pp. 49–56, 2004.

[7] M. J. Chang, Y. G. Kang, C. B. Chang, S. C. Seong, and T. K. Kim, "The patterns of limb length, height, weight and body mass index changes after total knee arthroplasty," *The Journal of Arthroplasty*, vol. 28, no. 10, pp. 1856–1861, 2013.

[8] S. Tipton, J. Sutherland, and R. Schwarzkopf, "Change in limb length after total knee arthroplasty," *Geriatric Orthopaedic Surgery & Rehabilitation*, vol. 6, no. 3, pp. 197–201, 2015.

[9] V. Y. Ng, J. H. DeClaire, K. R. Berend, B. C. Gulick, and A. V. Lombardi, "Improved accuracy of alignment with patient-specific positioning guides compared with manual instrumentation in TKA," *Clinical Orthopaedics & Related Research*, vol. 470, no. 1, pp. 99–107, 2012.

[10] M. Zhu, J. Y. Chen, H. C. Chong et al., "Outcomes following total knee arthroplasty with CT-based patient-specific instrumentation," *Knee Surgery, Sports Traumatology, Arthroscopy*, vol. 25, no. 8, pp. 2567–2572, 2017.

[11] J. Parvizi, P. F. Sharkey, G. A. Bissett et al., "Surgical treatment of limb-length discrepancy following total hip arthroplasty," *The Journal of Bone and Joint Surgery-American Volume*, vol. 85, no. 12, pp. 2310–2317, 2003.

[12] A. B. Sabir, M. Faizan, M. Ishtiaq, L. Z. Jilani, S. Ahmed, and Z. H. Shaan, "Limb length discrepancy after total knee arthroplasty: unilateral versus bilateral, a comparative study at tertiary centre," *Journal of Clinical Orthopaedics and Trauma*, vol. 11, pp. S740–S745, 2020.

[13] J. Chinnappa, D. B. Chen, I. A. Harris, and S. J. MacDessi, "Predictors and functional implications of change in leg length after total knee arthroplasty," *The Journal of Arthroplasty*, vol. 32, no. 9, pp. 2725–2729.e1, 2017.

[14] E. Sariali, C. Kajetanek, and Y. Catonné, "Comparison of custom cutting guides based on three-dimensional computerized CT-scan planning and a conventional ancillary system based on two-dimensional planning in total knee arthroplasty: a randomized controlled trial," *International Orthopaedics*, vol. 43, no. 11, pp. 2529–2538, 2019.

[15] P. Hinarejos, J. Sánchez-Soler, J. Leal-Blanquet, R. Torres-Claramunt, and J. C. Monllau, "Limb length discrepancy after total knee arthroplasty may contribute to suboptimal functional results," *European Journal of Orthopaedic Surgery & Traumatology*, vol. 30, no. 7, pp. 1199–1204, 2020.

[16] S. H. Kim, S.-M. Rhee, J.-W. Lim, and H.-J. Lee, "The effect of leg length discrepancy on clinical outcome after TKA and identification of possible risk factors," *Knee Surgery, Sports*

Traumatology, Arthroscopy, vol. 24, no. 8, pp. 2678–2685, 2016.

[17] M. Romeo, G. Rovere, L. Stramazzo, F. Liuzza, L. Meccariello, and L. Camarda, "Single use instruments for total knee arthroplasty," *Medicinski Glasnik*, vol. 18, pp. 316–320, 2021.

[18] S. Sabharwal, C. Zhao, J. McKeon, T. Melaghari, M. Blacksin, and C. Wenekor, "Reliability analysis for radiographic measurement of limb length discrepancy," *Journal of Pediatric Orthopaedics*, vol. 27, no. 1, pp. 46–50, 2007.

[19] A. Aaron, D. Weinstein, D. Thickman, and R. Eilert, "Comparison of orthoroentgenography and computed tomography in the measurement of limb-length discrepancy," *The Journal of Bone & Joint Surgery*, vol. 74, no. 6, pp. 897–902, 1992.

[20] B. Gurney, C. Mermier, R. Robergs, A. Gibson, and D. Rivero, "Effects of limb-length discrepancy on gait economy and lower-extremity muscle activity in older adults," *The Journal of Bone and Joint Surgery-American Volume*, vol. 83, no. 6, pp. 907–915, 2001.

7

A Review of Total Hip Arthroplasty Comparison in FNF and OA Patients

Jakub Szczesiul[1,2] **and Marek Bielecki**[1,2]

[1]*Department of Orthopedic, Traumatology and Hand Surgery, Medical University of Białystok, Białystok, Poland*
[2]*Department of Orthopedic, Traumatology and Hand Surgery, Uniwersytecki Szpital Kliniczny w Białymstoku, Białystok, Poland*

Correspondence should be addressed to Jakub Szczesiul; jakub.szczesiul@umb.edu.pl

Academic Editor: Panagiotis Korovessis

Background. Worldwide, total hip arthroplasty (THA) has become one of the most commonly performed surgical procedures. Femoral neck fracture (FNF) and osteoarthritis (OA) are two of the medical conditions necessitating a hip replacement, most frequently carried out. The preoperative and postoperative pathways for patients suffering from these two diseases differ, yet worldwide, many national healthcare systems underestimate or misinterpret the (more than nuanced) care plan differences of the two. *Factors and Criteria.* Analyzed material was gathered from studies published between 2013 and 2019. Various strands of data demographics, comorbidities, and complications, as well as treatment outcomes, were tabulated to compare and contrast THA patients suffering from FNF and OA to collate their findings. Outcomes were cross-checked and validated for reliability and then were presented in a table format. *Results.* All five retrospective cohort studies fitted the required criteria for inclusion in this work, four US-based study groups and one European-based study group. Data were gathered from three separate databases. The "average" FNF patient is 76.8 years old. There was a 68.96% female probability. The "average" OA patient is 69.15 years old. There was a 5.24% female probability. 59.57% operated for athrosis, and only 34.63% operated for fracture which received grade lower than the third in the American Society of Anaesthesiologist (ASA) classification. There was more than 3 times higher prevalence of complications in the trauma group. FNF patients' hospitalization was approximately 3 days longer. On average, 3.7% of patients operated for trauma and 1.5% of patients with elective THA required a second surgery. 6.57% FNF and 2.93% OA patients had unplanned readmission. *Conclusions.* In general, patients who suffer a femoral neck fracture are an extremely fragile group. They require additional perioperative and postoperative care. To meet these desired expectations, more FNF cost-comprehensive systems need to be initiated.

1. Introduction

1.1. Rationale. Hip arthroplasty which may be divided into total hip arthroplasty (THA) and hemiarthroplasty (HA) is a procedure that allows to replace damaged parts of the hip joint, such as the femoral head and neck or hip acetabulum, with artificial ones. The materials that compose the components are mostly titanium, titanium-cobalt alloy, stainless steel, or ceramic and are characterized by good biocompatibility.

Total hip arthroplasty (THA), due to its application in both osteoarthritis (OA) and displaced femoral neck fracture (FNF), has become a frequent orthopedic procedure worldwide. Complex medical care that prolongs patient's lifespan which leads to increased incidence of fragility hip fracture [1–3] makes the procedure even more commonly utilized.

Intra-articular hip fracture rates among top three of all hip fractures [4]. FNF is characterized by poor healing which necessitates hip arthroplasty. New research shows the advantage of THA over hemiarthroplasty in FNF treatment in terms of clinical results and reoperation rate, despite a higher incidence of dislocation in THA [4–6]. Fortunately, the latest studies indicate that dual-mobility total hip arthroplasty (DM THA) nullifies the dislocation disadvantage, and thus, THA remains a preferred treatment method in FNF in active elderly patients [7, 8]. The same procedure is also performed to increase hip mobility and relieve pain in hip joint osteoarthrosis. Even though endoprosthesis components and the conduct of the operation do not differ in THA for FNF and OA, patients' demographics, comorbidities, complications, or treatment outcomes vary in both groups [9–14].

This paper aims to gather and summarize publications related to THA comparison between patients suffering from femoral neck fracture and hip osteoarthritis in order to improve the understanding of the differences between these two groups.

1.2. Objectives. This is a traditional narrative review of articles published since 2012 comparing FNF and OA patients undergoing THA. The objective was to compare (1) preoperational status, (2) perioperation procedures performed before and after the surgery, and (3) complication rate in those groups. Furthermore, this study intends to highlight (4) strengths and weaknesses of gathered evidence and (5) guidelines for future research.

2. Materials and Methods

2.1. Data Source. The PubMed/MEDLINE database was used to gather observational studies regarding the comparison of THA in FNF and OA. Article selection was conducted using words "*total hip arthroplasty comparing,*" "*osteoarthritis and femoral neck fracture,*" and "*osteoarthritis and proximal femoral fracture.*" In order to meet inclusion criteria, the paper published date should not be older than 2012, study design should be observation study with retrospective cohort; also, a comparison of both groups' epidemiology and postoperative outcome was mandatory. The last search was carried out in June 2021 and resulted in finding 5 studies, including publications written by Schairer et al. [9], Charette et al. [10], Adam et al. [11], Qin et al. [12], and Le Manach et al. [13]. The selection process was illustrated on the graph (Figure 1).

The articles were written based on the data from 3 different databases. Three of them utilize the National Surgical Quality Improvement Program (NSQIP) database, one the National Hospital Discharge Database (NHDS), and one the French Hospital Discharge Database (FHDD). Four of the selected studies were based on the American and one on the European population (Table 1). Data concerning the patients' demographics, comorbidities, complications, and treatment outcomes were extracted.

2.2. Study Population. In all studies, patient populations were gathered based on the International Statistical Classification of Diseases and Health Related Problems (ICD 9) procedures. Authors utilized ICD 9 715.15, with the assist of CPT 2710 to determine patients' groups. Reoperation, polytrauma, and hip cancer cases were excluded from research. Even though each publication is a retrospective cohort study, the authors present different approaches to data selection, statistical analysis, or group observation period. For example, only Sasson et al. and Le Manach et al. decided to establish an age cutoff limit at 45 years. There were no data regarding minimal age research inclusion in the remaining works. THA as treatment for either FNF or OA was examined as the binary variable. In addition, in all listed studies, demographic data such as age, body mass, and comorbidities were included. Moreover, information concerning length of stay, home dismissal, and unplanned readmission was provided. Last but not least, some articles presented other additional data such as blood loss, post-operation function status, operation duration, preoperation transfusions, and type of anesthesia.

2.3. Statistical Analysis. Information concerning epidemiology, comorbidities, perioperation procedures, and complications was compared. Arithmetic average, standard deviation, and variance were calculated. A majority of gathered data were presented in tables. Additional analyses were performed on population matching cohorts. Results were described via diagrams.

3. Results

Factors that were studied in mentioned publications can be divided into four groups: demographic, comorbidities, complications, and outcome. The approaches in data collection chosen by the authors were not identical, yet similarities in their study design allow some degree of data comparison.

Patients' demographic: based on elaborated research, an average femoral fracture patient is 76.8 years old, and 68.96% of them are female. 55.24% OA patients were women, and OA patient average age was 69.15 years (Table 2). In Charette's work, there were no data concerning average age; instead, patients were divided into additional groups, with age above and below 70.

Patient medical records show a higher prevalence of comorbidities in FNF groups with the exception of obesity, which was more common in OA groups (Table 3). Most of the research papers used the ASA score to evaluate patient preoperative risk factors. The exception was Sasson et al. and Le Manach et al. Sasson et al. utilized the Deyo comorbidity score, and in research from France, no physical status classification has been used. The authors tabulated most common comorbidities in OA/FNF patients including their frequency instead. Based on publications written by Charles et al. and Charette et al., on average, 34.63% of patients undergoing surgery for femoral neck fracture and 59.57% of arthrosis patients were classified as ASA I + II. 65.37% treated for FNF and 40.03% operated for OA were classified as ASA III + IV. Research shows a higher prevalence of all comorbidities in the FNF group with the exception of obesity, although hypertension, according to some research studies [12, 14], may also be more common in the OA patient group.

Factors taken into consideration upon complication assessment in the discussed publications are not uniform; therefore, some data cannot be compared. Moreover, four out of five authors performed propensity matching on the queried groups. A. Sasson et al. calculated mortality in FNF

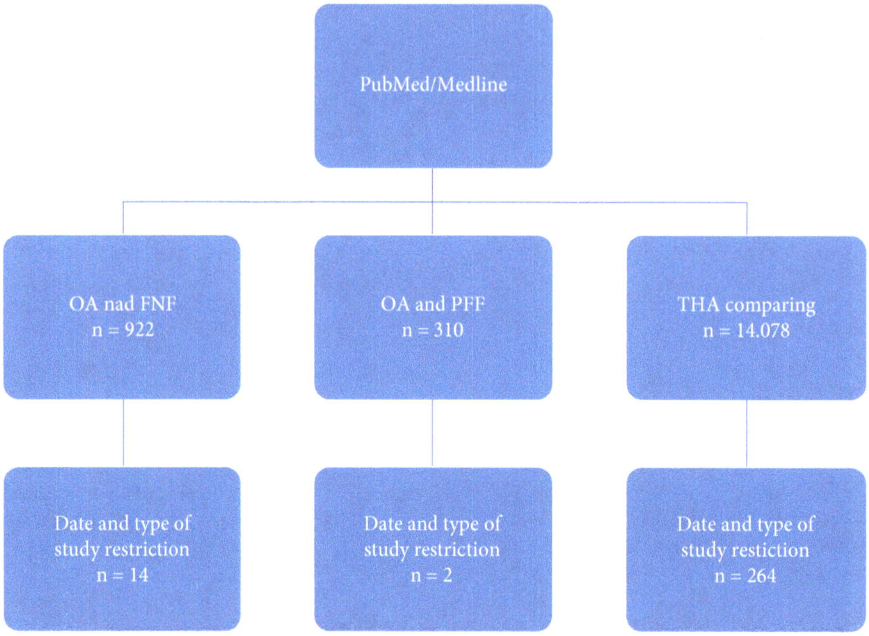

FIGURE 1: Results of scientific research findings based on the used phrase. OA: osteoarthrosis; FNF: femoral neck fracture; PFF: proximal femur fracture; THA: total hip arthroplasty.

to be 1.8% and in OA to be 0.2%, risk of pulmonary embolus in FNF to be 0.8% and in OA to be 0.3%, and risk of infection in FNF to be 1.7% and in OA to be 0.3%. Dislocation rate is also seven times higher in the fracture population, which is also more prone to unstable luxation [15]. Complications described above are restricted to hospitalization, and no propensity score matching was performed on these data. C.D. Qin et al. stated that 11.1% of FNF and 3% of patients with OA suffer in-hospital complications. After matching the cohorts, the numbers were 10.7% for FNF and 4% for OA patients. The study also indicates a significant difference in function status after the surgery (2% vs. 9.2%) in the matched population. Y. Le Manach et al. also compared postoperative outcomes in unmatched and matched study populations. In-hospital mortality was rated 3.42% and 0.18% in the unmatched population and 1.82% and 0.31 in the matched cohort in FNF and OA, respectively. The authors detailed myocardial infarction (0.36% vs. 0.22%), heart failure (5.22% vs. 0.77%), stroke (0.39% vs. 0.15%), renal failure (0.65% vs. 0.30%), and sepsis (0.27% vs. 0.09%), and the data consider the matched population study. Wiliam W. et al. in publication from 2016 described overall complication rate in the propensity score-matched cohort as 15% vs. 6% and surgical complication rate as 4% vs. 2% for FNF vs. OA populations. Chalette R. S. et al. also conducted research employing the propensity matching method. Their findings compared to the results of William W. et al. are demonstrated in Table 4.

In outcome analysis, all researchers took into consideration length of stay in-hospital and nonhomebound discharge and, except for Dr. Sasson, performed reoperations (Table 5). Moreover, in two publications, an additional endpoint, reoperation rate, was included. Based on the studies, the average length of stay for patients with FNF is almost 8 days, while OA patients stay in the ward only for 5 days on average. More than 67% of patients with hip fracture were discharged to another medical or caring facility, whilst 60% operated for hip osteoarthrosis went back home after the procedure. The described trends may also be a risk factor. According to Michael et al., a discharge to inpatient facilities after total hip arthroplasty is associated with increased postdischarge morbidity [16]. Often, requirement for additional postoperative care was described in Qin et al.'s study. Before the procedure, 9% of FNF and only 2% of OA patients were classified as functional dependent [13]. Readmissions are also more common for the trauma group. More than 6.5% of fractures had additional hospitalizations, and they were twice as much as for primary THA. Furthermore, based on the publication from 2016 to 2019, on average, 3.5% of FNF patients and 1.5% of OA patients required reoperation. It may be related to the increasing probability of periprosthetic fracture in the trauma group as both populations' level of BMD differs not only in the postoperation period but also in the preoperation period [17–19].

3.1. Significance. Based on elaborated research,

(i) average FNF patient is 7.64 years older than the OA patient.

(ii) There is statistically significant predominance to a female gender in the trauma group.

(iii) Fracture patients display a higher prevalence of comorbidities with the exception of obesity to which the primary THA group is more prone to.

(iv) FNF patients usually require longer hospitalizations and more frequent blood transfusions.

Table 1: Study design comparison.

Author, publication year	Study period	Patient group	Study design	Database	Population matching	Observation period
Sasson A., 2012/2013	1990–2007	174.641 FNF 2.160.061 OA	Retrospective cohort	NHDS	No	Hospitalization
Wiliam W., 2016	2007–2013	953 FNF 41.739 OA	Retrospective cohort	NSQIP	Yes	30 days after discharge
Le Manach Y., 2015	2010–2013	319.804 FNF 371.191 OA	Retrospective cohort	FHDD	Yes	Hospitalization + readmission 72 h
Charles D., 2016	2011–2014	1.580 FNF 58.302 OA	Retrospective cohort	NSQIP	Yes	30 days after discharge
Charette R. S., 2019	2008–2016	4.266 FNF 135.013 OA	Retrospective cohort	NSQIP	Yes	30 days after discharge

Table 2: Demographic comparison.

Author, publication year	Patient group	Average age	Female gender
Sasson A., 2012/2013	174.641 FNF 2.160.061 OA	79.1 FNF 68.4 OA	75.3% FNF 55.0% OA
Wiliam W., 2016	953 FNF 41.739 OA	73.4 FNF 65.0 OA	58.3% FNF 55% OA
Le Manach Y., 2015	319.804 FNF 371.191 OA	81.7 FNF 70.2 OA	74.8% FNF 55.6% OA
Charles D., 2016	1.580 FNF 58.302 OA	73.0 FNF 66.0 OA	67.9% FNF 55.8% OA
Charette R. S., 2019	4.266 FNF 135.013 OA	—	68.5 FNF 54.8 OA

Table 3: Comorbidities' comparison.

Publication	Classification	FNF	OA	Obesity*
Sasson A., 2012/2013	DCS none DCS M + S	55.1% 44.9%	75.9% 24.1%	No data No data
Le Manach Y., 2015	No ASA classification			FNF 2.1% OA 10.3%
Wiliam W., 2016	ASA I + II ASA III + IV	35,00% 65,00%	60,00% 40,00%	FNF 21% OA 45%
Charles D., 2016	ASA I + II ASA III + IV	35.3% 64.7%	60.5% 39.5%	FNF 25.7** OA 30.3**
Charette R. S., 2019	ASA I + II ASA III + IV	33.6% 66.4%	58.2% 41.8%	FNF 23.8% OA 46.3%

*Patient body mass index above 30 kg/m^2. **Average BMI in the FNF/OA population.

Table 4: Selected complications' comparison.

Complication	Group	Study	
		William W. (%)	Chalette R. S. (%)
Mortality	FNF OA	3 0	1.8 0.3
Wound infection	FNF OA	1.5 1.4	1 1
Respiratory complications	FNF OA	3 0	1 0.3

Table 5: Outcome comparison.

Outcome	Publication Disease	Sasson A., 2012/ 2013	Wiliam W., 2016	Le Manach Y., 2015	Charles D. Qin, 2016	Charette R. S., 2019
Readmission	FNF	No data	4%*	0.44%***	7.7%	8%
	OA	No data	2%*	1.22**	3.3%	3.5%
Nonhomebound discharge	FNF	79.3%	67%*	65.2%	63.4%	61%
	OA	49.2%	55%*	40%	25.9%	22%
Average length of stay (days)	FNF	9.1 days	6 days	12.1 days	4.5 days	53.8%**
	OA	5.1 days	4 days	7.8 days	3 days	7.5%**
Reoperation	FNF	No data	3%*	No data	No data	4.4%
	OA	No data	1%*	No data	No data	2%

*Matched cohort value. **More than 5 days. ***Within 72 hours.

(v) Trauma group is more than 2 times more prone to complications including respiratory complications or even death than the OA group. Furthermore, the studies indicate that "fractures" required more frequent reoperations.

(vi) FNF patients display worse postoperation functional status and are more often discharged to another medical or caring facility.

4. Discussion

Five publications were included in this study, and despite varying approaches to the subject, they all agree on the fact that FNF and OA patient groups differ in many ways. One could say that the type of treatment might be the only common feature. It is noticeable in demographics, comorbidities, and laboratory results, as well as in postoperative outcomes or complications [14, 20]. Authors of all mentioned publications agree that patients with hip fracture require additional care and have poorer prognosis than primary THA patients. Schairer et al. [10] indicated that patient death after surgically treated hip fracture is almost 10 times more probable than after hip OA operation. That study also compared complication frequency in both groups and showed almost 3 times higher prevalence of trauma in patients. Other authors described similar observations. Poor treatment outcome can be related to FNF patient group senile age and numerous comorbidities, but R.S. Charette et al. in their study [12] conducted propensity matching and multivariate analysis and came to a conclusion that hip fracture is an independent risk factor. Since the groups and their main diseases differ, despite similar surgical treatment, distinct in-hospital and often posthospital care is required. According to William W. et al., the trauma group needs, on average, 10 times more blood transfusions and 2 more days of preoperative preparations than the primary THA group [11]. Taking length of hospital stay into consideration, the percentage of nonhomebound discharged patients, and other mentioned factors, FNF patients appear more cost-intensive. Unfortunately, most medical facilities are paid for procedures; therefore, both groups are paid for in a similar fashion. This reasoning may indicate unjust THA financing policies whether it is a bundle payment or restricted by a hospital-government contract on the defined number of hip arthroplasty procedures. The problem was presented in previous subject-related publications [9–13], and all authors agree that a different system should be established. Additional studies should be held to determine the cost of prolonged THA hospitalization with particular emphasis on FNF patients.

The study has several limitations. Firstly, data in analyzed studies were not uniform. Secondly, study construction differed between publications. Observation period, population matching, and researched complications were not homogenous; therefore, calculations based on the data may only exhibit trends. Finally, no full statistical analysis was performed on the gathered material.

In summary, THA provides optimal treatment for both OA and FNF in active elderly patients. Because mentioned diseases vary in many aspects, their treatment should benefit from a different perioperative approach. In order to maintain best medical care, a more cost-comprehensive system should be established, a system that would penalize facilities performing THA for FNF instead for OA.

References

[1] B. Gullberg, O. Johnell, and J. Kannis, "Wordwide projections for hip fracture," *Osteoporosis International*, 1997.

[2] M. D. Young Lu and H. S. Uppal, "Hip fractures: relevant anatomy, classification, and biomechanics of fracture and fixation," *Geriatr Orthop Surg Rehabil*, 2019.

[3] H. Blain, C. Pascale, N. Portero-Muzy, F. Bonnel, and F. Canovas, "Cortical and trabecular bone disruption in the femoral neck in osteophorosis and osteoarthritis," *Bone*, vol. 43, 2018.

[4] L. Natália Zalc, M. Lucas da Ponte, N. David Gonçalves, F. Brandão de Andrade e Silva, K. E. Kojima, and S. Jorge Santos, "Femoral neck fracture Garden I and II. Evaluation of the deviation in lateral view," *Acta Ortopedica Brasileira*, vol. 25, 2017.

[5] F. Wang, H. Zhang, Z. Zhang, C. Ma, and X. Feng, "Comparison of bipolar hemiarthroplasty and total hip arthroplasty for displaced femoral neck fractures in the healthy elderly: a meta-analysis," *BMC Musculoskeletal Disorders*, vol. 16, 2015.

[6] L. Yu, Y. Wang, and J. Chen, "Total hip arthroplasty versus hemiarthroplasty for displaced femoral neck fractures: meta-analysis of randomized trials," *Clinical Orthopaedics and Related Research*, 2012.

[7] B. BoukebousP, B. R. ZahiC, and A. P. Guillon, "Comparison of dual mobility total hip arthroplasty and bipolar arthro-

plasty for femoral neck fractures: a retrospective case-control study of 199 hips Orthopaedics & Traumatology," *Surgery & ResearchVolume*, vol. 104, no. 3, 2018.

[8] C. W. Jones, I. De Martino, R. D'Apolito, A. A. Nocon, P. K. Sculco, and T. P. Sculco, "The use of dual-mobility bearings in patients at high risk of dislocation," *The Bone & Joint Journal*, vol. 101, 2019.

[9] W. W. Schairer, J. M. Lane, D. A. Halsey, R. Iorio, E. P. Douglas, and S. Alexander, *Total Hip Arthroplasty For Femoral Neck Fracture Is Not A Typical Drg 470: A Propensity-Matched Cohort Study*, The Association of Bone and Joint Surgeons, Park Ridge, IL, USA, 2016.

[10] R. S. Charette, M. Sloan, and G.-C. Lee, "Not all hip arthroplasties are created equal increased complications and re-admissions after total hip arthroplasty for femoral neck fractures compared with osteoarthritis," *The Bone & Joint Journal*, vol. 101, 2019.

[11] S. Adam, M. D'Apuzzo, S. Stephen, J. Cass, and T. Mabry, "Total hip arthroplasty for femoral neck fracture: comparing in-hospital mortality, complications, and disposition to an elective patient population," *The Journal of Arthroplasty* vol. 28, 2013.

[12] C. D. Qin, M. M. Helfrich, D. W. Fitz, M. A. Oyer, K. D. Hardt, and D. W. Manning, "Differences in post-operative outcome between conversion and primary total hip arthroplasty," *The Journal of Arthroplsty*, vol. 33, 2017.

[13] Y. Le Manach, G. Collins, M. Bhandari, B. Amal, and J. Boddaert, "Outcomes after hip fracture surgery compared with elective total hip replacement," *Journal of the American Medical Association*, vol. 314, 2015.

[14] S. Landro de Freitas, P. Fernando, R. Tiango Aguiar, and G. Felipe Silva, "Clinical, labolatory and densitometric comparison of patients with coxarthrosis and femoral neck fractures," *Revista do Colegio Brasileiro de Cirurgioes*, vol. 8, 2018.

[15] O. Wallner, A. Stark, O. Muren, T. Eisler, and O. Sköldenberg, "Unstable hip arthroplasties. A prospective cohort study on seventy dislocating hip followed up for four years," *SICOT* vol. 39, 2014.

[16] M. C. Fu, A. M. Samuel, K. Peter, H. Catherine, E. P. Douglas, and S. Alexander, "Discharge to inpatient facilities after total hip arthroplasty is associated with increased postdischarge morbidity," *The Journal of Arthroplasty*, vol. 32, 2017.

[17] T. Mann, T. Eisler, H. Bodén et al., "Larger femoral periphrostetic bone mineral density decrease following total hip arthroplasty for femoral neck fracture than for osteoarthritis: a prospective, observational cohort study," *Journal of Orthopaedic Research*, vol. 33, 2015.

[18] H. Lindahl, "Epidemiology of periphrostetic femur fracture around a total hip arthroplasty," *Injury*, vol. 38, 2007.

[19] B. D. Springer, C. D. Etkin, P. B. Shores, T. J. Gioe, D. G. Lewallen, and J. Kevin, "Bozic. Periopertive periphrostetic femur fractures are strongly correlated with fixation method: an anlysis from the American joint replacement registy," *The Journal of Arthroplasty*, vol. 34, 2019.

[20] C.-H. Rapin and R. Lagier, "Raised serum albumin in hip osteoarthrosis: a comparative study in women of some blood chemical parameters in aging and in cases of femoral neck fractures, osteoporotic vertebral crush fractures,and hip osteoarthrosisannal of rheumatic diseases," *Annals of the Rheumatic Diseases*, vol. 47, 1988.

8

A Preoperative Analytical Model for Patient-Specific Impingement Analysis in Total Hip Arthroplasty

Yolanda Gu,[1,2] Jim Pierrepont,[2] Catherine Stambouzou,[2] Qing Li,[1] and Jonathan Baré[3]

[1]*School of Aerospace, The University of Sydney, Mechanical and Mechatronic Engineering, Building J07, Sydney, NSW 2006, Australia*
[2]*Optimized Ortho, 17 Bridge Street, Pymble, NSW 2073, Australia*
[3]*Melbourne Orthopaedic Group, 33 The Avenue, Windsor, VIC 3191, Australia*

Correspondence should be addressed to Jim Pierrepont; jim.pierrepont@coringroup.com

Guest Editor: Yasushi Oshima

Prosthetic impingement is important to consider during total hip arthroplasty planning to minimise the risk of joint instability. Modelling impingement preoperatively can assist in defining the required component alignment for each individual. We developed an analytical impingement model utilising a combination of mathematical calculations and an automated computational simulation to determine the risk of prosthetic impingement. The model assesses cup inclination and anteversion angles that are associated with prosthetic impingement using patient-specific inputs, such as stem anteversion, planned implant types, and target Range of Motion (ROM). The analysed results are presented as a range of cup inclination and anteversion angles over which a colour map indicates an impingement-free safe zone in green and impingement risk zones in red. A validation of the model demonstrates accuracy within +/- 1.4° of cup inclination and anteversion. The study further investigated the impact of changes in stem anteversion, femoral head size, and head offset on prosthetic impingement, as an example of the application of the model.

1. Introduction

Dislocation is one of the most common complications leading to revision surgery after Total Hip Arthroplasty (THA), accounting for almost one-quarter (21%) of all revision procedures [1]. Component mal-positioning has long been recognised as a major cause of dislocation [2–5]. Although spontaneous dislocation can occur due to poor soft tissue balance, prosthetic impingement, due to mal-positioned components, commonly precedes dislocation.

In a cup retrieval study performed by Marchetti et al., 80% of cups revised due to dislocation showed evidence of prosthetic impingement [6]. Recurrent prosthetic impingement between the femoral neck and acetabular liner can cause severe component wear due to the high stress concentration at the impingement site, producing wear debris [7]. This wear debris may result in an increased risk of osteolysis [8]. In Marchetti et al.'s study, prosthetic impingement was observed in all retrieval groups including loosening, infection, osteolysis and miscellaneous cases, highlighting the importance of an impingement-free motion to the clinical outcome of THA. Due to the numerous undesirable effects of early impingement on the stability and longevity of the prosthetic hip, it is deemed necessary to place the components in a position that avoids prosthetic impingement whilst allowing maximum hip range of motion (ROM).

Acetabular "safe zones" have been introduced by various authors to assist with cup alignment and to minimise post-operative complications. Well-known safe zones, such as those published by Lewinnek [4], Esposito et al. [9], and Callanan et al. [10] are often used as gold standard in THA. However, despite the implementation of these "safe zones", postoperative dislocation rates remain the same [11]. In contemporary clinical studies, combined anteversion of the acetabular and femoral components, and not cup orientation alone, has been correlated with dislocation [12–15]. These more recent investigations have emphasised a need for an individualised target for cup orientation rather than a generic range applicable to all patients.

Motion capture, laboratorial simulators, and computational models are common methods of measuring range of motion of the hip [16–18]. These traditional methods can provide accurate analyses of the ROM of the hip with live subjects, generic bone models, or patient-specific bone models. However, these analyses are resource- and time-consuming and require significant setup. It is for these reasons that the above-mentioned methods are unviable for preoperative or intraoperative investigation on a large scale.

An analytical ROM model has been proposed by Yoshimine et.al. [19] and Hisatome & Doi [2] to calculate theoretical prosthetic impingement of the hip. Analytical models are faster to run and require less prework compared to traditional methods. However, analytical models are limited by their simplicity and key assumptions limit the accuracy of the model. The ROM model described in this study utilises a combination of computational simulations and analytical methods, which are accurate and efficient to run.

The aim of this study is to develop and validate a robust and accurate analytical model to assess the cup inclination and anteversion angles that are associated with prosthetic impingement using patient-specific inputs.

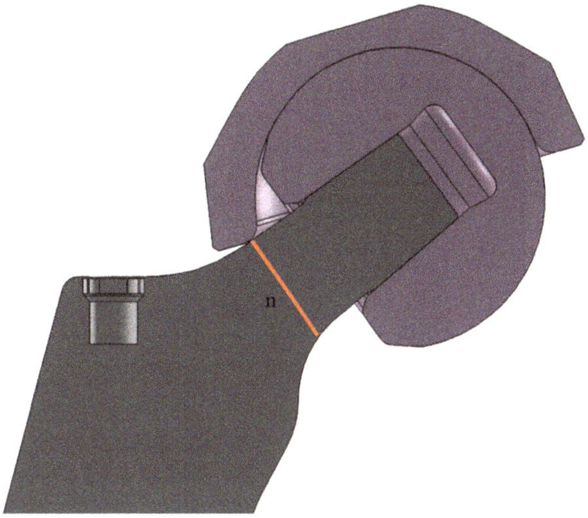

FIGURE 1: Stem neck width (n) at the impingement level.

2. Method

2.1. Model Development. Hisatome and Doi proposed a mathematical formula to calculate the theoretical range of motion using seven factors including head radius (r), cup depth (d), cup inclination (α) and anteversion (β), stem neck angle from the transverse plane (a), stem anteversion (b), and neck width at the impingement level (n) [2]. The first six factors are defined from implant design drawings and measurements. The last factor, neck width at the impingement level, varies for different stems and at different impingement positions. Hisatome and Doi assume all stem necks are cylindrical in shape, i.e., that neck width is a constant value at all stem positions. However, the neck width varies significantly in modern trapezoidal stem designs, and the assumption of a constant neck width will significantly affect the model accuracy. The model presented in this study improves on Hisatome and Doi's work by considering neck width as a variable that differs for different stem types and impingement positions.

Hisatome provided a mathematical formula to calculate the prosthetic hip range of motion in certain activities, i.e., pure flexion, extension, internal rotation at 90° flexion, and external rotation. The impingement model in this study allows for customised inputs to define the target ROM test conditions. The proposed model offers two combined target ROM conditions: (1) user-defined degree of Internal Rotation (IR) at any Flexion (FL) and (2) user-defined degree of External Rotation (ER) at any Extension (EX). The IR_FL test is associated with anterior prosthetic impingement in flexion, and the ER_EX test is associated with posterior prosthetic impingement in extension. The derivation of how to calculate the cup orientations that satisfy the user-defined target ROM (IR_FL and ER_EX) is detailed in the Appendix.

An automated computational simulation is used to calculate the stem neck width (n) at the impingement level (Figure 1) in Solidworks (Dassault Systèmes, US). The 3D geometry of the acetabular and stem components are imported into Solidworks. The centre of rotation of the acetabular and stem components are placed at the origin of the assembly. The stem component is placed at −40° to 60° of anteversion in 20° increments and 6° of natural femur adduction. The stem component is simulated to perform flexion/extension and then internal rotation/external rotation. The acetabular component can rotate about the stem component in a range of 0° to 60° inclination and anteversion. The cup orientation is measured using Murray's radiographic definitions [20]. The automated simulation records the cup inclination and anteversion angles, and the stem neck width when any collision is detected. The results are saved in a database for use in the proposed model.

Even with an automated simulation, and running only discrete values of stem anteversion, this is a time-consuming process. In order to run the impingement analysis at any stem anteversion, 'Thin Plate Spline Interpolation' was used to calculate the neck width at all cup and stem positions, utilising the simulated neck width values. The simulated data was plotted with cup inclination and anteversion on the X and Y axes, and neck width on the Z axis in Matlab (Mathworks, US) (Figure 2). Through the interpolated surface, the stem neck width can be calculated for any given cup and stem position in all cases with the same implant type. By utilising the neck width simulator and surface interpolation combined, the neck width at any given cup and stem position can be simulated robustly and accurately. The simulated neck width can then be placed in the formula given in the Appendix and cup orientations that satisfy the target ROM conditions can be calculated. The cup inclination and anteversion which fulfil the target ROM conditions are plotted as impingement boundaries. For ease of visualisation, the area that satisfies the ROM conditions is displayed in green and the area that does not satisfy the ROM conditions is displayed in red.

The proposed impingement model generates two impingement boundaries for any given set of target ROM conditions (IR@FL and ER@EX). Figure 3 illustrates an example of the output of the model with impingement

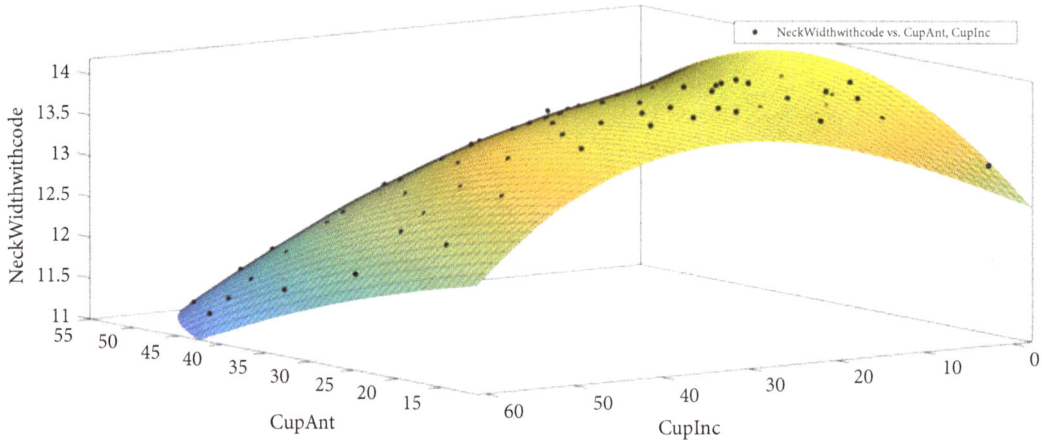

FIGURE 2: Surface interpolation of stem neck width.

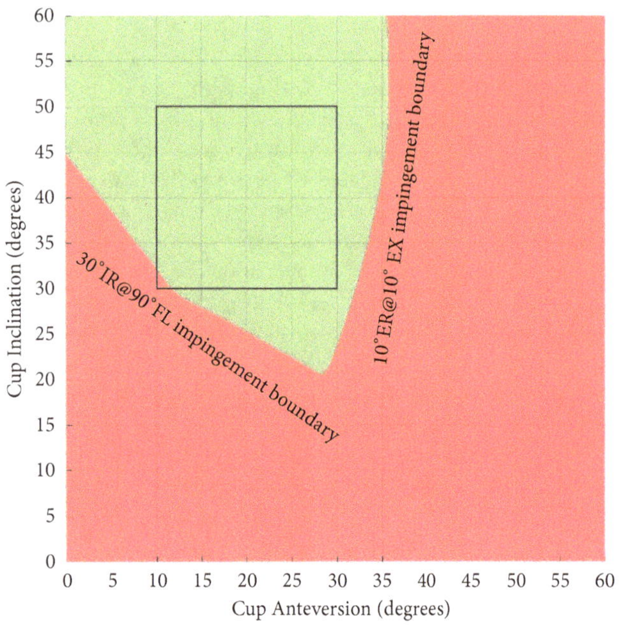

FIGURE 3: Impingement plot at 30° IR @ 90° FL and 10° ER @ 10° EX.

testing condition of 30°IR@90°FL and 10°ER@10°EX. The diagonal curve represents the 30°IR@90°FL impingement boundary. Cup orientations on the left-hand side of this boundary are at risk of prosthetic impingement in flexion. The vertical curve represents the 10°ER@10°EX impingement boundary. Cup orientations on the right-hand side of this boundary are at risk of prosthetic impingement in extension. The green cup orientations between these two boundaries satisfy the impingement conditions tested, and no impingement is detected. The cup orientations in red do not satisfy the impingement testing conditions as impingement is detected. A square black box is drawn on the graph for ease of comparison to the coloured area. The box highlights an area with 10° to 30° of cup anteversion and 30° to 50° of cup inclination which overlaps with commonly accepted cup positions [4, 10, 21].

Using the formula proposed in the Appendix, the cup orientations that satisfy any target ROM conditions can be calculated. The proposed model was investigated with the target ROM of 30°IR@90°FL and 10°ER@10°EX as an example. In order to test the application of the model in preoperative planning scenarios, three parameters (stem anteversion, femoral head size, and femoral head offset) were investigated to see how each parameter affects the prosthetic ROM. All other input parameters were set to the default values: neck-shaft angle = 125°, stem flexion = 0°, and stem adduction = 6°.

2.2. Model Validation. An alternative CAD model was used to verify that the proposed analytical model can accurately calculate the cup inclination and anteversion at impingement. The worst-case implant combinations that would provide the least accurate results were selected to validate the proposed model.

The worst-case implant size was determined with a combination of maximum head size which engaged with the shortest head offset. This resulted in the impingement to occur at the most lateral position of the stem (i.e., closer to the stem shoulder and therefore with the greatest difference in stem neck geometry (Figure 4)). This gives results furthest from the simulated impingement boundaries and therefore is the worst case for the accuracy test. The proposed model utilises the impingement boundaries in the neck width database, which was generated using 20° increments of stem anteversion, and then interpolated the impingement boundaries for other stem anteversions using the Thin Plate Spline Interpolation. Stem anteversions which would result in maximum deviation on the interpolated solution were selected for testing. It was hypothesised that the maximum deviation on the interpolated solution lies at the point which is the maximum distance away from any two exact solutions from the interpolation. The stem anteversion was placed at −40°, −20°, 0°, 20°, 40°, and 60° in the neck width database,

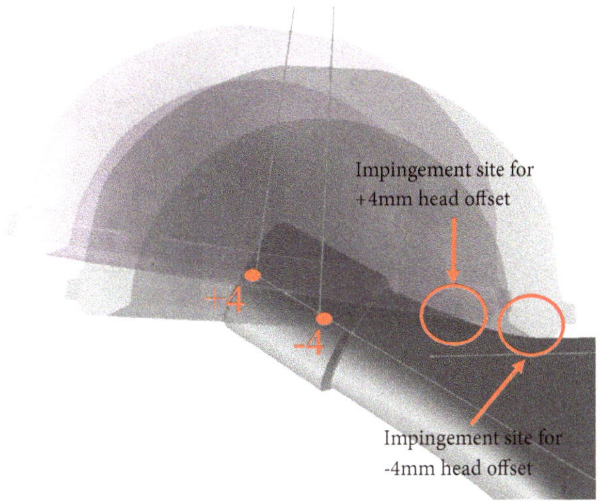

Figure 4: 40mm polyethylene liner engaging at -4mm head offset compares to engaging at +4mm offset.

Table 1: Maximum difference in cup orientation, at impingement in flexion and impingement in extension, between the proposed impingement model and an independent CAD model.

	Cup Anteversion	Cup Inclination
Maximum difference in flexion	1.1°	1.4°
Maximum difference in extension	1.4°	1.0°

Table 2: Neck width range for four stems investigated in this study.

Stems	Neck width range in mm (Avg)
Stem 1	11.3 – 22.2 (14.7)
Stem 2	10.9 – 17.3 (13.5)
Stem 3	11.0 – 18.2 (13.7)
Stem 4	10.9 – 20.3 (13.7)

and thus stem anteversions −30°, −10°, 10°, 30°, and 50° were selected for the accuracy test.

The implant geometries were imported into Solidworks and placed at the positions defined above. The liner was free to rotate about its centre of rotation. Using the interference detection function in Solidworks, the cup inclination and anteversion at which the acetabular component impinges with the stem can be recorded. The recorded cup inclination and anteversion in Solidworks were compared with the simulated results to determine the accuracy of the proposed model.

3. Results

The accuracy of the analytical model was assessed against the CAD model with worst case implant combinations. The cup orientation boundaries that were created by the proposed model and the CAD model were compared. The results show the maximum difference between the two models is 1.4° in both cup inclination and anteversion (Table 1).

In order to show how the neck width can vary at different impingement levels on the neck, four different stems were analysed within the neck width database. As shown in Table 2, the stem neck width varies significantly with different impingement locations. This suggests that using a constant neck width value is too simplistic to provide an accurate impingement analysis. The proposed model utilised a combination of an automated simulator and surface interpolation to create a database containing the neck width of the stem. Substituting the neck width database into the mathematical formula allowed the quick analysis of the prosthetic impingement model. By gaining computational efficiency in this way, the model can be used as an accurate preoperative planning tool or as a general tool to study how implant parameters impact the prosthetic ROM.

Figures 5–7 demonstrate how the prosthetic impingement can be impacted by stem anteversion, femoral head size, and femoral head offset using Stem 2 from Table 2 as an example. Similar trends can be observed with other types of stems which have a trapezoidal neck design.

As can been seen from Figure 5, as the stem anteversion increases, the impingement-free (green) zone shifts towards the low cup anteversion area, suggesting high stem anteversion must be combined with low cup anteversion in order to reduce the risk of prosthetic impingement, and vice versa. There is no significant difference in the area of the green zone at each stem anteversion. This finding agrees with the combined anteversion concept which states radiographic cup anteversion and stem anteversion are linearly correlate [2, 22, 23]. This further highlights the point that an acetabular safe zone should not be considered independent of stem anteversion.

The impingement safe zone generated by the proposed model is also affected by femoral head size. As the femoral head increases, the green zone gets larger, suggesting that a larger femoral head results in more cup component positions which satisfy the impingement testing condition (Figure 6), when all other parameters are kept constant. This agrees with previous studies that suggest that larger femoral head sizes allow for a wider range of acceptable implant orientations [24]. With a 40 mm head, the impingement-free area increases significantly compared to smaller heads. Other factors, such as wear rate and trunnionosis, should also be taken into account when selecting head sizes. Based on the implants assessed in this study, a 28 mm head should be avoided where possible as the impingement-free area decreases significantly.

Femoral head offset is a common parameter to consider when planning patient's leg length, offset, or soft tissue tension during THA. However, it can be overlooked during impingement analysis. The proposed model allows the impact of different head offsets on the prosthetic impingement to be considered. In the case of the stem tested (Stem 2), short (-4mm) and extra-long (+8mm) head offsets showed a smaller impingement-free zone (green area) compared to neutral (+0mm) and long (+4mm) head offsets (Figure 7), especially in the common cup orientation range (highlighted in black

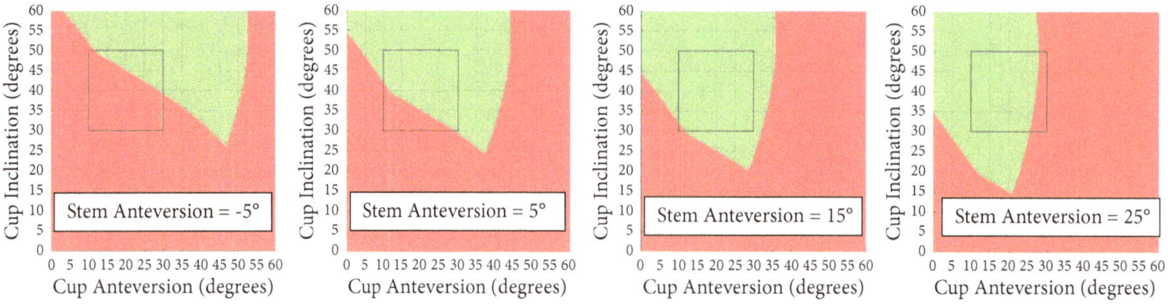

FIGURE 5: Impingement with different stem anteversion for Stem 2.

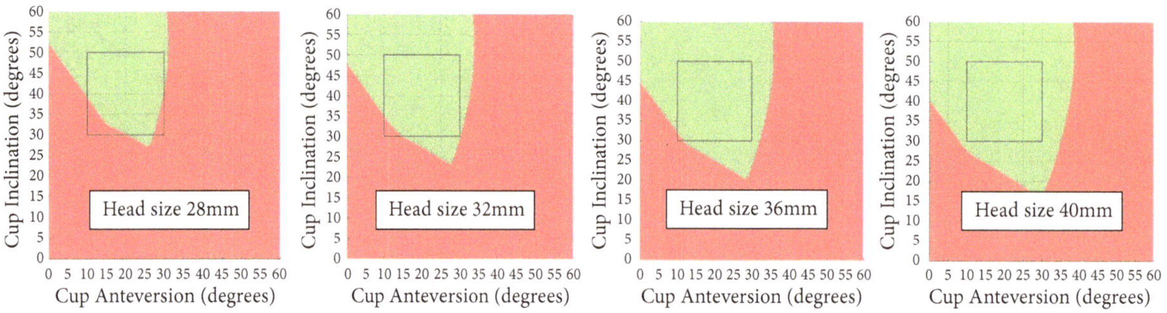

FIGURE 6: Impingement with different head sizes. At stem anteversion of 10° for stem 2.

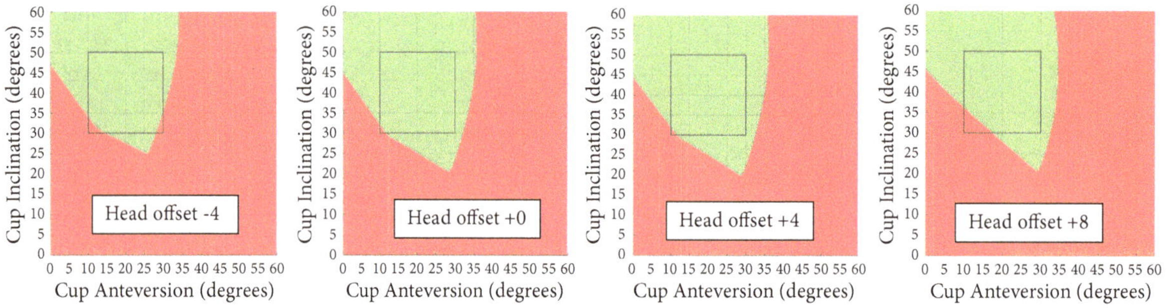

FIGURE 7: Impingement with different head offset for stem 2.

box). The femoral head offset is related to the stem neck width at the impingement level. Generally speaking, the shorter the offset, the wider the neck width at the impingement site, and consequently the smaller the hip range of motion (earlier impingement). However, in the case of extra-long (+8) head offset, impingement occurs at the level of the stem trunnion, which is usually wider than the stem neck. This results in extra-long head offset being less favourable than standard or long head options when trying to maximise prosthetic ROM (Figure 8).

4. Discussion

The present study introduced an analytical model for analysing prosthetic impingement in THA. The model involves a mathematical formula in combination with an automated neck width simulator which allows the model to take into account implant-specific neck width variations to accurately determine optimal cup orientations that are free from risk of prosthetic impingement. The model requires a one-off pre-generation of the neck width profile database for the stem of interest using the automated neck width simulator prior to the use of the model. Combined with the pre-generated neck width database and the proposed formula, the model is able to provide a zone of cup orientations that satisfy any user defined flexion and extension testing conditions, combined with any internal rotation or external rotation. The output of the model is presented as a colour map for ease of visualisation.

Even though the proposed model is capable of testing the prosthetic impingement at any user defined target ROM conditions, the question of which target ROM suits each individual patient is yet to be solved. Different target ROMs have been suggested by different groups. Incavo et al. studied passive ROM of eight cadaveric hips and suggested subjects can reach an average of 20° in extension and 24° in external

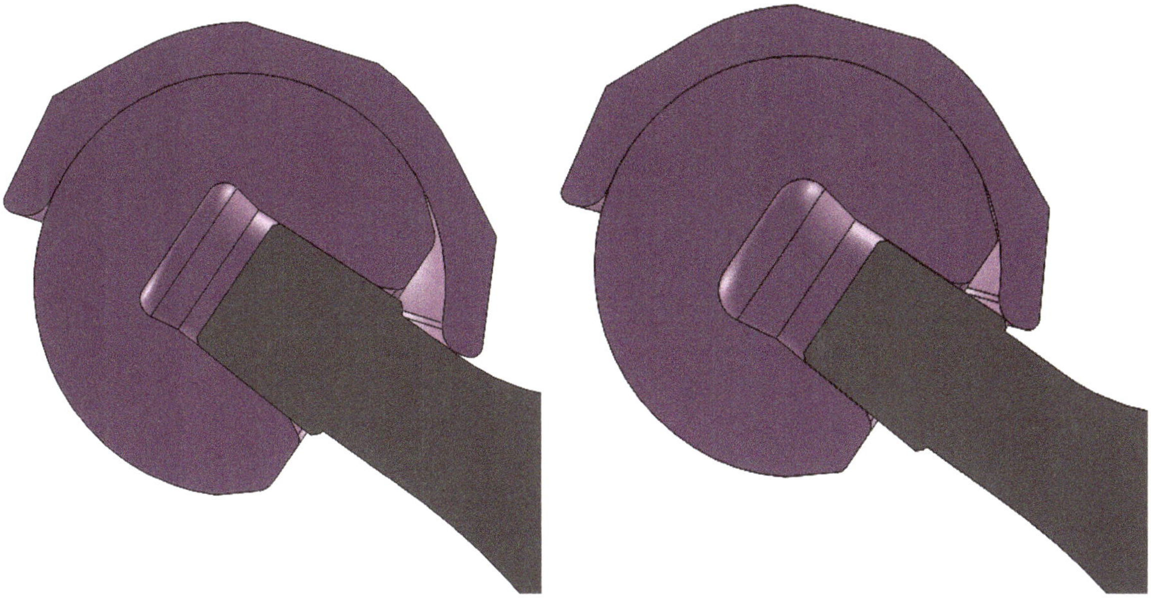

FIGURE 8: (Left) Liner impinges at stem neck with a +4mm offset head. (Right) Liner impinges at stem trunnion with a +8mm offset head.

rotation [25]. Similar cadaveric studies conducted by Miki et al. reported passive movement of the femur can reach up to 113° in flexion, 75° of internal rotation, 34° in extension and 36° of external rotation [26]. Only single movement and no combined movement of the femoral component were conducted in both studies. Yoshimine et al. [19] provided their combined motion ROM formula with 45° of internal rotation at 90° flexion, and Hisatome & Doi's [2] model is built based on 60° of internal rotation at 90° flexion. Both models use 30° of extension for their posterior impingement test; no combined extension and external rotation was tested. The combined motion tested in this study (30°IR@90°FL and 10°ER@10°EX) is smaller than suggested by previous authors for the following two reasons: (1) the neck width simulated from the actual stem geometry in our model is much larger than 10 mm (used in both Hisatome and Yoshimine's model). This results in fewer cup orientations that can satisfy the target ROM in our model. This also highlights the sensitivity of the stem neck width on the available ROM. The neck width of the actual stem should be used for more accurate results. (2) The previous studies suggested target ROMs were based on the results from cadaveric hips or intraoperative navigation data which did not isolate the femoral movement; i.e., pelvic movement was not taken into account during measurement of the femoral ROM. This results in overestimation of the femur movement as some of the movement observed should be attributed to the pelvis. The proposed model can accommodate different combined target ROM and was tested with 30° IR @ 90° FL, 10° ER @ 10° EX. Having customisable target ROM conditions enables the tool to accommodate inputs and test conditions on a patient-specific basis.

Similar to findings from previous studies, our model also highlights the importance of considering combined anteversion of the acetabular and femoral components. Widmer provided a simplified formula to achieve optimal ROM which suggests the sum of cup anteversion and 0.7 times the stem anteversion should be equal to 37° [22]. Similarly, Hisatome and Doi used their model and suggested cup anteversion and 0.7 times the stem anteversion should equal to 42° [2]. Other authors such as Jolles et al. and Dorr et al. suggested target ranges for combined anteversion which are 40°-60° and 25°-50°, respectively [12, 23]. Despite the various mathematical formulae or guidelines recommended in these studies, there is still a lack of general consensus of an optimal combined version. This is because the optimal combined version is multifactorial. As suggested in this study, stem version, head size, neck offset, and stem types (specifically neck width and neck angle) can all impact which cup orientations satisfy the targeted ROM. The impingement-free cup orientations determined by this model are customised for each individual and for the implant types/sizes modelled. The proposed analytical model allows different implants and positions to be input into the model and robustly calculates the range of impingement-free cup orientations.

There are a few limitations to the proposed model. First, the neck width simulator requires the specific implant geometry to be analysed prior to use. This limits the model to be used only with the implants available in the pregenerated database. More implants can be added into the database upon availability of the implant geometry. Secondly, the combined motion provided in this model is limited to the two mentioned above (IR@FL and ER@EX). Abduction and adduction of the femur were not considered in this model as it was believed that the amount of abduction and adduction was small during daily activities such as sitting and walking, in comparison to the other movements. Lastly, it is acknowledged that the functional outcome of a THA is multi-factorial and not only based on risk of

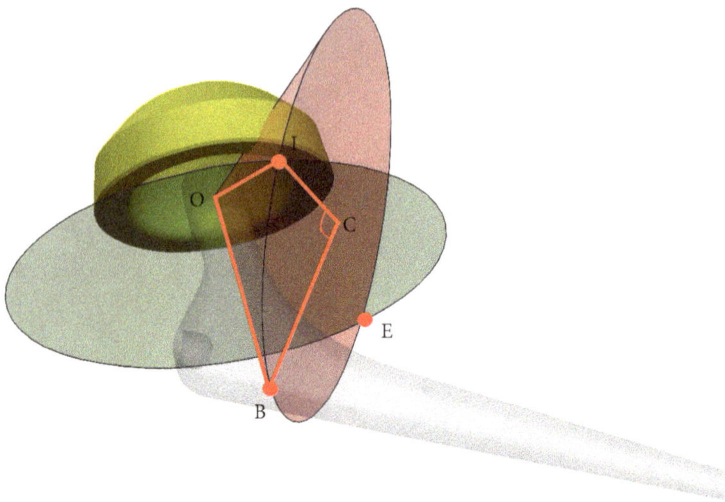

FIGURE 9: Cup cone and stem cone overlap. ∠BCI is the maximum internal rotation angle at the defined flexion angle.

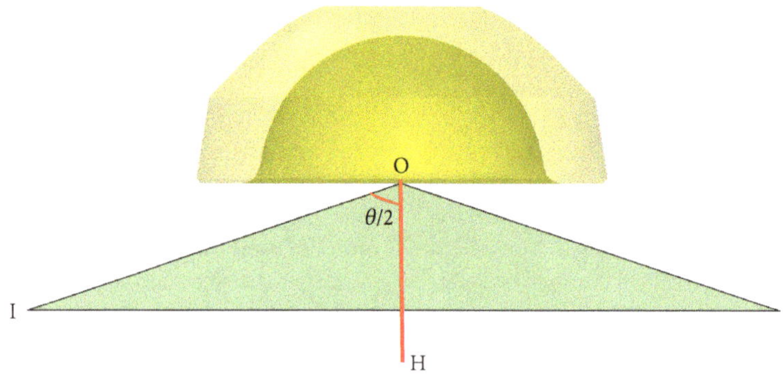

FIGURE 10: Cup cone.

prosthetic impingement. The cause of other phenomena, such as bony impingement, contact joint force, and component wear, will also significantly impact the functional outcome and longevity of the THA [9, 15, 27]. The proposed model should not be used in isolation, but rather, it should be used in combination with other analysis tools for preoperative THA planning.

This study describes an analytical model that determines a cup orientation "safe zone" for avoiding prosthetic impingement, based on accurately derived implant parameters. The model tests combined rotations of flexion/internal rotation and extension/external rotation, the limits of which can be customised. The model has demonstrated improved accuracy over other published impingement models and can be used as an investigational tool to assess the impact of varying implant parameters, in additon to preoperative planning in THA.

Appendix

The concept of creating the IR_FL formula is to calculate the maximum rotation of the stem at a defined degree of flexion via finding the intersection point I (INTRflx, INTRfly, INTRflz) of the cup rotation cone and stem rotation cone (Figure 9). The cup rotation cone is a right circular cone with a unit generatrix which is formed by rotating the stem component inside the cup. The orientation of the cup cone changes with changes in cup inclination and anteversion angle (Figure 10). By applying vector analysis to the cup cone, we can get the following two equations:

$$|I| = \text{INTRflx}^2 + \text{INTRfly}^2 + \text{INTRflz}^2 = 1 \tag{A.1}$$

$$\begin{aligned} &\text{INTRflx} * \sin(\beta) + \text{INTRfly} * \sin(\alpha) * \cos(\beta) \\ &\quad - \text{INTRflz} * \cos(\alpha) * \cos(\beta) = \cos\left(\frac{\theta}{2}\right) \end{aligned} \tag{A.2}$$

where α and β are cup inclination and anteversion, respectively. θ is the oscillation angle which can be calculated by $\theta = 360° - 2*\sin^{-1}(n/2r) - (180° - 2*\sin^{-1}((r-d)*r))$, where n is the neck width, r is the head radius, and d is the head centre offset from the liner centre.

The stem rotation cone is another right circular cone with a unit generatrix formed by rotating the stem at defined

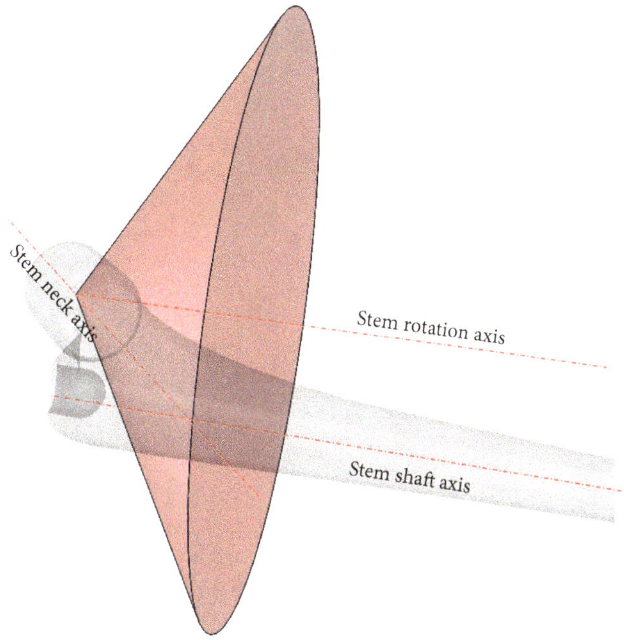

FIGURE 11: Stem cone.

flexion angle (Figure 11). By applying vector analysis to the stem cone, we can get the following equation:

$$\text{INTRflx} * \sin(\text{FL}) - \text{INTRflz} * \cos(\text{FL}) = \sin(a) \quad (\text{A.3})$$

where a is the angle between stem neck axis to transverse plane.

The maximum internal rotation angle is equal to $\angle BCI$, where B is the initial position of the stem and C is the base centre of the stem cone (Figure 9). By solving (A.1), (A.2), and (A.3) simultaneously, the coordinates of I (INTRflx, INTRfly, INTRflz) can be solved. Subsequently, $\angle BCI$ can be calculated and this is the maximum internal rotation (Max_IR) of the stem before impingement occurs.

$$\begin{aligned}\text{Max\_IR} &= \angle \text{BCI} \\ &= \text{acos}\Big(((\text{INTRflx} - \sin(a) * \sin(\text{FL})) * (\sin(a) * \sin(\text{FL}) - \cos(a) * \sin(b) * \cos(\text{FL}) - \sin(a) * \sin(\text{FL})) \\ &\quad + \text{INTRfly} * \cos(a) * \cos(b) + (\text{INTRflz} + \sin(a) * \cos(\text{FL})) * (-\cos(\text{FL}) * \sin(a) - \sin(\text{FL}) * \cos(a) * \sin(b) + \sin(a) * \cos(\text{FL}))) \times ((\cos(a))\ \hat{}\ 2)^{-1}\Big)\end{aligned} \quad (\text{A.4})$$

where a is the angle between stem neck axis to transverse plane and b is the angle between stem neck axis to coronal plane which projected onto transverse plane (stem anteversion).

The same concept can be applied to calculate the maximum external rotation of the stem at any defined extension angle.

$$\begin{aligned}&\text{Max\_ER} \\ &= \text{acos}\Big(((\text{EXTRexx} + \sin(a) * \sin(\text{EX})) * (-\sin(a) * \sin(\text{EX}) - \cos(\text{EX}) * \sin(b) * \cos(a) + \sin(a) * \sin(\text{EX})) \\ &\quad + \text{EXTRexy} * \cos(a) * \cos(b) + (\text{EXTRexz} + \sin(a) * \cos(\text{EX})) * (-\cos(\text{EX}) * \sin(a) + \sin(\text{EX}) * \sin(b) * \cos(a) + \sin(a) * \cos(\text{EX}))) \times ((\cos(a))\ \hat{}\ 2)^{-1}\Big)\end{aligned} \quad (\text{A.5})$$

where Max_ER is the target maximum external rotation defined by the user and EX is the target extension angle defined by the user. EXTRexx, EXTRexy, and EXTRexz are the coordinates of intersection point of the cup rotation cone and stem rotation cone when stem is in extension, a is the angle between stem neck axis to transverse plane, and b is the angle between stem neck axis to coronal plane which projected onto transverse plane (stem anteversion).

References

[1] Australian Orthopaedic Association National Joint Replacement Registry (AOANJRR), "Hip, Knee & Shoulder Arthroplasty: 2018 Annual Report," Tech. Rep., AOA, Adelaide, Australia, 2018.

[2] T. Hisatome and H. Doi, "Theoretically optimum position of the prosthesis in total hip arthroplasty to fulfill the severe range of motion criteria due to neck impingement," *Journal of Orthopaedic Science*, vol. 16, no. 2, pp. 229–237, 2011.

[3] M. Higa, H. Tanino, M. Abo, S. Kakunai, and S. A. Banks, "Effect of acetabular component anteversion on dislocation mechanisms in total hip arthroplasty," *Journal of Biomechanics*, vol. 44, no. 9, pp. 1810–1813, 2011.

[4] G. E. Lewinnek, J. L. Lewis, R. Tarr, C. L. Compere, and J. R. Zimmerman, "Dislocations after total hip-replacement arthroplasties," *The Journal of Bone & Joint Surgery*, vol. 60, no. 2, pp. 217–220, 1978.

[5] Australian Orthopaedic Association National Joint Replacement Registry (AOANJRR), "Hip, Knee & Shoulder Arthroplasty: 2017 Annual Report," Tech. Rep., AOA, Adelaide, Australia, 2017.

[6] E. Marchetti, N. Krantz, C. Berton et al., "Component impingement in total hip arthroplasty: frequency and risk factors. A continuous retrival analysis series of 416 cup," *Orthopaedics & Traumatology, Surgery & Research*, 2011.

[7] K. Onda, S. Nagoya, M. Kaya, and T. Yamashita, "Cup-neck impingement due to the malposition of the implant as a possible mechanism for metallosis in metal-on-metal total hip arthroplasty," *Orthopedics*, vol. 31, no. 4, p. 396, 2008.

[8] D. R. Pedersen, J. J. Callaghan, and T. D. Brown, "Activity-dependence of the "safe zone" for impingement versus dislocation avoidance," *Medical Engineering & Physics*, vol. 27, no. 4, pp. 323–328, 2005.

[9] C. I. Esposito, W. L. Walter, A. Roques et al., "Wear in alumina-on-alumina ceramic total hip replacements: a retrieval analysis of edge loading," *The Journal of Bone & Joint Surgery (British Volume)*, vol. 94, no. 7, pp. 901–907, 2012.

[10] M. C. Callanan, B. Jarrett, C. R. Bragdon et al., "The john charnley award: Risk factors for cup malpositioning: Quality improvement through a joint registry at a tertiary hospital," *Clinical Orthopaedics and Related Research*, vol. 469, no. 2, pp. 319–329, 2011.

[11] M. P. Abdel, P. von Roth, M. T. Jennings, A. D. Hanssen, and M. W. Pagnano, "What safe zone? The vast majority of dislocated THAs are within the Lewinnek safe zone for acetabular component position," *Clinical Orthopaedics and Related Research*, vol. 474, no. 2, pp. 386–391, 2016.

[12] B. M. Jolles, P. Zangger, and P.-F. Leyvraz, "Factors predisposing to dislocation after primary total hip arthroplasty: a multivariate analysis," *The Journal of Arthroplasty*, vol. 17, no. 3, pp. 282–288, 2002.

[13] L. D. Dorr and J. J. Callaghan, "Death of the Lewinnek "Safe Zone"," *The Journal of Arthroplasty*, vol. 34, no. 1, pp. 1-2, 2019.

[14] M. Komeno, M. Hasegawa, A. Sudo, and A. Uchida, "Computed tomographic evaluation of component position on dislocation after total hip arthroplasty," *Orthopedics*, vol. 29, no. 12, pp. 1104–1108, 2006.

[15] J. W. Pierrepont, C. Z. Stambouzou, B. P. Miles et al., "Patient Specific component alignment in total hip arthroplasty," *Reconstructive Review*, vol. 6, no. 4, 2016.

[16] T. F. McCarthy, V. Alipit, J. Nevelos, R. K. Elmallah, and M. A. Mont, "Acetabular cup anteversion and inclination in hip range of motion to impingement," *The Journal of Arthroplasty*, vol. 31, no. 9, pp. 264–268, 2016.

[17] P. P. Prabhakar, Q. Chen, F. Schultz, J. Y. Lazennec, and K.-N. An, "Automated range-of-motion device for total hip arthroplasty prosthesis," *Journal of Musculoskeletal Research*, vol. 10, no. 3, pp. 151–155, 2006.

[18] T. D. Brown and J. J. Callaghan, "Impingement in total hip replacement: mechanisms and consequences," *Current Orthopaedics*, vol. 22, no. 6, pp. 376–391, 2008.

[19] F. Yoshimine and K. Ginbayashi, "A mathematical formula to calculate the theoretical range of motion for total hip replacement," *Journal of Biomechanics*, vol. 35, no. 7, pp. 989–993, 2002.

[20] D. Murray, "The definition and measurement of acetabular orientation," *The Journal of Bone & Joint Surgery (British Volume)*, vol. 75-B, no. 2, pp. 228–232, 1993.

[21] D. E. McCollum and W. J. Gray, "Dislocation after total hip arthroplasty: causes and prevention," *Clinical Orthopaedics and Related Research*, no. 261, pp. 159–170, 1990.

[22] K. H. Widmer and B. Zurfluh, "Compliant positioning of total hip components for optimal range of motion," *Journal of Orthopaedic Research*, vol. 22, no. 4, pp. 815–821, 2004.

[23] L. D. Dorr, A. Malik, M. Dastane, and Z. Wan, "Combined anteversion technique for total hip arthroplasty," *Clinical Orthopaedics and Related Research*, vol. 467, no. 1, pp. 119–127, 2009.

[24] A. Bunn, C. W. Colwell Jr., and D. D. D'Lima, "Effect of head diameter on passive and active dynamic hip dislocation," *Journal of Orthopaedic Research*, vol. 32, no. 11, pp. 1525–1531, 2014.

[25] S. J. Incavo, M. T. Thompson, J. E. Gold, R. V. Patel, K. D. Icenogle, and P. C. Noble, "Which procedure better restores intact hip range of motion: total hip arthroplasty or resurfacing? a combined cadaveric and computer simulation study," *The Journal of Arthroplasty*, vol. 26, no. 3, pp. 391–397, 2011.

[26] H. Miki, W. Yamanashi, T. Nishii, Y. Sato, H. Yoshikawa, and N. Sugano, "Anatomic hip range of motion after implantation during total hip arthroplasty as measured by a navigation system," *The Journal of Arthroplasty*, vol. 22, no. 7, pp. 946–952, 2007.

[27] K.-H. Widmer, "Containment versus impingement: finding a compromise for cup placement in total hip arthroplasty," *International Orthopaedics*, vol. 31, supplement 1, pp. S29–S33, 2007.

9

Proposed Geometrical Tool for Cases of Laterally Adapted Tibial Tubercle during Total Knee Replacement

Umaima R. Khairy,[1] **Sadiq J. Hamandi**,[1] **and Ahmed S. Abid Ali**[2]

[1]*Biomedical Engineering Department, College of Engineering, Al-Nahrain University, Baghdad, Iraq*
[2]*Orthopedics Department, College of Medicine, Al-Nahrain University, Baghdad, Iraq*

Correspondence should be addressed to Umaima R. Khairy; umaimadabbagh@yahoo.com

Academic Editor: Panagiotis Korovessis

The alignment of tibial component in total knee replacement operation must be achieved in three planes to ensure optimum results. In coronal plane, the alignment depends on three anatomical landmarks. These landmarks are tibial tuberosity, leg shin, and midtalar point. In eastern community, people get used to sit cross-legged which causes additional tension in the quadriceps muscle which is attached distally to the tibial tuberosity. This tension causes adaptation of the tuberosity laterally. Tuberosity adaptation causes the three anatomical landmarks being not collinear. In this work, eight cases of lateral adapted tubercle were diagnosed of this condition before the surgery and their X-ray images after the surgery were checked regarding tibial alignment. Tibial alignment has been checked by measuring the medial proximal tibial angle (MPTA) which is the angle between the mechanical tibial axis and the tibial component plateau. MPTAs for the eight cases were (86.9°–93.6°). Three cases had MPTA less than 90° indicating varus alignment and five of them had MPTA more than 90° indicating valgus alignment. A geometrical tool was designed using the DesignSpark Mechanical software as a proposed solution to solve the adaptation problem. The tool can give a method for fixing the tibial component precisely without any varus\valgus malalignment.

1. Introduction

During total knee replacement surgery, in order to resect the tibial plateau correctly, a block should be placed satisfactorily in three planes near the tibial plateau. Then, the block would act as a saw guide to make the cut. The block for the left joint is shown in Figure 1 with the surgical saw notch also illustrated.

Ensuring correct placement of the block necessitates using some anatomical landmarks and anatomical aspects regarding the three planes (sagittal, coronal, and transverse planes), as in Table 1.

The block is held by the extramedullary (EM) guide; then, placing the extramedullary guide correctly would ensure correct block placement. The extramedullary guide is shown in Figure 2.

Laterally adapted tibial tubercle is a cause of many reasons. One of them is internal tibial torsion.

Internal tibial torsion is a deformity in the alignment of knee joint causing tibial torsion along its longitudinal axis [1, 2].

The tibia is internally rotated (medial rotation of the shin) in patients with tibial torsion. Diagnosis is made clinically with no need for imaging [3]. The evaluation of tibial rotation depends on several anatomical landmarks, one of them is the tibial tuberosity [2, 4]. In Asians, the upper end of the tibia exhibits more external rotation (i.e., the tibial shaft exhibits more intorsion). So, another reason that may cause lateral adaptation of tibial tubercle is cross-legged posture in Asian culture which is a frequent habit while sitting on the floor, as shown in Figure 3. This posture involves a complex combination of movements of the lower

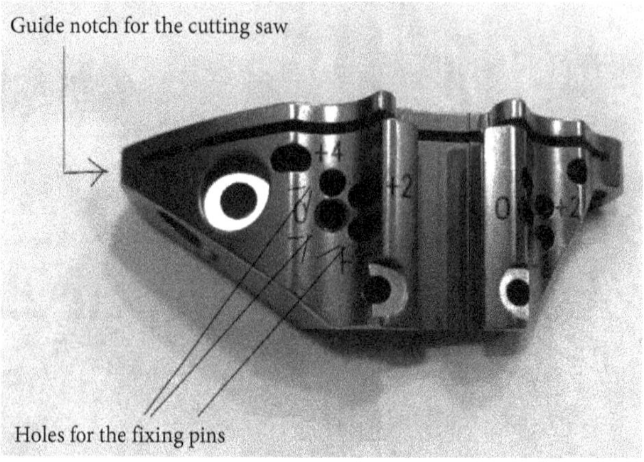

Figure 1: Tibial cutting blocks for left knees.

Table 1: Tibial component alignment in three planes.

Plane of alignment	Anatomical correct alignment	Technical concept to ensure the alignment
Sagittal	Tibial plateau slopes posteriorly 7°–10°	The cutting block has a slope of 7° and the guide rod should be one finger wide from the leg shin proximally and two fingers distally
Coronal	Patella tracked with the tibial tuberosity, leg shin, and midtalar point (MPTA is 90°)	The guide should be aligned to these three landmarks (medial third of tibial tuberosity for best patellar tracking [1], leg shin for a cut that is perpendicular to the tibial mechanical axis, and midtalar point [2])
Transverse	The joint line is the obvious landmark	Shifting the block vertically until the cut on the most defected side (right or left) is 2 mm

limb joints. At the hip, there is flexion (80° to 101°), external rotation (36° to 52°), and abduction (30° to 57°); at the knee joint, there is flexion (130° to 142°) and internal rotation (17° to 34°), and at the ankle, there is minimal planter flexion [3, 5].

Figure 4 illustrates a case intended for total knee replacement (TKR) with lateral adapted tibial tubercle.

Cinotti in 2013 studied the effect of tibial torsion on total knee replacement and specifically on extramedullary tibial cut guide fixation regarding distal position. They used the center of the intermalleolar distance at the ankle joint as anatomical landmark. Their results state that the center of the ankle joint was shifted laterally by 9–11 mm compared to the proximal axis. Mathematical calculations showed that a 10 mm displacement led to a varus cut of 4.4°. They concluded that the EM guide should be aligned more medially at the distal ankle for cases with tibial torsion to avoid varus implant malalignment [6]. Hernandez-Vaquero and his team in 2018 measured the tibial torsion angle before and after knee replacement to reveal if knee replacement could lessen torsion of the tibia. They found that joint replacement can lessen tibial torsion by approximately 2° (from 17.76° to 15.36° on average) but cannot cancel it [7]. Mizu-uchi et al. in 2006 studied the effect of ankle joint rotation on the tibia cut using the extramedullary cutting guide. They included fifty-three osteoarthritic knees in their study. These joints had external ankle rotation diagnosed using CT scans before the operation. The rotation diagnosis was defined by measuring the angle between proximal tibial plateau axis and distal ankle axis. The extramedullary guide distal end was placed in front of the center of the ankle joint, and the proximal end was placed on the line of the extended anteroposterior axis of the proximal part of the tibia. After the surgery, the tibial coronal alignment was varus (0.5° to 5.1°) for all cases. As a conclusion, if extramedullary alignment guide is used for cases of external ankle rotation, varus alignment of the tibial component can occur [8]. Jörg Lützner et al. in 2010 made an investigation about the tibial tuberosity landmark regarding fixing the cutting guide on the tuberosity medial border or medial third. They found that the mismatch is greater when the cutting guide was fixed according to the medial border than the medial third. They found that the best part of the tuberosity to be followed is the medial third of the tuberosity [1]. During the last few years, researchers investigated solving the tibial alignment problem by using the patient-specific instrumentation (PSI). Kwon et al. in 2017 saw that the surgical operation time was less using the PSI (63.9 ± 13.6 min) compared to CI (82.8 ± 24.9 min), but regarding the alignment, they proved that both techniques conduct to the same results [9]. Kosse et al. in 2018 also proved that both techniques give the same results regarding stability and alignment after they examined 42 patients pre- and postoperatively after 6 weeks and 3 and 12 months and took CT images to evaluate the joint alignment and rotation [10].

In cases of lateral adapted tibial tubercle intended for total knee replacement, an alternative decision should be made regarding coronal tibial alignment for varus fixation to be avoided. One of the three coronal landmarks mentioned in Table 1 would be compromised for this purpose. Tibial

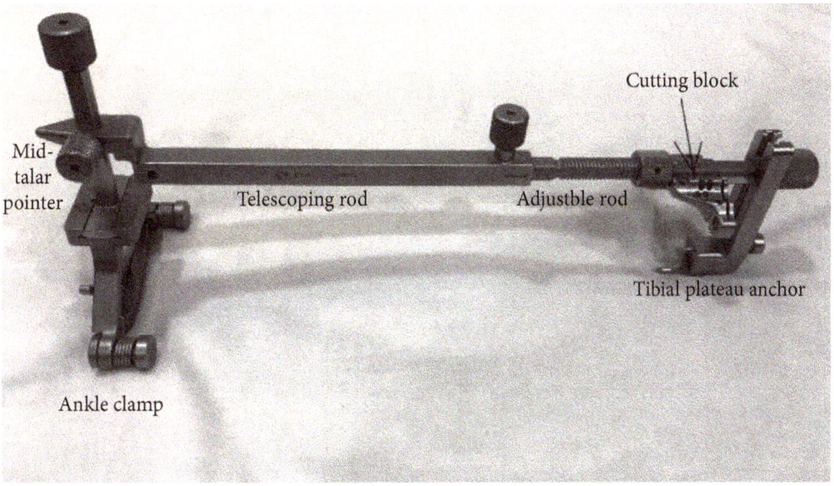

(a)

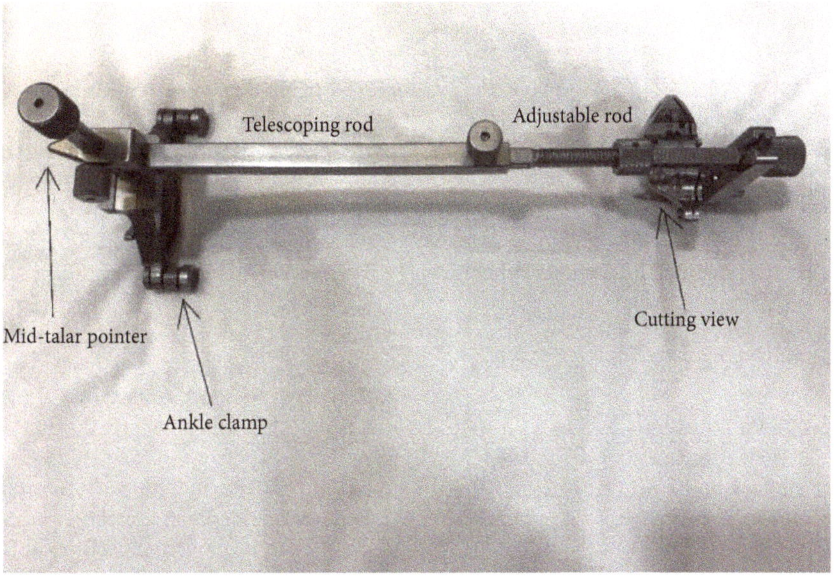

(b)

FIGURE 2: The extramedullary cutting guide. (a) Side view. (b) Top view.

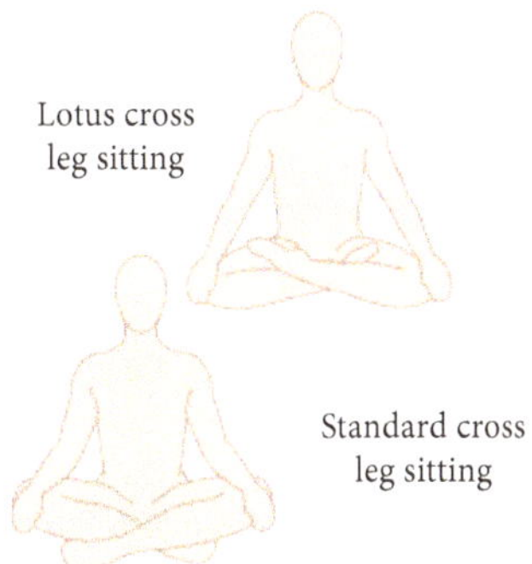

FIGURE 3: Cross-leg sitting (standard and lotus positions) [2].

tuberosity needs to be followed to ensure correct patellar tracking, since patellar tendon is attached to it. Tibial shin is a parallel guide to the extramedullary rod to ensure perpendicular tibial cut to the tibial shaft. So, midtalar point is the landmark to be neglected by the design presented in this study. This design proposed in this research is a

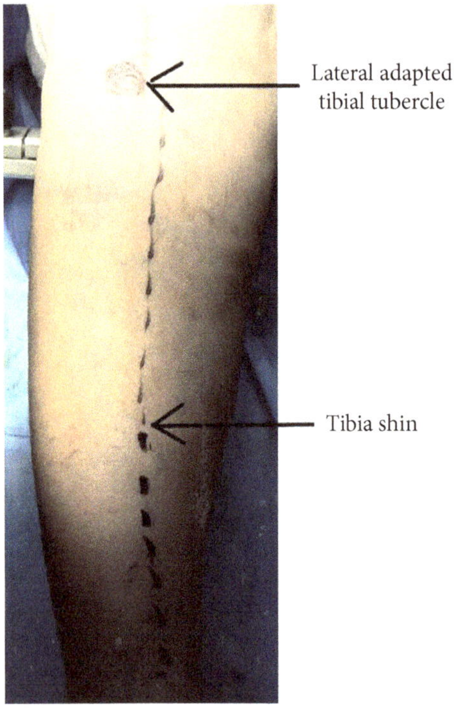

Figure 4: Case with lateral adapted tibial tubercle.

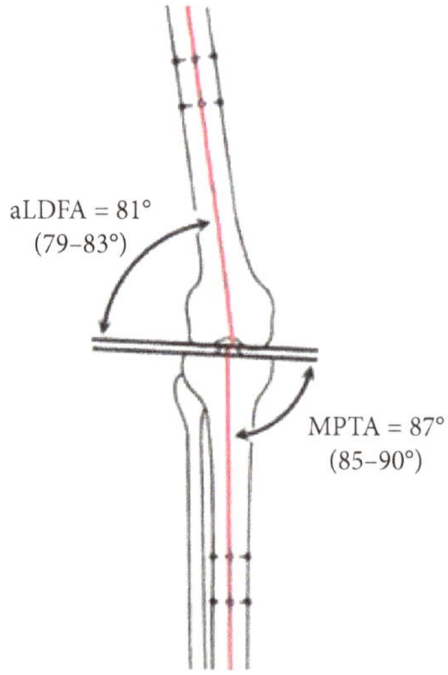

Figure 5: aLDFA and MPTA in normal knee joint.

suggested solution for cases of lateral adapted tibial tubercle intended for total knee replacement surgery.

2. Subjects

Eight cases of internal tibial torsion were studied with their knees need to be replaced. Their ages were in the range 51–75 years. Six of them were females and two were males. Their MPTAs measured before the knee replacement surgery were on average 87° (80°–94°).

3. Method

Independent alignment of the femur and tibia is measured by calculating the angles between their horizontal surfaces with their mechanical axes. These angles are named LDFA (lateral distal femoral angle, normally 87°) and MPTA (medial proximal tibial angle, normally 87°), as in Figure 5.

The aLDFA (81°) corresponds to (anatomical lateral distal femoral angle) which means that it is measured between the anatomical femoral axis and the femoral condylar horizontal surface; adding the 6° to that angle yields the mLDFA (mechanical lateral distal femoral angle). The MPTA (87°) corresponds to (medial proximal tibial angle) meaning that it is measured between the mechanical axis of the tibia and the proximal horizontal tibial plateau [6, 11].

During joint replacement surgery, tibial component generally is implanted perpendicular to the mechanical axis of the tibia in the coronal plane (medial proximal tibial angle (MPTA) 90° rather than 87°) rather than the normal 3° varus avoiding the unintended excessive varus alignment after replacing. The femoral component usually is implanted in 5 to 6 degrees of anatomical valgus and neutral to the mechanical axis (the amount necessary to reestablish a neutral mechanical axis of the limb), so distal femur cut is performed perpendicular to femur mechanical axis and the anatomical lateral distal femoral angle (aLDFA) aimed at 84° rather than 83° for the same reason as tibia. After the surgery, MPTA measurement should be 90° as optimum alignment, ±3° alignment deviation may have to be accepted.

The EM guide is fixed in coronal plane according to three landmarks, tibial tuberosity, tibial shin, and midtalar point. In cases of lateral adapted tibial tubercle, the EM should be placed proximally with lateral tibial tuberosity and parallel to the tibial shin for the reasons that have been cleared in Table 1.

This research included a presentation of eight adapted tibial tubercle cases, a clarification of their MPTAs before and after the surgery, and an illustration of the effect of their tubercle state on the tibial component alignment after the replacement.

Also, the study included designing a new geometrical tool that is meant to be used for those cases intended for knee replacement surgeries. This geometrical tool was proposed as a complementary guide with the extramedullary tibial guide and they both may work together to ensure better tibial cut and improved MPTAs after the replacement.

The working principle of the designed geometrical tool is that it holds another shaft that adheres along the tibial shin and in the same time parallel to the EM guide, as in Figures 6 and 7.

First, the surgeon fixes the EM guide to the tibial tuberosity. Then, he fixes the tool to the EM guide and keeps regulating the EM long rod at the ankle junction until the shaft is aligned parallel to the tibial shin, as illustrated in Figure 8.

The designed tool is composed of three parts. Two of them are holders (numbered 1 and 2 in Figure 9) that hold the shaft bridge. The third part is the shaft bridge (in Figure 9, it is numbered as 3) that holds the shaft along the tibial shin. The tool shown in Figure 9 has been 3D printed as a prototype using the 3D printing material St-PLA.

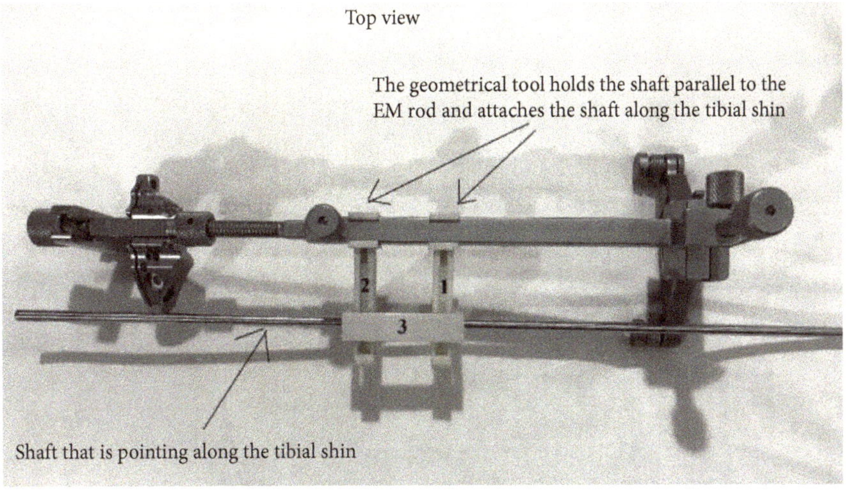

FIGURE 6: The EM guide with the left cutting block and the geometrical tool prepared to be used for left knees.

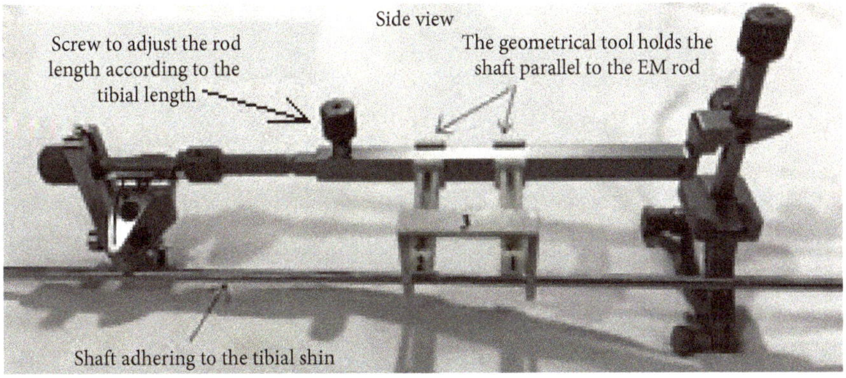

FIGURE 7: The geometrical tool (numbered 1, 2, and 3) fixed to the original tool.

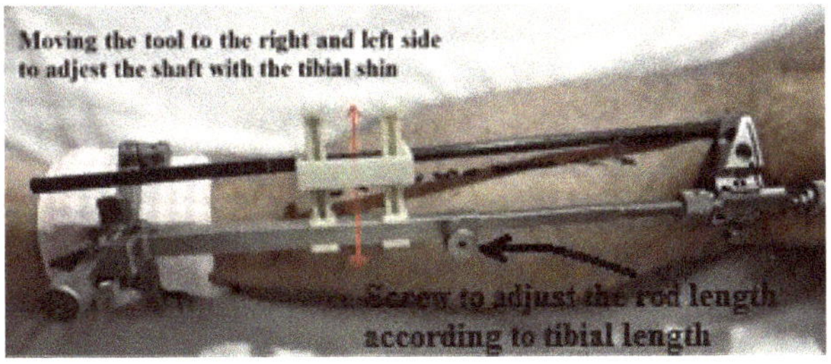

FIGURE 8: Fixing the tool properly.

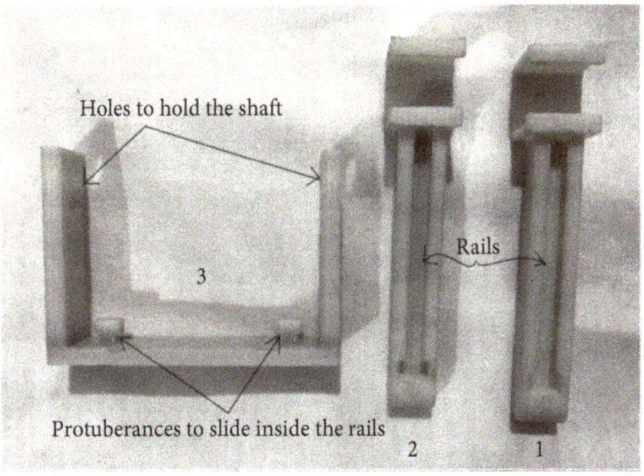

FIGURE 9: St-PLA prototype of the geometrical tool parts.

Each holder has a rail in which the shaft bridge slides along via a protuberance. The purpose of this connection is to accommodate with different stages of lateral tibial tuberosity adaptation.

The geometrical tool is designed to be symmetrical for both side usage. It can be used for both the right and left knees, as shown in Figure 10.

4. Results

Ten cases intended for primary total knee replacement surgery have been included in this study for tibial tuberosity adaptation clinical examination. Eight out of ten were diagnosed with tibial tuberosity adaptation. The other two cases had normal knees with collinear tuberosity, shin, and midtalar point.

For all these eight cases, the medial proximal tibial angle (MPTA) has been measured by postoperative X-ray image as an indication for tibial component alignment after the replacement surgery. The X-ray image has been inserted into ImageJ software through which the angle has been measured, as shown in Figure 11.

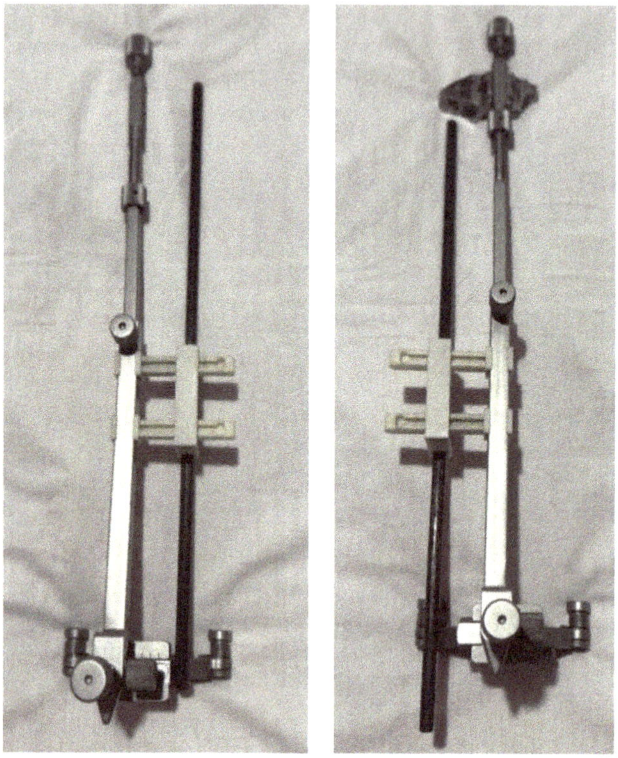

(a) (b)

FIGURE 10: The tool can be fixed for both right and left sides. (a) Right leg. (b) Left leg.

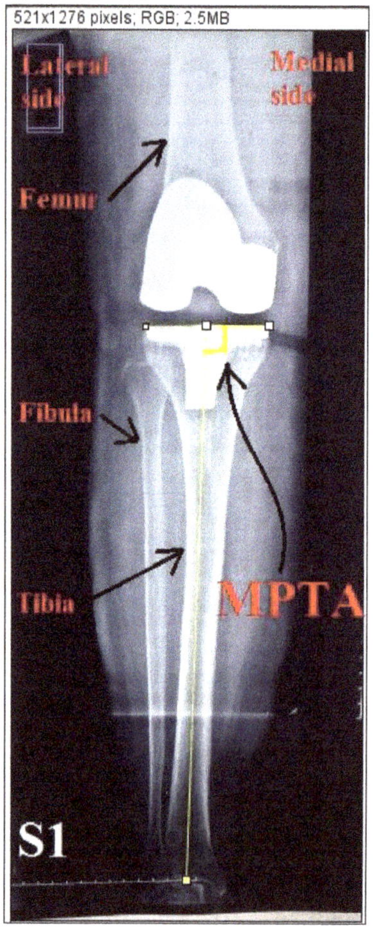

FIGURE 11: MPTA measurement using ImageJ software.

TABLE 2: MPTAs of subjects' knees after the surgery.

Subject number	Gender	MPTA after surgery (°)	MPTA before surgery (°)	Knee side
S1	Female	91.871	94	Right
S2	Female	92.286	86	Right
S3	Female	91.443	86	Right
S4	Female	86.927	86	Left
S5	Female	88.755	80	Right
S6	Male	89.567	83	Left
S7	Male	93.415	87	Right
S8	Female	94.562	86	Right

The angle measurement is done by drawing a line along the tibial plateau and a line along the mechanical axis of the tibia (the line connecting center of the tibial plateau and the midtalar point), and then the angle is the one between these two lines. MPTAs of all eight subjects are shown in Table 2.

5. Discussion and Conclusions

Knee replacement reduced the alignment deviation by comparing the MPTA before and after the surgery. Yet, the MPTA measurements after the surgery for the eight studied cases revealed a serious need for alignment improvement in fixing the tibial component of the knee implant. The intended MPTA is 90° for optimum tibial alignment. The mean alignment deviation from the 90° is 2.31° (ranging from minimally 0.54° to maximally 4.5°). Three of the cases (S4, S7, and S8) had an alignment of more than ±3° deviation which is beyond the acceptable range. It can be seen from the results that the gender and knee side have no effect on the MPTA results. Yet, MPTAs of all cases can be improved to reach the optimum 90°. The tool provides a parallel relation between the EM guide and tibial shin, since the holders are designed to be perpendicular to the EM rod and the shaft holder is perpendicular to the shaft. This parallel relation is the needed condition to ensure perpendicular tibial cut to the mechanical tibial axis and, as a result, 90° MPTA. The proposed geometrical tool designed in this study can provide this parallel condition and consequently solve this alignment problem.

References

[1] J. Lützner, F. Krummenauer, K. Günther, and S. Kirschner, "Rotational alignment of the tibial component in total knee arthroplasty is better at the medial third of tibial tuberosity than at the medial border," *BMC Musculoskeletal Disorders*, vol. 11, no. 1, 2010.

[2] W. N. Scott, *Insall and Scott Surgery of the Knee*, Elsevier, Amsterdam, Netherlands, 2018.

[3] A. S. Gonzales, A. Y. Saber, G. Ampat, and M. D. Mendez, *Intoeing*, StatPearls Publishing, Treasure Island, FL, USA, 2020.

[4] S. J. Hamandi and D. M. Ruken, "Biomechanical study with kinematic and kinetic descriptions of the effect of high-heeled shoes in healthy adult females based on gait analysis," *IOP Conference Series: Materials Science and Engineering*, vol. 671, no. 1, 2020.

[5] B. M. Arun, A. K. Sharma, and S. V. Marawar, *Tibial Torsion in Non-arthritic Indian Adults: A Computer Tomography Study of 100 Limbs*, Springer, Berlin, Germany, 2008.

[6] G. Cinotti, P. Sessa, A. D. Rocca, F. R. Ripani, and G. Giannicola, "Effects of tibial torsion on distal alignment of extramedullary instrumentation in total knee arthroplasty," *Acta Orthopaedica*, vol. 84, no. 3, pp. 275–279, 2013.

[7] D. Hernandez-Vaquero, A. Noriega-Fernandez, S. Roncero-Gonzalez, A. A. Sierra-Pereira, and M. A. Sandoval-Garcia, "Total knee replacement modifies the preoperative tibial torsion angle-similar results between computer-assisted and standard technique," *Annals of Translational Medicine*, vol. 6, no. 7, p. 113, 2018.

[8] H. Mizu-uchi, S. Matsuda, H. Miura, H. Higaki, K. Okazaki, and Y. Iwamoto, "The effect of ankle rotation on cutting of the tibia in total knee arthroplasty," *The Journal of Bone and Joint Surgery-American Volume*, vol. 88A, no. 12, pp. 2632–2636, 2006.

[9] O. R. Kwon, K. T. Kang, J. Son, D. S. Suh, D. B. Heo, and Y. G. Koh, "The effect of patient-specific instrumentation incorporating an extramedullary tibial guide on operative efficiency for total knee arthroplasty," *BioMed Research International*, vol. 2017, Article ID 2034782, 7 pages, 2017.

[10] N. M. Kosse, P. J. C. Heesterbeek, J. J. P. Schimmel, G. G. Van Hellemondt, A. B. Wymenga, and K. C. Defoort, "Stability and alignment do not improve by using patient-specific instrumentation in total knee arthroplasty: a randomized controlled trial," *Knee Surgery, Sports Traumatology, Arthroscopy*, vol. 26, no. 6, pp. 1792–1799, 2018.

[11] J. J. Cherian, B. H. Kapadia, S. Banerjee, J. J. Jauregui, K. Issa, and M. A. Mont, "Mechanical, anatomical, and kinematic axis in TKA: concepts and practical applications," *Current Reviews in Musculoskeletal Medicine*, vol. 7, no. 2, pp. 89–95, 2014.

10

Comparison of Functional Outcome of Total and Unicompartmental Knee Arthroplasty Using Computer-Assisted Patient-Specific Templating

Atef Mohamed Morsy,[1] Emad Gaber Elbana,[1] Ahmed Gaber Mostafa,[1] Mark Ashraf Edward,[2] and Mahmoud A. Hafez[2]

[1]*The Orthopaedic Department, Beni-Suef University, Beni-Suef, Egypt*
[2]*The Orthopaedic Department, Faculty of Medicine, October 6 University, Giza, Egypt*

Correspondence should be addressed to Mahmoud A. Hafez; mhafez@msn.com

Academic Editor: Benjamin Blondel

Background. Knee arthroplasty surgeries are in ever-increasing demand. With unicompartmental knee arthroplasty (UKA), patients may benefit from a higher range of flexion and a better Knee Society Score (KSS). *Aim.* In this study, we compared the short-term clinical outcomes of total knee arthroplasty (TKA) and UKA using the patient-specific templating (PST) technique. *Methods.* Two groups of 20 knees each were divided into UKA and TKA groups depending on the Oxford criteria of UKA. Only patients with medial compartmental osteoarthritis were included. KSS, functional knee score (FKS), and ROF were assessed preoperatively and at 6 months postoperatively. *Results.* The TKA group has shown a significant improvement compared to the UKA group in KSS (MD = 39.35 vs. 31.2, respectively, $p = 0.003$). Both TKA and UKA have shown no significant difference concerning both the FKS (MD = 32 and 31.75, respectively, $p = 0.926$) and ROF (MD = 10.25 and 7.25, respectively, $p = 0.072$). *Discussion.* The higher improvement of KSS in the TKA group can be attributed to the fact that patients in the TKA had significantly worse KSS preoperatively. Also, the small improvement in ROF in the UKA group might be related to their wider preoperative ROF. *Conclusion.* Preoperatively, the TKA group had lower KSS and ROF compared to UKA. The improvement of KSS from preoperative to postoperative was more significant in TKA. However, the TKA group has shown less range of flexion postoperatively.

1. Introduction

Unicompartmental osteoarthritis (OA) targets mainly the medial compartment rather than the lateral aspect of the patellofemoral joint. Almost half of these patients are suitable for unicompartmental knee arthroplasty (UKA) [1]. The current operative treatment modalities of advanced osteoarthritis are total knee arthroplasty (TKA) and unicompartmental knee arthroplasty (UKA). However, replacing all the affected and nonaffected surfaces is considered the gold standard procedure [2, 3]. On the other hand, many surgeons argue the superiority of UKA in unicompartmental cases to spare the undamaged compartments, despite having higher revision rates when compared to TKA [2, 4].

Patient-specific instrumentation (PSI) used in UKA or TKA can decrease the intraoperative time drastically, which consequently would reduce the intraoperative and postoperative complications. This is possible through the preoperative use of a CT scan or MRI to determine the size of the implant [5, 6]. There are many logistic difficulties to use PSI in Egypt; consequently, we developed a hospital-based PSI protocol under the name of patient-specific templating (PST). This protocol requires CT imaging, a dedicated engineer to design the implants, and a small 3D printer. Although previous studies have investigated the effectiveness of PSI [7], comparing the effectiveness of this technique in both UKA and TKA was not performed before.

In this study, we aim to record the short-term outcomes of TKA and UKA using PST in terms of the Knee Society Score (KSS) [8, 9], functional knee score (FKS) [8, 9], and the range of flexion (ROF).

2. Methods

We performed anon-randomized controlled trial on a total of 40 patients, all of whom received patient-specific templating (PST) TKA or UKA. Patients were assigned into two groups of equal sizes (20 participants in each group). Patients of group 1 received TKA, while those of group 2 received UKA. The process of patients' enrollment in the study is shown in Figure 1. The basic patients' characteristics and demographics are given in Table 1.

Our PST is based on commercially available patient-specific instrumentation (PSI) but with some modifications. We use CT imaging to measure the size of the required implant and to print it using hospital-based 3D printers. Figures 2 and 3 show how templating was carried out. Figure 4 shows the UKA template after the implantation to facilitate the cutting guidance. Ethical approval was obtained from the ethical committee of the participating hospital. All patients consented to the surgical procedures and to participate in the study. We included adult patients with ages ranging between 40 and 75 of both sexes. Patients were asked about instability, underwent clinical examination for laxity and intact anterior cruciate ligament (ACL), and investigated with anteroposterior and lateral view knee X-ray to check for intact ACL, probable subluxation, and stage of the osteoarthritic bone erosion. Patients with a history of meniscal or ligamental tear, previous knee surgery, infected knee, severe varus deformities of more than 10 degrees, neurological impairment (e.g., Charcot's joint), or tricompartmental osteoarthritis were excluded. Revision cases were not included in our study. These inclusions/exclusions apply to both UKA and TKA groups. Patients' allocation into the TKA or UKA group depended on the Oxford criteria for UKA that included medial bone on bone, full-thickness lateral cartilage, intact ACL on lateral view X-ray, normal MCL on valgus stress view, and accepted patella-femoral joint in skyline X-ray. If the patient met the criteria, UKA was advised and performed. Otherwise, TKA was performed instead [10, 11].

In UKA and TKA, we used the Oxford partial knee system and the Vanguard knee system developed by Biomet, respectively. Details of the preoperative and postoperative assessment were documented. The clinical assessment included assessing the Knee Society Score (KSS) [8, 9], functional knee score (FKS) [8, 9], and the range of flexion (ROF). We also conducted a radiological assessment using a plain X-ray in the anteroposterior and lateral views preoperatively and postoperatively (Figure 5). Postoperative evaluation included KSS, FKS, ROF, and anteroposterior and lateral views knee X-ray. This study is not designed to examine the survival of the implants. Short-term follow-up was conducted at six months postoperatively.

Student's t-test and Pearson Chi-square parametric tests were used to highlight the differences between the two groups' demographic data. Data regarding age, sex, body mass index, degree, and side of varus deformity were obtained and entered using Microsoft Excel 2010. Statistical analyses were performed using IBM SPSS version 20. A p value of <0.05 was considered statistically significant.

3. Results

We included 40 patients in our study and distributed them into two groups of equal sizes. The mean duration of the follow-up was 7.4 months, ranging from 2 to 12 months. Two patients from the TKA group and one from the UKA group failed to follow-up at 6 months, but they were contacted by phone and reported any complications. Accordingly, the results of the comparison between the preoperative and postoperative values were based on 18 and 19 patients in the TKA and UKA groups, respectively.

Our study population has shown no significant difference between both groups concerning the age (64.5 vs. 61.3, respectively, $p = 0.223$), female sex (12 vs. 11, respectively, $p = 0.102$), or BMI (30.04 vs. 29.03, respectively, $p = 1.146$) (Table 1). Preoperatively, the TKA group had statistically significant lower KSS (46.35 vs. 54.10, respectively, $p = 0.001$) and lower ROF (97 vs. 107, respectively, $p = 0.001$) compared to UKA. Postoperatively, we have found that the absolute ROF in the UKA group was higher than the TKA group (122.25 vs. 107.25, respectively, $p = 0.001$). However, the change in ROF was higher in the TKA group with statistically insignificant results (10.25 vs. 7.25, respectively, $p = 0.075$). On the other hand, there was no statistically significant difference between the two groups postoperatively regarding the KSS and the FKS (Table 2).

We noticed that the TKA group has shown better results than the UKA group regarding the KSS (mean diff. = 39.35 and 31.2, respectively, $p = 0.003$). However, there was no significant difference between both groups concerning FKS (mean diff. = 32 and 31.75, respectively, $p = 0.926$) and ROF (mean diff. = 10.25 and 7.25, respectively, $p = 0.072$) (Table 3).

4. Discussion

In our study, we investigated the clinical differences in 40 patients undergoing medial UKA or TKA using PST. We have found a significant improvement in KSS in the TKA group over the UKA group. Nevertheless, when comparing the preoperative data, we have found that the UKA group had better values than the TKA group in both KSS and ROF. Both findings may be related to the significant improvement of KSS with TKA and the insignificant improvement of ROF in UKA. Unfortunately, adjusting for group differences before the initiation of this study was not feasible as the surgeons were compelled to adhere to the Oxford criteria for UKA [10, 11].

Similarly, in a systematic review of cohort studies, Kleeblad et al. agreed that range of motion (ROM) was higher in medial UKA patients compared to TKA patients,

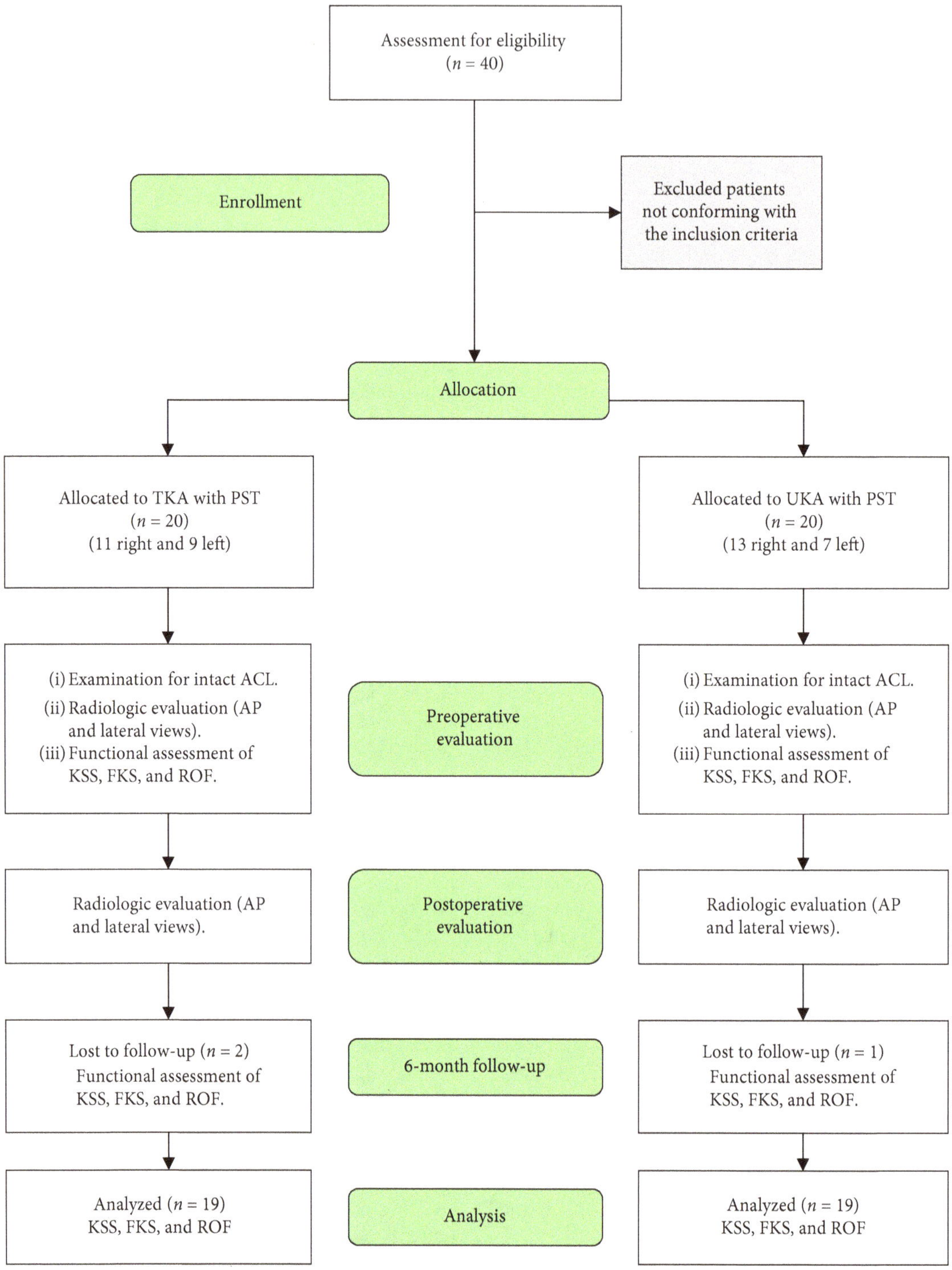

FIGURE 1: Flow diagram showing the recruitment process in the study. TKA, total knee arthroplasty; UKA, unicompartmental knee arthroplasty; PST, patient-specific templating; AP, anteroposterior; KSS, knee society score; FKS, functional score of knee society score; ROF, range of flexion.

while both groups had nearly the same overall function outcome scores [12]. On the other hand, Blevins et al. conducted a retrospective analysis of 150 medial UKAs using the MAKO® robotic interactive orthopedic arm (MAKO® Surgical Corp.) and 150 TKAs using either conventional or patient-specific cutting blocks. They found that the UKA group had less postoperative numeric pain rating scale (NPRS) score, higher KSS and FKSS, faster return to work, and higher mean Forgotten Joint Score (FJS). But a drawback to this study is that both comparative groups received neither the same technique nor the same instrumentation [13]. It is also worth mentioning that using different tibial trays in UKA has an impact on implant positioning. This was investigated by Escudier et al., and they found that using a

Table 1: Basic characteristics of the participants.

		Group 1 (TKA) $N = 20$	Group 2 (UKA) $N = 20$	p value
Age (years)	Mean ± SD	65.5 ± 6.00	63.95 ± 9.36	0.537
	Range	56–74	48–75	
Sex	Female	12 (60%)	11 (55%)	0.749
	Male	8 (40%)	9 (45%)	
BMI (kg/m^2)	Mean ± SD	30.04 ± 3.26	29.03 ± 2.18	0.259
	Range	24.1–35.6	25.4–32.7	
Side	Right	13 (65%)	11 (55%)	0.519
	Left	7 (35%)	9 (45%)	
Degree of varus deformity	Mean ± SD	7.5 ± 2.56	7.5 ± 2.56	1.000
	Range	5–10	5–10	
Polyethylene implant size (mm)	Mean ± SD	11.50 ± 4.05	5.45 ± 1.76	0.001
	Range	8–20	3–9	

TKA, total knee arthroplasty; UKA, unicompartmental knee arthroplasty; SD, standard deviation.

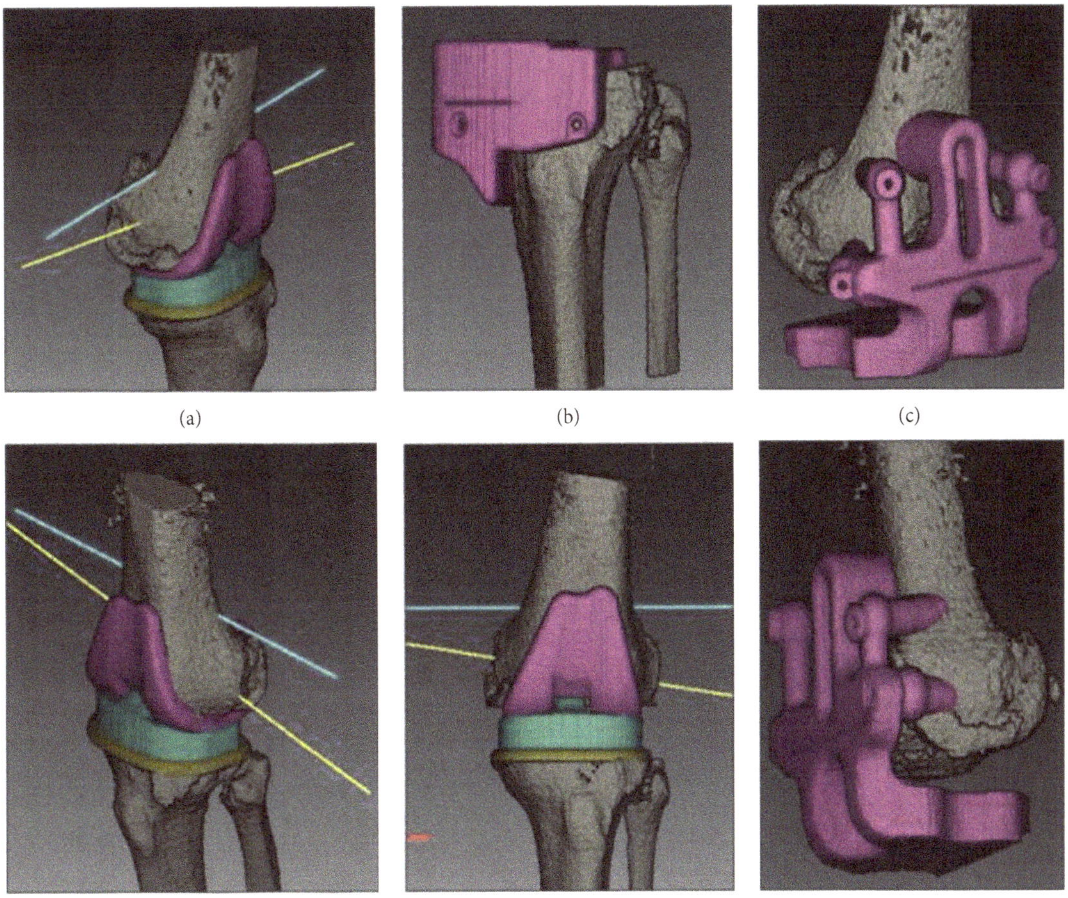

(a) (b) (c) (d) (e) (f)

Figure 2: TKA planning showing the sizing, alignment, and implant positioning that matches the patient's anatomy.

morphometric tibial tray is better than using a symmetric tibial tray in terms of decreasing the rate of overhand and improving the short-term clinical outcomes at one-year follow-up [14].

Another study published in 2017 found that UKA patients older than 75 years had less operative time and a shorter hospital stay. The initial recovery postoperatively was also better in the UKA group [15]. On the other hand, when comparing the annual revision rates of UKA and TKA, Kleeblad et al. in their systematic review found that UKA patients have a higher possibility of revision surgery [12]. In specific patients groups like severely obese patients, medial

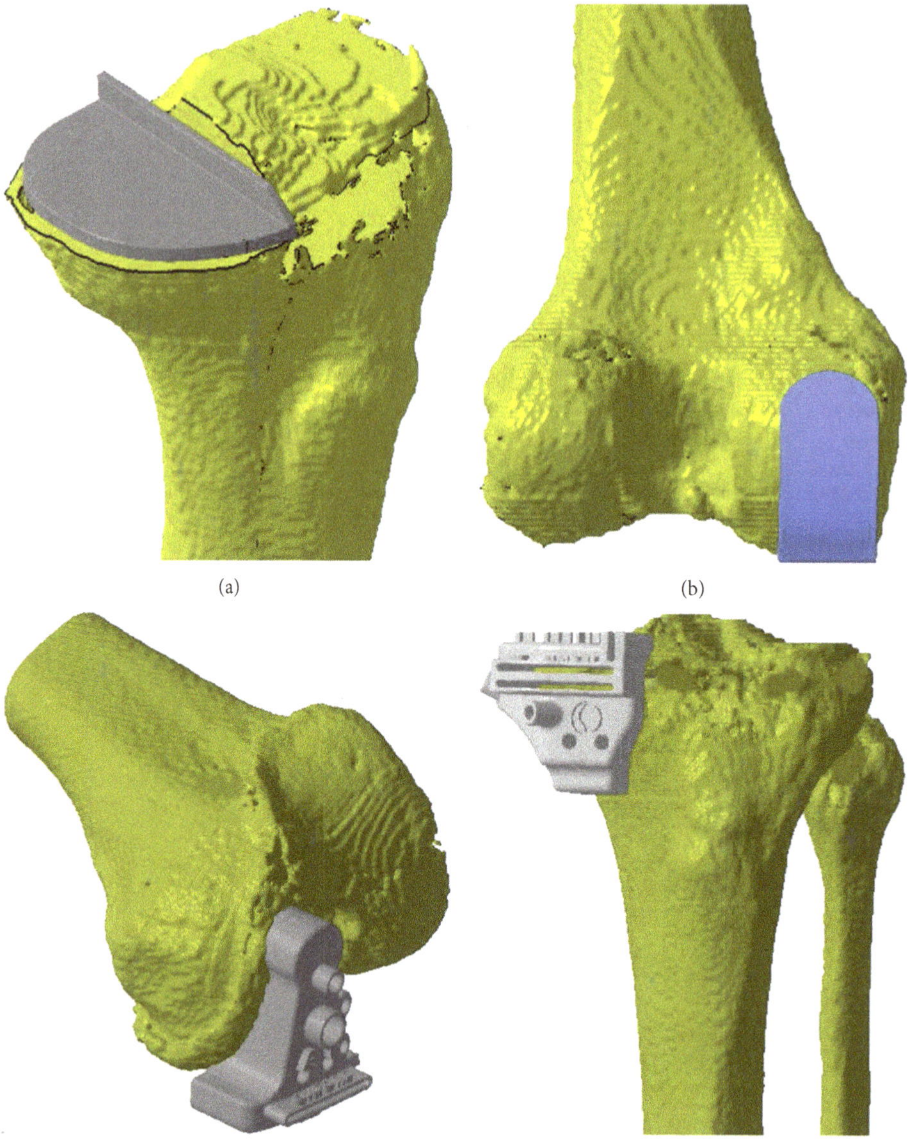

(a) (b)

(c) (d)

FIGURE 3: UKA planning showing the sizing, alignment, and implant positioning that matches the patient's anatomy.

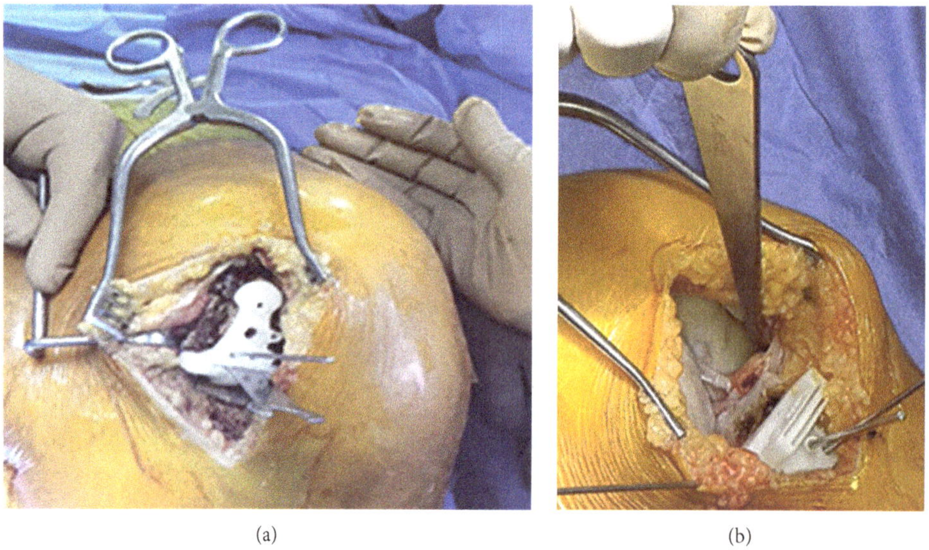

(a) (b)

FIGURE 4: The femoral (a) and tibial (b) components of the UKA patient-specific cutting guides.

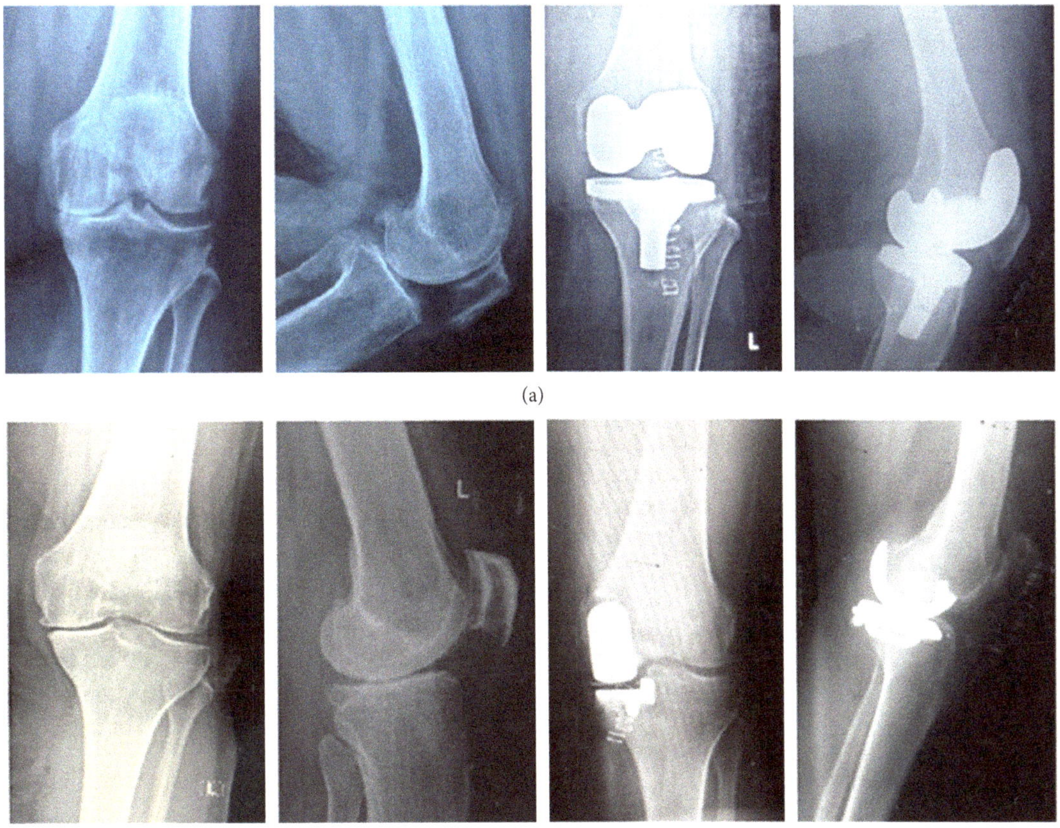

(a)

(b)

Figure 5: Preoperative and postoperative radiological assessment of two left knees of two female patients who undergone TKA (a) and UKA (b). Both patients had perfect operations with no complications.

Table 2: Comparison between TKA and UKA groups, preoperatively and postoperatively.

		Group 1 (TKA) $N = 18$	Group 2 (UKA) $N = 19$	p value
Preoperative assessment				
KSS	Mean ± SD	46.35 ± 7.92	54.10 ± 6.16	0.001
	Range	24–56	45–68	
FKS	Mean ± SD	42.00 ± 8.18	40.00 ± 7.43	0.423
	Range	30–55	30–55	
ROF	Mean ± SD	97.00 ± 9.38	115.00 ± 6.49	0.001
	Range	85–115	100–125	
Postoperative assessment at six months				
KSS	Mean ± SD	85.70 ± 6.28	85.30 ± 5.24	0.828
	Range	69–96	75–92	
FKS	Mean ± SD	74.00 ± 12.42	71.75 ± 10.04	0.532
	Range	55–95	55–90	
ROF	Mean ± SD	107.25 ± 8.38	122.25 ± 2.55	0.001
	Range	95–125	120–125	

TKA, total knee arthroplasty; UKA, unicompartmental knee arthroplasty; KSS, Knee Society Score; FKS, functional knee score; ROF, range of flexion; SD, standard deviation.

UKA was found to be more effective than TKA in improving functional knee scores and maintaining range of motion [16].

This study provides an insight into the possible outcomes of PST in UKA and TKA. It has shown that both operations provide great benefits to any patient with advanced medial compartmental osteoarthritis, regardless of age, sex, and preoperative assessment results. Nevertheless, some limitations may hinder the significance of this study. Our sample size is relatively small in comparison to other studies investigating arthroplasty; however, PST is not favored in many situations due to many logistic difficulties. Also, no

TABLE 3: Comparison of the difference between the postoperative and preoperative values of Knee Society Score, functional knee score, and the range of flexion in the two groups.

	Group 1 (TKA) $N=18$			Group 2 (UKA) $N=19$			p value
	Mean difference	SD	SE	Mean difference	SD	SE	
KSS	39.35	7.74	1.73	31.20	5.08	1.14	0.003
FKS	32.00	8.18	1.83	31.75	8.93	2.00	0.926
ROF	10.25	4.72	1.06	7.25	5.50	1.23	0.072

TKA, total knee arthroplasty; UKA, unicompartmental knee arthroplasty; KSS, Knee Society Score; FKSS, functional knee score; ROF, range of flexion; SD, standard deviation; SE, standard of error.

studies are comparing PSI used in UKA and TKA. Another limitation is the short follow-up duration. This study was designed to examine only short-term follow-up because reviewing the survival is outside the scope of this study. Moreover, finding more matching groups preoperatively, especially in ROM, KSS, FKS, and FJS, will help in deciding which operation provides better outcomes. In our case, we used the Oxford criteria for UKA [10, 11]. However, it must be pointed out that the indications of using which technique for a patient are different according to the patient's condition and the surgeon's preference. It might also be of value in future research to compare PSI in UKA to conventional instrumentation, not only from the outcome point of view but according to the surgical techniques, learning curve, and cost-effectiveness. Whenever possible, this comparison can expand to include TKA as well. Finally, assessing other outcomes such as the cost and complications will be beneficial as well.

5. Conclusion

In this manuscript, we aimed at providing an insight into the short-term clinical outcomes of UKA and TKA in patients with medial compartmental osteoarthritis. Preoperatively, the TKA group had lower KSS and ROF compared to UKA. The improvement of KSS from preoperative to postoperative was more significant in TKA. However, the TKA group has shown less range of flexion postoperatively. Both UKA and TKA appear to be good treatment options for medial compartment osteoarthritis. In our study, the differences between the functional outcome of UKA and TKA were not remarkable. This was because of the sedentary lifestyle of most of our patients. Another reason is there is no significant difference between the mean age of both TKA and UKA groups (65.5 and 63.95, respectively). Accordingly, we cannot generalize and state that unicompartmental provides better functionality because studies on conventional UKA did not fully support this claim either.

Abbreviations

UKA: Unicompartmental knee arthroplasty
TKA: Total knee arthroplasty
PST: Patient-specific templating
KSS: Knee Society Score
FKS: Functional knee score
ROF: Range of flexion
ROM: Range of motion
ACL: Anterior cruciate ligament
MCL: Medial cruciate ligament
AP: Anteroposterior
ECAR: Egyptian Community Arthroplasty Registry
NPRS: Numeric pain rating scale
FJS: Forgotten joint scores.

Additional Points

Clinical Correlation. Performing UKA instead of TKA in patients with unicompartmental knee osteoarthritis may provide slightly better joint functionality in some patients if done using PSI techniques.

Authors' Contributions

MAH developed the idea and with the help of MAE, wrote the protocol. The surgeries were performed by the first author with the help of AM, EGE, and AGM. Data collection and statistical analysis were performed by MAE. All authors reviewed the article.

Acknowledgments

The authors acknowledge the support of Mr. Abdelrahman M Makram (abd-makram@hotmail.com; ORCID: 0000-0003-2011-8092) from the Faculty of Medicine, October 6 University, who performed the literature review, wrote the manuscript, submitted the study for publication, and edited the manuscript according to the reviewer's comments.

References

[1] C. A. Willis-Owen, K. Brust, H. Alsop, M. Miraldo, and J. P. Cobb, "Unicondylar knee arthroplasty in the UK National Health Service: an analysis of candidacy, outcome and cost efficacy," *Knee*, vol. 16, no. 6, pp. 473–478, 2009.

[2] D. J. Beard, L. J. Davies, J. A. Cook et al., "Total versus partial knee replacement in patients with medial compartment knee osteoarthritis: the TOPKAT RCT," *Health Technology Assessment*, vol. 24, no. 20, pp. 1–98, 2020.

[3] A. V. Wiik, D. Nathwani, A. Akhtar, B. Al-Obaidi, R. Strachan, and J. P. Cobb, "The unicompartmental knee is

the preferred side in individuals with both a unicompartmental and total knee arthroplasty," *Knee Surgery, Sports Traumatology, Arthroscopy*, vol. 28, no. 10, pp. 3193–3199, 2019.

[4] A. J. Pearse, G. J. Hooper, A. Rothwell, and C. Frampton, "Survival and functional outcome after revision of a unicompartmental to a total knee replacement: the New Zealand National Joint Registry," *The Journal of Bone and Joint Surgery*, vol. 92, no. 4, pp. 508–512, 2010.

[5] M. P. Ast, D. Nam, and S. B. Haas, "Patient-specific instrumentation for total knee arthroplasty: a review," *Orthopedic Clinics of North America*, vol. 43, no. 5, pp. e17–22, 2012.

[6] W. C. Chan, E. Pinder, and M. Loeffler, "Patient-specific instrumentation versus conventional instrumentation in total knee arthroplasty," *Journal of Orthopaedic Surgery*, vol. 24, no. 2, pp. 175–178, 2016.

[7] A. Arirachakaran, P. Choowit, C. Putananon, S. Muangsiri, and J. Kongtharvonskul, "Is unicompartmental knee arthroplasty (UKA) superior to total knee arthroplasty (TKA)? a systematic review and meta-analysis of randomized controlled trial," *European Journal of Orthopaedic Surgery and Traumatology*, vol. 25, no. 5, pp. 799–806, 2015.

[8] J. N. Insall, L. D. Dorr, R. D. Scott, and W. N. Scott, "Rationale of the knee society clinical rating system," *Clinical Orthopaedics and Related Research*, vol. 248, pp. 13-14, 1989.

[9] S. Asif and D. S. Choon, "Midterm results of cemented press fit condylar sigma total knee arthroplasty system," *Journal of Orthopaedic Surgery*, vol. 13, no. 3, pp. 280–284, 2005.

[10] R. H. Emerson, O. Alnachoukati, J. Barrington, and K. Ennin, "The results of Oxford unicompartmental knee arthroplasty in the United States: a mean ten-year survival analysis," *Journal of Bone and Joint Surgery*, vol. 98, no. 10, pp. 34–40, 2016.

[11] S. C. Kozinn and R. Scott, "Unicondylar knee arthroplasty," *The Journal of Bone and Joint Surgery*, vol. 71, no. 1, pp. 145–150, 1989.

[12] L. J. Kleeblad, J. P. van der List, H. A. Zuiderbaan, and A. D. Pearle, "Larger range of motion and increased return to activity, but higher revision rates following unicompartmental versus total knee arthroplasty in patients under 65: a systematic review," *Knee Surgery, Sports Traumatology, Arthroscopy*, vol. 26, no. 6, pp. 1811–1822, 2018.

[13] J. L. Blevins, K. M. Carroll, J. A. Burger et al., "Postoperative outcomes of total knee arthroplasty compared to unicompartmental knee arthroplasty: a matched comparison," *Knee*, vol. 27, no. 2, pp. 565–571, 2020.

[14] J. C. Escudier, C. Jacquet, X. Flecher, S. Parratte, M. Ollivier, and J. N. Argenson, "Better implant positioning and clinical outcomes with a morphometric unicompartmental knee arthroplasty: results of a retrospective, matched-controlled study," *The Journal of Arthroplasty*, vol. 34, no. 12, pp. 2903–2908, 2019.

[15] H. Siman, A. F. Kamath, N. Carrillo, W. S. Harmsen, M. W. Pagnano, and R. J. Sierra, "Unicompartmental knee arthroplasty vs. total knee arthroplasty for medial compartment arthritis in patients older than 75 years: comparable reoperation, revision, and complication rates," *The Journal of Arthroplasty*, vol. 32, no. 6, pp. 1792–1797, 2017.

[16] Z. C. Lum, D. A. Crawford, A. V. Lombardi Jr. et al., "Early comparative outcomes of unicompartmental and total knee arthroplasty in severely obese patients," *Knee*, vol. 25, no. 1, pp. 161–166, 2018.

11

Immediate Physical Therapy following Total Joint Arthroplasty: Barriers and Impact on Short-Term Outcomes

Hunter Warwick, Andrew George, Claire Howell, Cynthia Green, Thorsten M. Seyler, and William A. Jiranek

Department of Orthopaedic Surgery, Duke University Hospital, Durham, NC 27710, USA

Correspondence should be addressed to Hunter Warwick; hunter.warwick@duke.edu

Academic Editor: Allen L. Carl

Background. Recent evidence suggests benefit to receiving physical therapy (PT) the same day as total joint arthroplasty (TJA), but relatively little is known about barriers to providing PT in this constrained time period. We address the following questions: (1) Are there demographic or perioperative variables associated with receiving delayed PT following TJA? (2) Does receiving immediate PT following TJA affect short-term outcomes such as length of stay, discharge disposition, or 30-day readmission? *Methods.* Primary TJA procedures at a single center were retrospectively reviewed. Immediate PT was defined as within eight hours of surgery. Demographic and perioperative variables were compared between patients who received immediate PT and those who did not. We identified an appropriately matched control group of patients who received immediate PT. Postoperative length of stay, discharge disposition, and 30-day readmissions were compared between matched groups. *Results.* In total, 2051 primary TJA procedures were reviewed. Of these, 226 (11.0%) received delayed PT. These patients had a higher rate of general anesthesia (25.2% versus 17.8%, p=0.006), later operative start time (13:26 [11:31-14:38] versus 9:36 [8:24-11:16], p<0.001), longer operative time (1.8 [1.5-2.2] versus 1.6 [1.4-1.8] hours, p=0.002), and higher overall caseload on the day of surgery (6 [4-9] versus 5 [4-8], p=0.002). A matched group of patients who received immediate PT was identified. There were no differences in postoperative length of stay or discharge disposition between matched immediate and delayed PT groups, but delayed PT (OR 4.54; 95% CI 1.61-12.84; p=0.004) was associated with a higher 30-day readmission rate. *Conclusion.* Barriers to receiving immediate PT following TJA included general anesthesia, later operative start time, longer operative time, and higher daily caseload. These factors present potential targets for improving the delivery of immediate postoperative PT. Early PT may help reduce 30-day readmissions, but additional research is necessary to further characterize this relationship.

1. Introduction

Total joint arthroplasty (TJA) is a highly successful surgical intervention, providing significant improvements in physical function and quality of life [1]. Given the rising demand and high costs associated with TJA [2, 3], an increasing focus is being placed on accelerated perioperative care to speed recovery, improve patient outcomes, and decrease costs [4, 5]. These programs emphasize preoperative patient education and counseling, multimodal perioperative analgesia, and aggressive postoperative rehabilitation [6].

Early postoperative physical therapy (PT) is a key component of accelerated perioperative care, and health systems are beginning to implement perioperative pathways that include early PT following TJA. However, there is little knowledge on the challenges associated with providing PT in this constrained time period. One study [7] identified late operative end time, defined as after 15:00, as a risk factor for not receiving PT on the same day as surgery. Still, 80% of patients who did not receive PT on the same day as surgery had an operative end time before 15:00, suggesting that there are additional factors at play. Identifying these barriers could hold implications for improving the delivery of early PT following TJA.

Several studies have demonstrated benefits of earlier postoperative PT after TJA, including decreased length of stay (LOS), reductions in cost, and clinical improvements in pain, range of motion, quadriceps and hamstring strength, gait, and balance [7–10]. However, several recent systematic reviews have questioned the quality of evidence supporting these benefits [11, 12]. Moreover, many of these studies examined enhanced perioperative pathways in general without investigating individual components such as early postoperative PT. Thus, it is important to examine the isolated effects of early PT on short-term postoperative outcomes.

In this study, we address the following questions: (1) Are there demographic or perioperative variables associated with receiving delayed PT following TJA? (2) Does receiving immediate PT following TJA affect short-term outcomes such as length of stay, discharge disposition, or 30-day readmission?

2. Methods

This retrospective study was performed at a single academic medical center from July 2015 to December 2017. All primary total hip and knee arthroplasty procedures performed at the center during this period were analyzed following appropriate Institutional Review Board approval. Patients below 18 years of age and patients undergoing nonelective TJA for traumatic or neoplastic etiologies were excluded from analysis.

The standard of care at our institution is for patients undergoing TJA to receive PT within eight hours of surgery. Thus, immediate PT was defined as being delivered within the eight-hour time period following the operation. Patients are encouraged to get out of bed and ambulate during the first visit, but each therapy session is tailored to an individual patient's needs and abilities and can range from bed exercises to walking stairs. Cases that did not receive immediate PT (delayed PT) were identified and compared to those that did (immediate PT).

Baseline and perioperative variables assessed included sex, age, body mass index (BMI), preoperative American Society of Anesthesiology (ASA) classification, insurance type, procedure performed, primary anesthesia type, procedure start time, operative time, and overall TJA caseload on the day of surgery. Information on specific comorbidities and postoperative complications was unavailable. Primary anesthesia type was classified as either general or regional. Regional anesthesia techniques included central neuraxial blockade, peripheral nerve blockade, and monitored anesthesia care. Patients receiving a combination of both general and regional anesthesia were classified as general. Operative time was from incision to closure. Caseload was defined as the total number of primary TJA cases performed at the institution on the day of the procedure. Location of and time to first PT session were also recorded for each procedure. Time to first PT session was defined as the time between leaving the operating room (OR) and the first PT session. For the Immediate PT group, we determined whether patients were able to ambulate during their initial PT session or not.

For the delayed PT group, medical records were reviewed to determine the reason for not receiving immediate PT. Several steps must occur in order for a patient to receive immediate PT. First, a physical therapist is assigned to each patient at the beginning of the day based on the operative schedule. Then, following surgery, anesthesia must sign off on the patient before 19:00, the order for PT must be activated by the nursing staff before 19:00, and the patient must agree to participate in PT. Our PT department does not target patients for immediate postoperative PT if anesthesia signs off or PT order activation occurs after 19:00. This sequence was assessed for each patient that did not receive immediate PT to determine the reason for delayed PT. If another reason was discovered on review, it was recorded. If all necessary steps were documented and no other reason was identified, it was classified as a "failure to see patient." For these cases and those where PT was not assigned, the PT staffing schedule was reviewed on the relevant date to determine whether there was adequate staffing or not.

In order to assess the relationship between immediate PT and short-term outcome measures, a control group of 669 procedures that received immediate PT was identified by three-to-one matching for sex, age, BMI, ASA classification, insurance type, procedure performed, anesthesia type, operative time, and caseload. The control group was not matched for procedure start time due to its close correlation with delayed PT. The maximum allowable absolute difference between propensity scores was 0.01. Number of PT sessions prior to discharge, postoperative LOS, discharge disposition, and 30-day readmissions were compared between matched groups. Postoperative LOS was defined as the time from leaving the OR to discharge. For postoperative variables found to be different between groups, we used repeated-measures logistic regression to predict the outcome while adjusting for procedure start time and ability to ambulate on the same day as surgery.

Categorical data were analyzed with the chi-squared or Fisher's exact test (expected cell counts <5) and displayed using counts with percentages. Continuous variables were tested for normality using the Kolmogorov-Smirnov test. Normal data were analyzed with the two-sample t-test and expressed as means ± standard deviation, and nonnormal data were analyzed with the Mann-Whitney U test and expressed as medians with 25th and 75th percentiles. Logistic regression models were used to predict delayed PT based on both the operative start time and overall caseload by determining the start time and caseload that maximized the area under the receiver operating characteristic curve, which also maximized the sensitivity and specificity for determining delayed PT. All tests were two-sided and a p value < 0.05 was considered statistically significant. All statistical analyses were performed using SAS v9 (SAS Institute, Cary, NC).

3. Results

In total, 2051 primary TJA procedures were performed at our institution from July 2015 to December 2017. Of these, 226 (11.0%) did not receive immediate PT. These cases had a higher rate of general anesthesia (25.2% versus 17.8%, p=0.006), later median operative start time (13:26 [11:31-14:38] versus 9:36 [8:24-11:16], p<0.001), longer median operative time (1.8 [1.5-2.2] versus 1.6 [1.4-1.8] hours, p=0.002), and higher median overall caseload (6 [4-9] versus 5 [4-8],

Table 1: Demographic and perioperative variables for immediate and delayed PT groups.

	Immediate PT (n=1826)	Delayed PT (n=226)	p value
Sex			
Female	53.3%	59.7%	0.065
Male	46.7%	40.3%	
Age	64.8±10.9	64.1±12.5	0.369
BMI	30.6±5.4	31.2±5.9	0.144
ASA			
I-II	44.2%	37.6%	0.061
III-IV	55.8%	62.4%	
Insurance Type			
Commercial	37.7%	33.6%	0.330
Medicare	58.5%	61.5%	
Medicaid	1.4%	2.7%	
Other	2.4%	2.2%	
Procedure			
TKA	63.2%	65.9%	0.418
THA	36.8%	34.1%	
Anesthesia Type			
General	17.8%	25.2%	0.006
Regional	82.2%	74.8%	
Median Procedure Start Time	9:36 [8:24-11:16]	13:26 [11:31-14:38]	<0.001
Median Operative Time (hours)	1.6 [1.4-1.8]	1.8 [1.5-2.2]	<0.001
Median Overall Caseload	5 [4-8]	6 [4-9]	0.002

Table 2: Reasons for delayed PT.

Reason	Number of Patients (%)
No PT Assigned	62 (27.4%)
Inadequate PT Staff	43 (19.0%)
Adequate PT Staff	19 (8.4%)
Late Order Activation	58 (25.7%)
Late Anesthesia Sign-Off	37 (16.4%)
Failure to See Patient	24 (10.6%)
Inadequate PT Staff	13 (5.8%)
Adequate PT Staff	11 (4.9%)
Failed Attempted PT Visit	41 (18.1%)
Pain	20 (8.8%)
Drowsiness	10 (4.4%)
Patient Unavailable	4 (1.8%)
Weakness	3 (1.3%)
Hypotension	2 (0.9%)
Nausea	1 (0.4%)
Language Barrier	1 (0.4%)
Post-Op Complication	4 (1.8%)

p=0.002) (Table 1). Data on operative time was not available for 66 patients and was excluded from analysis. The proportion of missing operative time data did not differ between groups (immediate PT: 3.2%, delayed PT: 3.5%; p=0.771).

A procedure start time after 11:30 (OR 12.09; 95% CI 8.71-16.77; p<0.001) and an overall daily caseload higher than six (OR 1.56; 95% CI 1.18-2.06; p=0.002) maximized the sensitivity and specificity of predicting delayed PT (procedure start time >11:30: sensitivity = 78.8%, specificity = 76.9%; overall caseload >6: sensitivity = 59.0%, specificity = 52.0%). Median time to first PT session was almost four times longer for the delayed PT group (18.4 [16.7-20.7] versus 4.8 [3.9-5.7] hours, p<0.001), and a lower percentage of these patients received their first PT session in the postanesthesia care unit (0.9% versus 18.4%, p<0.001). The most common reasons for delayed PT were missed PT assignment (n=62), late PT order activation (n=58), and failed attempted PT visit (n=41). The most common reasons for failed attempted visit were pain (n=20) and drowsiness (n=10). Postoperative complications (n=4) were a less common reason for delayed PT (Table 2).

Patients who received delayed PT were matched based on demographic and preoperative variables to a group of patients who received immediate PT. There were no differences in sex, age, BMI, ASA classification, insurance type, procedure performed, anesthesia type, operative time, or overall caseload between matched groups (Table 3). Patients who received delayed PT had a lower median number of PT sessions prior to discharge (3 [2-3] versus 3 [2-4], p<0.001) and an increased rate of unplanned 30-day readmission (7.6% versus 3.1%, p=0.004). No differences were observed in postoperative LOS or discharge disposition (Table 4).

Delayed PT, number of PT sessions before discharge, procedure start time, and ambulation on POD 0 were entered

TABLE 3: Demographic and perioperative variables for matched immediate and delayed PT groups.

	Immediate PT (n=669)	Delayed PT (n=223)	p value
Sex			
Female	59.2%	59.6%	0.906
Male	40.8%	40.4%	
Age	64.3±11.5	64.1±12.5	0.787
BMI	31.2±5.5	31.1±5.9	0.773
ASA			
I-II	40.2%	37.7%	0.502
III-IV	59.8%	62.3%	
Insurance Type			
Commercial	34.1%	33.6%	
Medicare	60.2%	61.9%	0.895
Medicaid	2.5%	2.2%	
Other	3.1%	2.2%	
Procedure			
TKA	64.7%	65.5%	0.840
THA	35.3%	34.5%	
Anesthesia Type			
General	25.0%	24.7%	0.929
Regional	75.0%	75.3%	
Median Operative Time	1.7 [1.5-2.1]	1.8 [1.5-2.1]	0.420
Median Overall Caseload	6 [4-9]	6 [4-9]	0.448

TABLE 4: Postoperative variables for matched immediate and delayed PT groups.

	Immediate PT (n=669)	Delayed PT (n=223)	p value
Median Postoperative LOS (hours)	48.6 [28.6-54.8]	46.9 [30.5-68.8]	0.750
Median PT Sessions Before Discharge	3 [2-4]	3 [2-3]	<0.001
Mean PT Sessions Before Discharge	3.3±1.7	2.9±1.8	
Discharge Disposition			
Home/Self Care	62.5%	59.2%	
Home Health Service	20.8%	24.2%	
SNF	15.2%	15.2%	0.819
Rehab Facility	1.3%	1.3%	
Expired	0.1%	0.0%	
30-Day Readmission	3.1%	7.6%	0.004

into a repeated-measures logistic regression model matched for baseline covariates to predict 30-day readmission. Delayed PT (OR 4.54; 95% CI 1.61-12.84; p=0.004) and number of PT sessions prior to discharge (OR 1.17; 95% CI 1.04-1.32; p=0.009) were associated with an increased 30-day readmission rate (Table 5).

4. Discussion

As perioperative care continues to become more expedited and health systems aim to implement programs to speed recovery and reduce costs, it is important to identify barriers to early rehabilitation and the potential impact on short-term outcomes. In this retrospective review of 2051 TJA procedures performed at a single institution, we found that the majority of patients (89%) received immediate postoperative PT. Patients who did not receive immediate PT were more likely to have a later procedure start time, general anesthesia, longer operative time, and a higher overall caseload on the day of surgery. We also found that patients who did not receive immediate PT had an increased rate of unplanned 30-day readmission.

This study is subject to the limitations of retrospective analysis. The clinical information collected is dependent on accurate and complete documentation. Also, there are multiple factors that can affect 30-day readmission following TJA [13–16]. We attempted to control for commonly reported factors, including age, sex, BMI, overall health

Table 5: ORs for 30-day readmission.

	OR (95% CI)	p value
Delayed PT	4.54 (1.61-12.84)	0.004
PT Sessions	1.17 (1.04-1.32)	0.009
Procedure Start Time	0.93 (0.02-43.97)	0.969
Ambulation POD 0	2.02 (0.70-5.82)	0.192

status, insurance type, anesthesia type, operative time, length of stay, and discharge location; however, inclusion of other factors such as specific comorbidities and postoperative complications, which were not available for our study, would have strengthened our analysis. Along the same lines, some institutions schedule patients with higher medical comorbidity or surgical complexity near the end of the day, which could confound our results; however, the protocol at our institution is to schedule more comorbid and complex primary TJA patients at the beginning of the day, which makes this potential issue less likely. Finally, our study was performed using data from a single academic center, and results may not be generalizable to other regions, institutions, or practice settings.

Previous reports have noted later operative end time as a risk factor for not receiving PT on the same day as surgery [7]. Similarly, we found that patients receiving delayed PT were more likely to have a later operative start time. The odds of not receiving immediate PT were 12 times higher for patients with a start time after 11:30. Interestingly, the majority of delayed PT cases were the result of logistical factors such as late order activation, late anesthesia sign-off, missed PT assignment, or failure to see the patient. These reasons accounted for 80% of delayed PT cases, while patient-level factors such as refusal to participate in PT and postoperative complications accounted for only 20%. Longer operative time and higher total caseload were also associated with a decreased likelihood of receiving immediate PT. Altogether, these findings emphasize the importance of operative scheduling and PT staffing in the consistent provision of early postoperative PT. Indeed, one study [17] found that a simple change in PT staffing hours resulted in an increased proportion of patients receiving PT on the same day as TJA from 64% to 85%.

Another risk factor for not receiving immediate PT following TJA was general anesthesia. Multiple studies have demonstrated the benefits of regional over general anesthesia in TJA, including decreased LOS, reduced postoperative complications, and decreased 30-day mortality [18–23]. Our study suggests the additional benefit of allowing earlier rehabilitation following surgery, highlighting the interdependence of the various aspects of advanced perioperative care. This is consistent with results from a systematic review [24] that found that, compared to general anesthesia, regional anesthesia reduced postoperative pain and facilitated rehabilitation for patients undergoing TKA. We did not distinguish between various regional anesthetic techniques in our study, but it is important to note that growing evidence suggests that adductor canal block specifically, when compared to femoral canal block, is superior for postoperative rehabilitation and ambulation [25, 26].

With recent trends showing a decrease in LOS and an increase in 30-day readmissions for primary TJA patients [27, 28], there is concern that accelerated perioperative care regimens may increase the risk of short-term readmission. However, several studies indicate that this may not be the case [29–32], and others suggest that accelerated clinical pathways could even decrease early readmission following TJA [6, 33]. We found that immediate PT, an important component of accelerated perioperative pathways, was associated with a decreased 30-day readmission rate. Early mobilization following TJA has been associated with improvements in short-term functional outcomes, pain scores, and health-related quality of life [34]. It has also been associated with a reduced risk of deep vein thrombosis, infection, and gastrointestinal and pulmonary complications [35]. Interestingly, we found the relationship between immediate PT and 30-day readmission to be independent of ambulation during the first PT session, suggesting that there may be benefit to early individualized PT regardless of patients' postoperative abilities. Still, our results are based on retrospective analysis and require confirmation with high-quality, prospective randomized trials.

Several studies have demonstrated an association between earlier postoperative PT and shorter LOS [7–10]. Interestingly, we did not observe a decrease in LOS for patients receiving immediate PT following TJA. However, postoperative LOS was shorter overall in our study compared to previous studies, likely reflecting institutional differences as well as a continuing trend toward accelerated perioperative care and earlier discharge [6, 27, 28, 36]. Our median postoperative LOS was two days for both immediate and delayed PT groups. In comparison, Chen et al. [7] reported an average postoperative LOS of three days for patients who received PT on the same day as surgery and four days for those who did not. As LOS for TJA procedures continues to decrease with overall advances in perioperative care, the incremental effect of earlier PT may become less influential. Nonetheless, with the growth of outpatient joint arthroplasty [37], this study suggests that there may be value in receiving PT prior to discharge.

5. Conclusion

In conclusion, a majority of patients were able to participate in immediate postoperative PT following TJA. Barriers to receiving immediate PT included general anesthesia, later operative start time, longer operative time, and higher daily caseload. These factors present potential targets for improving the delivery of immediate postoperative PT. Early PT may help reduce 30-day readmissions, but additional research is necessary to further characterize this relationship.

References

[1] C. J. M. Bachmeier, L. M. March, M. J. Cross et al., "A comparison of outcomes in osteoarthritis patients undergoing total hip and knee replacement surgery," *Osteoarthritis and Cartilage*, vol. 9, no. 2, pp. 137–146, 2001.

[2] T. K. Fehring, S. M. Odum, J. L. Troyer, R. Iorio, S. M. Kurtz, and E. C. Lau, "Joint replacement access in 2016: a supply side crisis," *The Journal of Arthroplasty*, vol. 25, no. 8, pp. 1175–1181, 2010.

[3] N. A. Wilson, E. S. Schneller, K. Montgomery, and K. J. Bozic, "Hip and knee implants: Current trends and policy considerations," *Health Affairs (Millwood)*, vol. 27, no. 6, pp. 1587–1598, 2008.

[4] K. Larsen, T. B. Hansen, P. B. Thomsen, T. Christiansen, and K. Søballe, "Cost-effectiveness of accelerated perioperative care and rehabilitation after total hip and knee arthroplasty," *The Journal of Bone & Joint Surgery*, vol. 91, no. 4, pp. 761–772, 2009.

[5] K. Larsen, O. G. Sørensen, T. B. Hansen, P. B. Thomsen, and K. Søballe, "Accelerated perioperative care and rehabilitation intervention for hip and knee replacement is effective: a randomized clinical trial involving 87 patients with 3 months of follow-up," *Acta Orthopaedica*, vol. 79, no. 2, pp. 149–159, 2008.

[6] K. R. Berend, A. V. Lombardi, and T. H. Mallory, "Rapid recovery protocol for peri-operative care of total hip and total knee arthroplasty patients," *Surgical Technology International*, vol. 13, pp. 239–247, 2004.

[7] A. F. Chen, M. K. Stewart, A. E. Heyl, and B. A. Klatt, "Effect of Immediate Postoperative Physical Therapy on Length of Stay for Total Joint Arthroplasty Patients," *The Journal of Arthroplasty*, vol. 27, no. 6, pp. 851–856, 2012.

[8] G. Tayrose, D. Newman, and J. Slover, "Rapid mobilization decreases length-of-stay in joint replacement patients," *Bulletin of the Hospital for Joint Diseases*, vol. 71, no. 3, pp. 222–226, 2013.

[9] N. S. Labraca, A. M. Castro-Sánchez, G. A. Matarán-Peñarrocha, M. Arroyo-Morales, M. Del Mar Sánchez-Joya, and C. Moreno-Lorenzo, "Benefits of starting rehabilitation within 24 hours of primary total knee arthroplasty: Randomized clinical trial," *Clinical Rehabilitation*, vol. 25, no. 6, pp. 557–566, 2011.

[10] M. C. Munin, T. E. Rudy, N. W. Glynn, L. S. Crossett, and H. E. Rubash, "Early inpatient rehabilitation after elective hip and knee arthroplasty," *Journal of the American Medical Association*, vol. 279, no. 11, pp. 847–852, 1998.

[11] A. L. Curry, M. T. Goehring, J. Bell, and D. U. Jette, "Effect of physical therapy interventions in the acute care setting on function, activity, and participation after total knee arthroplasty: a systematic review," *Journal of Acute Care Physical Therapy*, vol. 9, no. 3, pp. 93–106, 2018.

[12] K. G. Henderson, J. A. Wallis, and D. A. Snowdon, "Active physiotherapy interventions following total knee arthroplasty in the hospital and inpatient rehabilitation settings: a systematic review and meta-analysis," *Physiotherapy (United Kingdom)*, vol. 104, no. 1, pp. 25–35, 2018.

[13] S. M. Kurtz, E. C. Lau, K. L. Ong, E. M. Adler, F. R. Kolisek, and M. T. Manley, "Which Hospital and Clinical Factors Drive 30- and 90-Day Readmission After TKA?" *The Journal of Arthroplasty*, vol. 31, no. 10, pp. 2099–2107, 2016.

[14] R. C. Clement, P. B. Derman, D. S. Graham et al., "Risk factors, causes, and the economic implications of unplanned readmissions following total hip arthroplasty," *The Journal of Arthroplasty*, vol. 28, 8, pp. 7–10, 2013.

[15] A. J. Pugely, J. J. Callaghan, C. T. Martin, P. Cram, and Y. Gao, "Incidence of and risk factors for 30-day readmission following elective primary total joint arthroplasty: Analysis from the ACS-NSQIP," *The Journal of Arthroplasty*, vol. 28, no. 9, pp. 1499–1504, 2013.

[16] B. Zmistowski, C. Restrepo, J. Hess, D. Adibi, S. Cangoz, and J. Parvizi, "Unplanned readmission after total joint arthroplasty: rates, reasons, and risk factors," *The Journal of Bone & Joint Surgery*, vol. 95, no. 20, pp. 1869–1876, 2013.

[17] C. E. Pelt, M. B. Anderson, R. Pendleton, M. Foulks, C. L. Peters, and J. M. Gililland, "Improving value in primary total joint arthroplasty care pathways: changes in inpatient physical therapy staffing," *Arthroplasty Today*, vol. 3, no. 1, pp. 45–49, 2017.

[18] A. Perlas, V. W. Chan, and S. Beattie, "Anesthesia technique and mortality after total hip or knee arthroplasty: a retrospective, propensity score-matched cohort study," *Anesthesiology*, vol. 125, no. 4, pp. 724–731, 2016.

[19] B. A. Basques, J. O. Toy, D. D. Bohl, N. S. Golinvaux, and J. N. Grauer, "General compared with spinal anesthesia for total hip arthroplasty," *Journal of Bone and Joint Surgery - American Volume*, vol. 97, no. 6, pp. 455–461, 2015.

[20] M. A. Helwani, M. S. Avidan, A. Ben Abdallah et al., "Effects of regional versus general anesthesia on outcomes after total hip arthroplasty: A retrospective propensity-matched cohort study," *Journal of Bone and Joint Surgery - American Volume*, vol. 97, no. 3, pp. 186–193, 2015.

[21] S. G. Memtsoudis, X. Sun, Y. L. Chiu et al., "Perioperative comparative effectiveness of anesthetic technique in orthopedic patients," *Anesthesiology*, vol. 118, no. 5, pp. 1046–1058, 2013.

[22] A. J. Pugely, C. T. Martin, Y. Gao, S. Mendoza-Lattes, and J. J. Callaghan, "Differences in short-term complications between spinal and general anesthesia for primary total knee arthroplasty," *The Journal of Bone & Joint Surgery*, vol. 95, no. 3, pp. 193–199, 2013.

[23] W. J. Mauermann, A. M. Shilling, and Z. Zuo, "A comparison of neuraxial block versus general anesthesia for elective total hip replacement: a meta-analysis," *Anesthesia & Analgesia*, vol. 103, no. 4, pp. 1018–1025, 2006.

[24] A. J. Macfarlene, G. A. Prasad, V. W. S. Chan, and R. Brull, "Does regional anesthesia improve outcome after total knee arthroplasty?" *Clinical Orthopaedics and Related Research*, vol. 467, no. 9, pp. 2379–2402, 2009.

[25] S. C. Mudumbai, T. E. Kim, S. K. Howard et al., "Continuous adductor canal blocks are superior to continuous femoral nerve blocks in promoting early ambulation after TKA," *Clinical Orthopaedics and Related Research*, vol. 472, no. 5, pp. 1377–1383, 2014.

[26] N. A. Shah and N. P. Jain, "Is continuous adductor canal block better than continuous femoral nerve block after total knee arthroplasty? Effect on ambulation ability, early functional recovery and pain control: A randomized controlled trial," *The Journal of Arthroplasty*, vol. 29, no. 11, pp. 2224–2229, 2014.

[27] P. Cram, X. Lu, S. L. Kates, J. A. Singh, Y. Li, and B. R. Wolf, "Total knee arthroplasty volume, utilization, and outcomes among medicare beneficiaries, 1991-2010," *Journal of the American Medical Association*, vol. 308, no. 12, pp. 1227–1236, 2012.

[28] P. Cram, X. Lu, P. J. Kaboli et al., "Clinical characteristics and outcomes of medicare patients undergoing total hip arthroplasty, 1991-2008," *Journal of the American Medical Association*, vol. 305, no. 15, p. 1560, 2011.

[29] J. S. Vorhies, Y. Wang, J. H. Herndon, W. J. Maloney, and J. I. Huddleston, "Decreased length of stay after TKA is not associated with increased readmission rates in a national medicare sample," *Clinical Orthopaedics and Related Research*, vol. 470, no. 1, pp. 166–171, 2012.

[30] M. Raphael, M. Jaeger, and J. Van Vlymen, "Easily adoptable total joint arthroplasty program allows discharge home in two days," *Canadian Journal of Anesthesia*, vol. 58, no. 10, pp. 902–910, 2011.

[31] J. S. Vorhies, Y. Wang, J. Herndon, W. J. Maloney, and J. I. Huddleston, "Readmission and length of stay after total hip arthroplasty in a national medicare sample," *The Journal of Arthroplasty*, vol. 26, 6, pp. 119–123, 2011.

[32] H. Husted, K. S. Otte, B. B. Kristensen, T. Ørsnes, and H. Kehlet, "Readmissions after fast-track hip and knee arthroplasty," *Archives of Orthopaedic and Trauma Surgery*, vol. 130, no. 9, pp. 1185–1191, 2010.

[33] M. M. Dowsey, M. L. Kilgour, N. M. Santamaria, and P. F. M. Choong, "Clinical pathways in hip and knee arthroplasty: A prospective randomised controlled study," *Medical Journal of Australia*, vol. 170, no. 2, pp. 59–62, 1999.

[34] M. L. Guerra, P. J. Singh, and N. F. Taylor, "Early mobilization of patients who have had a hip or knee joint replacement reduces length of stay in hospital: A systematic review," *Clinical Rehabilitation*, vol. 29, no. 9, pp. 844–854, 2015.

[35] B. J. Kalisch, S. Lee, and B. W. Dabney, "Outcomes of inpatient mobilization: A literature review," *Journal of Clinical Nursing*, vol. 23, no. 11-12, pp. 1486–1501, 2014.

[36] C. L. Peters, B. Shirley, and J. Erickson, "The effect of a new multimodal perioperative anesthetic regimen on postoperative pain, side effects, rehabilitation, and length of hospital stay after total joint arthroplasty," *The Journal of Arthroplasty*, vol. 21, no. 6, supplement 2, pp. 132–138, 2006.

[37] J. M. Bert, J. Hooper, and S. Moen, "Outpatient Total Joint Arthroplasty," *Current Reviews in Musculoskeletal Medicine*, vol. 10, no. 4, pp. 567–574, 2017.

12

The Status of Assessments and Treatments for Osteoporosis in Patients 5 Years after Total Hip Arthroplasty: A Cross-Sectional Survey of 194 Post-THA Patients

Keiji Kamo,[1,2] Hiroaki Kijima,[2,3] Koichiro Okuyama,[1] Shin Yamada,[2] Natsuo Konishi,[2] Hitoshi Kubota,[2] Hiroshi Tazawa,[2] Naohisa Miyakoshi,[3] and Yoichi Shimada[2,3]

[1]*Akita Rosai Hospital, Japan*
[2]*Akita Hip Research Group, Japan*
[3]*Department of Orthopedic Surgery, Akita University Graduate School of Medicine, Japan*

Correspondence should be addressed to Keiji Kamo; keiji-kamo@par.odn.ne.jp

Academic Editor: Benjamin Blondel

Background. Assessments for osteoporosis in patients who have undergone total hip arthroplasty (THA) are very important with respect to the clinical results. However, few studies have investigated the status of the assessments and treatments for osteoporosis in post-THA patients. The purpose of this multicenter study was to investigate the status of assessments and treatments for osteoporosis in post-THA patients. *Methods.* The results of a self-report questionnaire and the medical records of 194 post-THA patients over 40 years of age who visited the outpatient departments of the five hospitals participating in the study were analyzed. *Results.* A total of 125 patients (64.4%) had been examined for osteoporosis, and 69 patients (35.6%) had never been assessed for osteoporosis. It was assumed, based on the questionnaire results, that 50 (40%) of the 125 patients should have been receiving treatment for osteoporosis. Forty-five (90%) of these 50 patients were actually taking medication for osteoporosis at the time of the investigation. Overall, a total of 58 (29.9%) patients were receiving treatment for osteoporosis. *Conclusions.* The present survey revealed that 64.4% of post-THA patients had been evaluated for osteoporosis. Moreover, while 40% of post-THA patients over 40 years of age may require treatment for osteoporosis, only 29.9% were actually receiving treatment.

1. Introduction

The proportion of elderly people is increasing globally. Of all the advanced countries, Japan is at the center of this aging society phenomenon. Yoshimura et al. have estimated that nearly 970,000 people (160,000 men, 810,000 women) ranging in age from 40 to 79 years develop osteoporosis in Japan annually [1]. While some racial differences are likely to be present, similar incidences of osteoporosis can be expected in other countries. The prevalence of degenerative hip disorders or traumatic disorders requiring surgical intervention is higher in the elderly population, and it is assumed that the number of older patients who choose to undergo THA to improve their quality of life will increase [2, 3]. Thus, orthopedic surgeons will likely use THA as a surgical intervention to treat these disorders much more frequently in the aging societies of the future.

Osteoporosis is one of the main causes of intraoperative periprosthetic femoral fracture and reduced initial stability of the implant in cementless THA [4, 5]. Osteoporosis also increases the chances of a periprosthetic fracture after THA with uncemented stem [5, 6]. A periprosthetic femoral fracture negatively affects not only the results of THA but also a mortality rate [6–8]. Thillemann et al. reported that the 10-year cumulative implant revision rate in primary THA patients with osteoporosis from the Danish Hip Arthroplasty Registry, in which the implant fixation technique of THA included cemented, uncemented, and hybrid fixation, was 8.3% [9], which is significantly higher than the rate in patients without osteoporosis. Therefore, the assessments and treatments for osteoporosis in patients who undergo THA, especially with uncemented stem, are crucial to improve or maintain the clinical results. While several studies have demonstrated the importance of the degree of osteoporosis in

Table 1: Questionnaire about assessments and treatments for osteoporosis given to post-THA patients.

Question	Answer
(1) Have you ever been evaluated for osteoporosis?	(a) Yes (b) No
(2) If you have been evaluated for osteoporosis, what was the result?	(a) Treatment required (b) No treatment required (c) Unknown
(3) Have you ever been treated for osteoporosis?	(a) Yes (b) No (c) I was previously being treated, but I am not being treated now.
(4) If you are being treated for osteoporosis, what kind of treatment are you receiving?	

patients who undergo THA, very little attention has been paid to the pre- and postoperative status of the assessments and treatments for osteoporosis. To the best of our knowledge, few reports have investigated osteoporosis in post-THA patients. The purpose of the present multicenter study involving five affiliated hospitals in Akita Prefecture, Japan, was to evaluate the status of assessments and treatments for osteoporosis in post-THA patients.

2. Materials and Methods

This cross-sectional study of the assessments and treatments for osteoporosis in post-THA patients was approved by the Ethics Committee of the authors' affiliated institutions. A total of 194 post-THA patients (246 hips) over 40 years of age who visited the outpatient department of the five participating hospitals between April and May 2016 were investigated. The status of assessments and treatments for osteoporosis were ascertained using a self-report questionnaire (Table 1) and the patients' medical records. All 194 patients were enrolled in this survey.

3. Results

The mean age of the patients was 70 years (range, 44–92 years), and there were 26 men and 168 women. The mean duration after THA was 62 months (1–408 months). Reasons for undergoing THA included osteoarthritis (163 cases), rheumatoid arthritis (8 cases), osteonecrosis of the femoral head (8 cases), hip fracture (7 cases), and rapidly destructive coxarthropathy (4 cases). The original diseases of the remaining four cases were not clearly recorded. In terms of the type of implant fixation technique, there were 183 uncemented, 5 cemented, and 6 hybrid fixation of THA in this survey.

Of the 194 patients who were enrolled in this survey, 125 (64.4%) patients reported that they had been evaluated for osteoporosis in the questionnaire. It was ascertained that 40.0% (50/125) of the patients assessed for osteoporosis required treatment, while 55.2% (69/125) did not. The remaining six patients answered "unknown" regarding their osteoporotic assessment. Ninety percent (45/50) of the patients that required osteoporotic treatment were taking medication at the time of the present survey. One patient (1/50) had never been treated for osteoporosis. Of the patients assessed for osteoporosis, 8.0% (4/50) had stopped receiving treatment before the time of the present investigation. Of the patients that were not evaluated for osteoporosis, 8.7% (6/69) were being treated for osteoporosis at the time of the present survey. In total, 58 (29.9%) of the 194 patients were being treated for osteoporosis at the time of the present survey. Bisphosphonate, vitamin D, selective estrogen receptor modulator, teriparatide, calcium, and denosumab were the medications being taken for treatment of osteoporosis in 33, 18, 9, 6, 5, and 4 cases, respectively. Of the 163 OA patients, 108 (66.3%) had been assessed for osteoporosis. Thirty-nine (36.1%) of the 108 patients assessed for osteoporosis reported that they were required treatment in the result of the assessment. Forty-six (28.2%) of the 163 OA patients were being treated for osteoporosis at the time of the present investigation. Of the remaining 31 patients who received THA for the other reasons, 17 (54.8%) had been assessed for osteoporosis. Eleven (64.7%) of the 17 patients assessed for osteoporosis reported that they were required treatment in the result of the assessment. Twelve (38.7%) of 31 THA patients for the other reasons were being treated for osteoporosis at the time of the present investigation.

4. Discussion

In the present survey, the status of assessments and treatments for osteoporosis in post-THA patients was investigated in five affiliated hospitals in Akita Prefecture, Japan. Results show that approximately two-thirds of the patients had been examined for osteoporosis, and that more than 40.0% of the patients required treatment for osteoporosis. However, only 29.9% (58/194) of the patients were actually undergoing treatment for osteoporosis. Previous studies have reported an incidence of osteoporosis of 25–28% in women with hip arthritis scheduled for or undergoing THA [10, 11]. The present survey included patients that were followed up for an average of 5 years after THA. To our knowledge, although previous studies have described preoperative status, no other study has described the postoperative assessments of osteoporosis or osteoporosis treatment. The patients in the present study were older and the prevalence of osteoporosis was higher than in past reports [10]. It is speculated that, given the length of the follow-up period (mean, 62 months; range, 1–408 months), some patients without osteoporosis at the time of THA may have developed osteoporotic conditions by the time of the survey. Consequently, it is crucial to examine the status of osteoporosis not only at the time of THA surgery, but also throughout the period of post-THA follow-up.

In previous studies related to THA and osteoporosis medication, Yamasaki et al. reported that risedronate reduced periprosthetic bone resorption after cementless THA [12]. Iwamoto et al. reported that alendronate monotherapy and combined therapy using alendronate and alfacalcidol both prevent periprosthetic bone mineral density loss after THA [13]. In addition, a few reports have demonstrated that bisphosphonate use is associated with a lower risk for revision surgery in patients with osteoporosis undergoing primary THA [13, 14]. Therefore, treatment for osteoporosis in patients that have undergone THA is very important for improving the long-term results of THA.

In the present study, while approximately 40% of patients were considered to need osteoporotic treatment, only 30% were being treated for osteoporosis at the time of the investigation. This discrepancy must not be overlooked. It is assumed that some patients (about 10%) that were being followed up as outpatients after THA were neither diagnosed with nor being treated for osteoporosis despite presenting with osteoporotic conditions.

Approximately 90% of the patients diagnosed with conditions requiring treatment for osteoporosis were actually receiving treatment for osteoporosis. This indicates that adherence to osteoporosis therapies is extremely good when patients who have undergone THA are informed that they have osteoporosis and require treatment. Six patients (8.7%) among the patients who had not been evaluated for osteoporosis were receiving treatment for osteoporosis. It is speculated that patients receiving long-term steroids are treating osteoporosis for the prevention of osteoporosis. Gleeson et al. reported that periodic follow-up interaction between patients and health care professionals appeared to be beneficial for improving adherence and persistence with osteoporosis medications [15]. Patients that have had THA are required to visit the hospital regularly for radiographs of their hips. It is speculated that this periodic follow-up of patients after THA improves their adherence to osteoporosis therapies.

Patients who underwent or are scheduled for THA will inevitably age, so it is essential that these patients receive the appropriate osteoporotic treatment at the appropriate time. Regarding the adherence of patients to osteoporosis therapies after THA, there is a possibility that the pre- and postoperative assessments of osteoporosis indirectly improve the long-term results of THA.

The present study had several limitations. First, this investigation only used a questionnaire and medical records. Second, the method used for osteoporotic assessment was unknown. Osteoporosis should be diagnosed based on the presence of a fragility fracture and measurements of bone mineral density [16]. However, the results of this research clarified the current situation regarding the evaluation of and treatment for osteoporosis in patients who underwent THA within the previous 5 years. Future studies should investigate whether treatment for osteoporosis prevents periprosthetic fractures and improves the long-term results of THA.

In conclusion, more than 40% of patients over the age of 40 years who underwent THA may require treatment for osteoporosis. However, less than 30% of patients were being treated for osteoporosis, as only about two-thirds of patients were actually evaluated for osteoporosis. Because the adherence to osteoporosis therapies in post-THA patients is very good, thorough evaluation of osteoporosis after THA may lead to better long-term results of THA.

References

[1] N. Yoshimura, S. Muraki, H. Oka et al., "Epidemiology of lumber osteoporosis and osteoarthritis and their causal relationship-is osteoarthritis a predictor for osteoporosis or vice versa?: The Miyama study," *Osteoporosis International*, vol. 20, no. 6, pp. 999–1008, 2009.

[2] D. J. Culliford, J. Maskell, D. J. Beard, D. W. Murray, A. J. Price, and N. K. Arden, "Temporal trends in hip and knee replacement in the United Kingdom: 1991 to 2006," *The Bone & Joint Journal*, vol. 92, no. 1, pp. 130–135, 2010.

[3] T. Yuasa, K. Maezawa, M. Nazawa, and K. Kaneko, "Cementless total hip arthroplasty in patients aged ≥80 years," *Journal of Orthopaedics*, vol. 13, no. 1, pp. 29–32, 2016.

[4] H. T. Aro, J. J. Alm, N. Moritz, T. J. Mäkinen, and P. Lankinen, "Low BMD affects initial stability and delays stem osseointegration in cementless total hip arthroplasty in women: a 2-year RSA study of 39 patients," *Acta Orthopaedica*, vol. 83, no. 2, pp. 107–114, 2012.

[5] M. Lindberg-Larsen, C. C. Jørgensen, S. Solgaard, A. G. Kjersgaard, H. Kehlet, and Lundbeck Foundation Centre for Fast-Track Hip and Knee Replacement Collaborative Group, "Increased risk of intraoperative and early postoperative periprosthetic femoral fracture with uncemented stems. 7,169 total hip arthroplasties from 8 Danish centers," *Acta Orthopaedica*, vol. 88, no. 4, pp. 390–394, 2017.

[6] M. R. Streit, C. Merle, M. Clarius, and P. R. Aldinger, "Late peri-prosthetic femoral fracture as a major mode of failure in uncemented primary hip replacement," *The Journal of Bone & Joint Surgery (British Volume)*, vol. 93, no. 2, pp. 178–183, 2011.

[7] T. Bhattacharyya, D. Chang, J. B. Meigs, D. M. Estok II, and H. Malchau, "Mortality after periprosthetic fracture of the femur," *The Journal of Bone & Joint Surgery*, vol. 89, no. 12, pp. 2658–2662, 2007.

[8] V. Bottai, G. Dell'Osso, F. Celli et al., "Total hip replacement in osteoarthritis: the role of bone metabolism and its complications," *Clinical Cases in Mineral and Bone Metabolism*, vol. 12, no. 3, pp. 247–250, 2015.

[9] T. M. Thillemann, A. B. Pedersen, F. Mehnert, S. P. Johnsen, and K. Søballe, "Postoperative use of bisphosphonates and risk of revision after primary total hip arthroplasty: a nationwide population-based study," *Bone*, vol. 46, no. 4, pp. 946–951, 2010.

[10] T. J. Mäkinen, J. J. Alm, H. Laine, E. Svedström, and H. T. Aro, "The incidence of osteopenia and osteoporosis in women with hip osteoarthritis scheduled for cementless total joint replacement," *Bone*, vol. 40, no. 4, pp. 1041–1047, 2007.

[11] J. Glowacki, S. Hurwitz, T. S. Thornhill, M. Kelly, and M. S. LeBoff, "Osteoporosis and vitamin-D deficiency among postmenopausal women with osteoarthritis undergoing total hip arthroplasty," *The Journal of Bone & Joint Surgery—American Volume*, vol. 85, no. 12, pp. 2371–2377, 2003.

[12] S. Yamasaki, K. Masuhara, K. Yamaguchi, T. Nakai, T. Fuji, and Y. Seino, "Risedronate reduces postoperative bone resorption after cementless total hip arthroplasty," *Osteoporosis International*, vol. 18, no. 7, pp. 1009–1015, 2007.

[13] N. Iwamoto, Y. Inaba, N. Kobayashi et al., "The effectiveness of mono or combined osteoporosis drug therapy against bone mineral density loss around femoral implants after total hip arthroplasty," *Journal of Bone and Mineral Metabolism*, vol. 32, no. 5, pp. 539–544, 2014.

[14] M. Khatod, M. C. S. Inacio, R. M. Dell, S. A. Bini, E. W. Paxton, and R. S. Namba, "Association of Bisphosphonate use and risk of revision after THA: outcomes from a US total joint replacement registry," *Clinical Orthopaedics and Related Research*, vol. 473, no. 11, pp. 3412–3420, 2015.

[15] T. Gleeson, M. D. Iversen, J. Avorn et al., "Interventions to improve adherence and persistence with osteoporosis medications: a systematic literature review," *Osteoporosis International*, vol. 20, no. 12, pp. 2127–2134, 2009.

[16] S. Soen, M. Fukunaga, T. Sugimoto et al., "Diagnostic criteria for primary osteoporosis: year 2012 revision," *Journal of Bone and Mineral Metabolism*, vol. 31, no. 3, pp. 247–257, 2013.

13

Knee–Hip–Spine Syndrome: Improvement in Preoperative Abnormal Posture following Total Knee Arthroplasty

Yasushi Oshima,[1] Nobuyoshi Watanabe,[2] Norishige Iizawa,[1] Tokifumi Majima,[1] Mitsuhiro Kawata,[3] and Shinro Takai[1]

[1]*Department of Orthopaedic Surgery, Nippon Medical School, 1-1-5 Sendagi, Bunkyo-ku, Tokyo 113-8603, Japan*
[2]*Department of Orthopaedic Surgery, Kyoto Kujo Hospital, 10 Karahashi Rajomoncho, Minami-ku, Kyoto 601-8453, Japan*
[3]*School of Health Sciences, Bukkyo University, 7 Higashitoganoo-cho, Nakagyo-ku, Kyoto 604-8418, Japan*

Correspondence should be addressed to Yasushi Oshima; y-oshima@nms.ac.jp

Academic Editor: Panagiotis Korovessis

An ergonomic upright body posture is maintained by the alignment of the spine, pelvis, and lower extremities, and the muscle strength of body trunk and lower extremities. The posture varies with age because of the degenerative changes in the involved structures and the weakening of the muscles. The compensatory mechanisms underlying these changes have recently been evaluated, and the loss of lumbar lordosis results in spinal kyphosis, pelvic retroversion, hip extension, knee flexion, and ankle dorsiflexion. These mechanisms are referred to as the hip–spine and knee–spine syndromes. The spine, hip, and knee are anatomically connected, and the pain and discomfort of the lower back, hip, and knee frequently arise due to degenerative changes of these structures. Thus, these mechanisms are considered as the knee–hip–spine syndrome. Spinal fusion, total hip arthroplasty, and total knee arthroplasty are the surgical procedures for severe degeneration, and their clinical outcomes for the affected sites are promising. However, despite surgeries, other structures may degenerate and result in complications, such as proximal junctional kyphosis and hip dislocation, following spinal fusion. Therefore, it is necessary to evaluate each patient under specific conditions and to treat each section while considering associations between the target structure and entire body. The purpose of this article is to introduce postural maintenance, variations with age, and improvements with surgical interventions of spine, hip, and knee as the knee–hip–spine syndrome.

1. Introduction

An ergonomic upright body posture is maintained by the alignment of the spine, pelvis, and lower extremities with the support of the muscles of the body trunk and lower extremities, and this posture varies with age because of degeneration of the involved structures and weakening of the muscles. In the advent of an aging society, abnormal posture with body balance disorders is a serious issue because it leads to decline in activities of daily living and health-related quality of life (QOL).

In the last few decades, treatments involving surgical procedures have been developed as specialized interventions for adult spinal deformity (ASD), osteoarthritis of the hip (hip OA), and osteoarthritis of the knee (knee OA). More recently, mechanisms underlying interactions among the spine, hip, and knee as well as compensatory mechanism underlying their deformities have been elucidated. In addition, similar medical conditions have been speculated to arise from different segments. For instance, spinal deformity results in spinal kyphosis; however, progressions of hip and knee OA may lead to the abnormal global sagittal alignment of the body.

Therefore, the purpose of this article is to summarize the current understanding of associations of the spine, pelvis, hip, and knee with the global and abnormal body postures and to explain postural improvements with surgical interventions, including our clinical outcomes of postural variations following total knee arthroplasty (TKA).

2. Body Posture

In 1994, Dubousset put forth the concept of "the cone of economy," which refers to the upright body posture maintained by the skeletal muscle strength of the body trunk and lower extremities and the alignment of the skeletal structures, including the head, spine, pelvis, and lower extremities. Body posture has been considered the chain of balance, with the body being balanced as an inverted pendulum in the standing position such that both feet on the floor act as the fulcrum connecting the ankles, knees, hips, pelvis, spinal segments, and head. The body sways to maintain balance while standing as the shape of a cone, and the body posture remains stable with minimal energy expenditure when the cone size is narrow. In contrast, the body becomes unstable and the energy expenditure increases when the cone size is large as the body trunk is positioned peripherally of the cone. Thus, when the trunk extends beyond cone, supportive devices, such as cane or crutch, are necessary to prevent fall [1].

3. Global Alignment

Body alignment is an important index of body balance in static and dynamic conditions, and it is known to vary with age. The ideal alignment of the body is considered to match C7 plumb line, which is the center of the gravity of the body trunk, and the center of the sacral vertical line in the coronal plane. C7 plumb line passes thought the posterior of the rotational center of the hip in the sagittal plane [2, 3]. In the previous study, the global sagittal alignment of 40-year-old healthy individuals was extensively investigated using a three-dimensional X-ray device [4]; the authors reported that the head was almost on the gravity line, as determined using a force plate as a vertical line from the center of gravity. Moreover, the cervical, thoracic, and lumbar regions of the spine showed lordosis, kyphosis, and lordosis in the normal adult posture, respectively. T7 was the posterior apex of the spine and was 5.0 cm posterior to the gravity line, while L4 was 0.6 mm anterior to the gravity line. The hip center was 1.4 cm anterior to the gravity line, whereas the knee and ankle centers were 2.4 mm and 4.8 cm posterior to the gravity line, respectively. When the ideal alignment of these segments is disrupted due to degenerative change of the involving structures, the underlying compensatory mechanisms preserve the body balance. Otherwise, the body becomes instable and loses balance.

4. Fall

The frequency of fall increases with age. Approximately 30% of the individuals older than 65 years of age fall more than once a year. Falls were reported to account for 10% of the emergency room visits and 6% of the hospital admissions [5].

Compared with those who did not fall, individuals who suffered falls showed reportedly poorer body balance, spinal sagittal alignment, muscle strength, and gait speed [6]. Falls in older people, especially in those with osteoporosis, may cause fractures, including vertebral compression as well as proximal femoral and distal radius fractures. Majority of these fractures can easily occur as low-energy injuries with fall from standing height. In older individuals who suffered proximal femoral fracture, 1-year incidence of second hip contralateral fractures was 2.7%–9% [7, 8] and 1-year mortality was approximately 10% [9].

Therefore, preventing falls via strategies involving exercises is crucial considering the higher overall 30-day mortality rate of older patients than that of younger patients following bone fractures [10, 11].

5. Sagittal Vertical Axis (SVA) and Sagittal Malalignment

On the contrary to coronal alignment, global sagittal alignment and pelvic version are associated with health-related QOL in terms of pain and disability [12]. Thus, many studies have focused on global sagittal alignment.

SVA, defined as the horizontal distance from the posterosuperior corner of S1 to the plumb line dropped from the center of the body at C7, is one of the indices of the sagittal body balance. A positive SVA indicates a plumb line passing anteriorly to the front of the sacrum, while a negative SVA indicates a plumb line passing through or behind the sacrum.

SVA of adolescents is significantly more negative than that of adults [13]. Thereafter, SVA has been reported to increase with age [2, 4]. Higher SVA values indicate forward bending the body trunk, resulting in low back pain, difficulty in touching the top of the shelf, and performing routine tasks, all of which lead to restricted activities of daily living. Consequently, back muscle strength is reduced, and the vertebral spine motion is limited. The vision is directed downwards, which impairs the ability to grasp the circumstances quickly and may lead to imbalance, walking disturbances, and falls [6, 12, 14].

SVA is an index of a stable standing posture, in which the femur is fixed and the gluteus maximus is contracted such that the pelvis is tilted posteriorly [15]. Thus, SVA is an indicator of changes due to the actions of compensatory mechanisms of the pelvis, hip, and knee [16, 17]. However, in the dynamic status, the femur is not fixed and the pelvis may tilt anteriorly [18]. Therefore, additional indices must be applied to dynamic alignment while performing normal activities.

6. ASD

Degenerative spinal kyphoscoliosis of the coronal and sagittal alignments occurs with degeneration of the facet joints and/or spinal discs, vertebral compression fractures, and weakening of the lumbodorsal muscles. Reduced lumbar lordosis (LL: the sagittal Cobb angle measured between the superior end plate of L1 and the superior end plate of S1) and excessive spinal kyphosis are associated with increased intradiscal pressure, which may cause low back pain [19]. Approximately 60% of the older individuals are considered to present with ASD; however, some patients with abnormal posture do not show any spinal deformities [20].

According to the Scoliosis Research Society-Schwab Classification, ASD is characterized by coronal curves of 4 types: type T, a thoracic major curve of >30° (apical level of T9 or higher); type L, a lumbar or thoracolumbar major curve of >30° (apical level of T10 or lower); type D, a double-major curve, with each curve >30°; and type N (normal), no coronal curve >30° (i.e., no major coronal deformity) [20]. Moreover, sagittal alignment is characterized through 3 modifiers: (1) the difference between the angle of the pelvic incidence (PI: the angle between the line drawn perpendicular to the sacral end plate at its midpoint and the line drawn from the midpoint of the sacral end plate to the midpoint of the bicoxofemoral axis) and LL; (2) the pelvic tilt (PT: the angle between the line connecting the midpoint of the sacral end plate to the midpoint of the bicoxofemoral axis and the vertical); and (3) SVA (SVA > 40 mm indicates poor sagittal alignment).

Variations in the spinal alignment are related to the pelvis position as a compensatory mechanism. When LL increases, the pelvis tilts anteriorly and thoracic kyphosis (TK) increase as a reciprocal change. In contrast when LL decreases, the pelvis tilts posteriorly and TK increase and the knee flexes. However, when this mechanism cannot maintain body posture, the thoracic and lumbar kyphosis increase, the body bends forward, and the gravity line moves forward, giving rise to severe abnormal posture with the stretching of the erector spinae muscles and chronic low back pain [2].

The pelvis has a fundamental role as the main regulator of the chain of correlation between the spine and lower extremities in this compensatory mechanism. Thus, the parameters LL, PT, sacral slope (SS; the tangent line to the superior endplate of S1 and the horizontal plane), and PI (the sum of PT and SS, which does not change with patient position, activity, age, or structural deformity) are important in the evaluation of the relationship between the spine and pelvis [12, 21].

7. Hip and Knee OA

OA is the most common form of arthritis and involves inflammation and major structural changes of the joints, causing pain and functional disabilities.

The risk of knee OA increases with age, with the global prevalence of radiographically confirmed symptomatic knee OA estimated to be 3.8%. In contrast, the incidence of hip OA is less than that of knee OA, with the global age-standardized prevalence of symptomatic radiographically confirming hip OA being 0.85% [22].

Coxitis knee is defined as the secondary knee OA, which occurs due to hip OA. Originally, coxitis knee was believed to be related to hip disease. However, adduction contracture of the hip and discrepancies of leg length have been regarded as the main etiologies of coxitis knee [23]. Of note, although an important symptom of hip and knee OA, coxitis knee affects the coronal alignment of the body posture to a greater extent rather than the sagittal alignment for the body posture.

8. Hip–Spine Syndrome

The concept of hip-spine syndrome, in which the spinal and hip diseases are related and/or concomitant, was first proposed in 1983 [24]. This syndrome was classified into 4 groups: simple, complex, secondary, or misdiagnosed hip–spine syndrome.

Subsequently, the association between spinal alignment and hip was studied. Nonetheless, it is necessary to evaluate hip pathology and spinal alignment in hip OA treatment [25].

In the coronal plane, spinal scoliosis shifts the center of the body gravity line, and the mechanical load increases on one side of the hip and results in hip pain of the affected side. In this situation, the compensatory mechanism of the pelvis is activated, with the gluteus maximus being responsible for the reciprocal movement of the spine and pelvis.

On the other hand, the sagittal alignment progresses to spinal kyphosis and pelvic retroversion with age. In such cases, the loading area of the acetabulum reduces and the load per unit area increases significantly; this is considered to be the mechanism of the progression of primary hip OA. When the hip develops a fixed flexion deformity, there may be an associated loss of LL. Thus, in patients with severe hip OA, the body trunk bends forward, resulting in low back pain and sagittal malalignment. In contrast, in acetabular dysplasia of the hip, which is one of the main causes of secondary hip OA, the front coverage area of the acetabulum remains anatomically small. Thus, the compensatory mechanism activates pelvic anteversion, leading to increased LL and SS [25] and eventually resulting in vertebral disk dislocation, foraminal stenosis, radiculopathy, and low back pain [26]. In this situation, the compensatory mechanism is not activated when the spine too undergoes degenerative changes and the hip OA may thus progress.

Since symptoms of lumbar radiculopathy of L3 root nerve greatly vary from thigh pain to hip and/or knee pain, they may appear similar to pain due to hip or knee OA [27]. Thus, lumbar disease might be mistreated as hip and/or knee diseases. Therefore, lumbar diseases should be considered in nonrespondents of hip and knee OA treatment [28].

9. Knee–Spine Syndrome

In the sagittal alignment, spinal kyphosis induces pelvic retroversion, hip extension, knee flexion, and ankle dorsi-flexion as compensation mechanisms [12]. These mechanisms increase the load on the knee joint and lead the progression of knee OA.

A study evaluating compensatory mechanisms of knee OA in older patients reported that knee flexion in mild knee OA was mainly compensated with the lumbar spine to reduce LL and move C7 plumb line forward [29]. Moreover, sagittal balance was not compensated by the lumbar spine only in severe knee OA; the hip was flexed and the pelvis was anteverted with significant forward spinal inclination, resulting in an unbalanced status.

Spinal compensatory abilities are limited for knee flexion because older patients might have spinal deformity, and the flexibility of the spine may be poor [17, 29]. In this condition, the head goes forward, SVA increases, and sagittal malalignment leads to low back pain. Interestingly, knee flexion contracture can lead to loss of LL and anterior sagittal shift in young individuals without any spinal pathology, although it does not influence the pelvis [17].

Tsuji et al. described a correlation between sacral inclination and patella-femoral pain, which is related to changing of lumbar alignment as the knee–spine syndrome [30]. After that, the relationship between the knee and spine involving pelvis has been examined. Murata et al. also evaluated the correlation between the restriction of knee extension and loss of LL [31]. Lumbar malalignment is common in patients older than 70 years of age; however, such restriction of knee extension is predominantly found in patients older than 60 years of age. Therefore, knee OA may occur first, followed by spinal deformity. Harato et al. suggested knee flexion contracture significantly influenced three-dimensional trunk kinematics and would lead to spinal imbalance [32]. Moreover, Tauchi et al. demonstrated the relationship between increased spinal inclination and knee OA as the knee–spine syndrome [33].

10. Spinal Fusion Surgery and Alignment

Loss of LL with age is a common cause of sagittal malalignment of the spine. When the body trunk is located peripherally to the shape of the cone along with markedly increase SVA, surgical interventions with spinal osteotomy and fusion have been applied to improve the abnormal posture. Although the surgical algorithmic approaches for ASD have not been established, a postoperative SVA of <50 mm has been suggested as an optimal target [21, 34]. Aggressive correction of the malignment in older patients increases the risk of proximal junctional kyphosis and treatment failure. However, inflexible deformities generally require more aggressive approaches to achieve adequate correction. Thus, careful planning with operative alignment target and determining spinal flexibility are important to obtain successful outcomes [21].

11. THA and Alignment

Implantation of the acetabular cup in the ideal orientation is necessary to reduce edge loading and to avoid articular impingent; the malposition of prostheses in THA accelerates polyethylene wear and increases risk of hip dislocation. Traditionally, the anteroposterior view of the radiography has been applied to evaluate the cup positioning and implantation of the prosthesis within the safe zone. However, patients with normal standing cup orientation occasionally experience dislocation. Therefore, a new idea of the functional orientation of the acetabular cup has been developed recently, wherein the sagittal pelvic kinematics is involved [35, 36].

Pelvic retroversion progresses with age regardless of THA, and the risk of superior edge loading and anterior hip dislocation increases with hip extension. Patients with sagittal deformities are at an increased relative risk of dislocation and THA revision [37]. Moreover, spinal fusion following THA increases the risk of hip dislocation, particularly involving the fusion of the sacrum. Anterior impingement of the hip in deep hip flexion may be the risk factor for posterior THA dislocation while in stand up from the chair because the pelvis is surgically fixed [38–40]. Moreover, THA following spinal fusion is associated with a high risk of hip posterior dislocation because the pelvis is not posteriorly tilted, which may occur even in the sitting position [35].

Therefore, different reactions of the pelvis in individual patients need to be carefully considered during THA to prevent postoperative hip dislocation. More studies regarding cup positioning are necessary; however, restoration of normal sagittal balance and consideration of patient-specific pelvic kinematics are speculated to be critical [14, 36].

12. TKA and the Alignment

Muscle weakness of the lower extremities and restriction of knee extension in knee OA have been considered to be associated with loss of LL and abnormal posture [31]. However, malalignment of the lower extremities and limited range of motion of the knee, particularly extension, can be improved by TKA. Thus, effects of the spinopelvic alignment following TKA were evaluated, and SS was reported to increase postoperatively in the preoperative knee contracture of >10° [41].

Recently, effects of TKA on sagittal malalignment and variations in the alignment of the spine, pelvis, and lower extremity following TKA were assessed prospectively in our institution [42]. In the present study, the hip flexion was defined as the angle between the femoral shaft and vertical line in the standing position, and SVA ≤ 40 mm was considered normal. Patients with primary knee OA, who were scheduled to undergo primary TKA, were enrolled. However, patients with arthritis secondary to another etiology, such as rheumatoid arthritis, trauma, and previous surgical interventions to the knee, were excluded. Moreover, patients with hip and ankle OA, cranial nerve diseases, and severe spinal deformity were excluded. The study was approved by an institutional review board, and informed consent for participation was obtained from all patients. We observed different patterns of postural changes as well as hip and knee angles following TKA. Three typical cases are presented.

Maintained Normal SVA with the Extension of the Hip and Knee Joints. A case of 69-year-old man who underwent right TKA: the preoperative roentgenographic parameters of SVA, TK, LL, PI, PT, SS, hip flexion, and knee flexion were 14.8 mm, 34°, 40°, 52°, 20°, 32°, 7°, and 18°, respectively (Figure 1(a)). Preoperative SVA was normal and hip and knee joints were flexed while standing. At 12 months after TKA, the parameters of SVA, TK, LL, PI, PT, SS, hip flexion, and knee flexion became 0 mm, 35°, 45°, 55°, 23°, 32°, 1°, and 8°, respectively (Figure 1(b)). These results indicated that SVA remained normal with the extension of hip and knee joints. Some of the patients with the preoperative normal SVA showed that the hip and knee positions tended to extend, lumbar lordosis was decreased, and SVA was increased; however, SVA was still almost within the normal range after TKA.

Abnormal SVA in spite of the Extension of the Hip and Knee Joints. A case of 72-year-old woman who underwent bilateral TKA as a two-stage surgery: the preoperative parameters of SVA, TK, LL, PI, PT, SS, hip flexion, and knee flexion were 75.0 mm, 23°, 23°, 58°, 35°, 23°, 6°, and 17°, respectively (Figure 2(a)). Postoperative evaluations were performed after

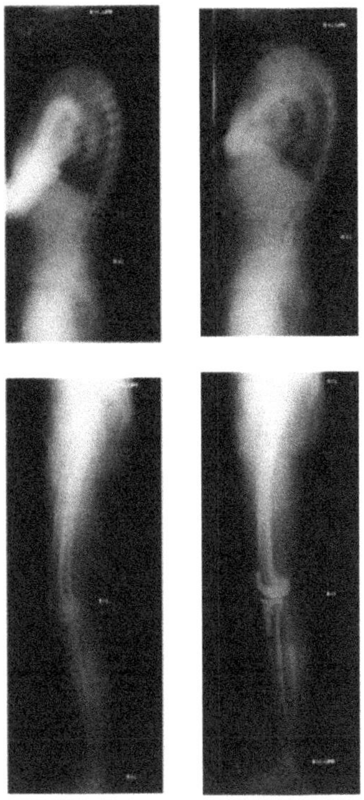

(a) (b)

FIGURE 1: A case of normal SVA with the extension of knee joint (a) before and (b) after the surgery.

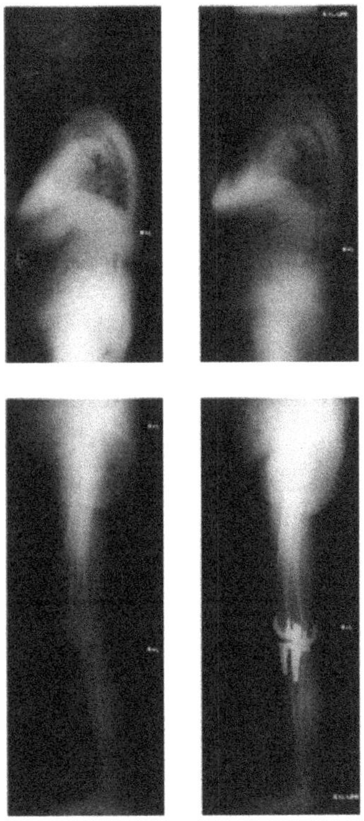

(a) (b)

FIGURE 2: A case of improved abnormal SVA with the extension of knee joint (a) before and (b) after the surgery.

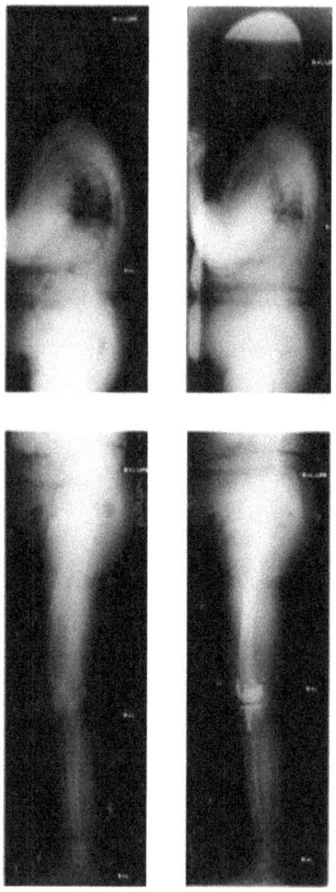

(a) (b)

FIGURE 3: A case of the improved SVA with the extension of hip and knee joints (a) before and (b) after the surgery.

19 and 6 months of right and left TKA, respectively. Postoperative parameters of SVA, TK, LL, PI, PT, SS, hip flexion, and knee flexion became 49.7 mm, 21°, 25°, 54°, 35°, 19°, 5°, and 10°, respectively (Figure 2(b)). Some of the patients with the preoperative abnormal SVA showed that the hip and knee tended to extend; however, pelvic posterior tilt was not improved and SVA was increased, or PT and SVA were increased.

Decreased SVA with the Extension of the Hip and Knee Joints. A case of 74-year-old woman who underwent left TKA: preoperative parameters of SVA, TK, LL, PI, PT, SS, hip flexion, and knee flexion were 70.5 mm, 58°, 57°, 58°, 25°, 33°, 8°, and 17°, respectively (Figure 3(a)). At 12 months after TKA, the parameters of SVA, TK, LL, PI, PT, SS, hip flexion, and knee flexion became 28.4 mm, 50°, 55°, 57°, 23°, 34, 4°, and 7°, respectively (Figure 3(b)). Thus, most patients with the preoperative abnormal SVA showed that the hip and knee became extended, lumbar lordosis increased, and pelvic posterior tilt decreased even after the short-time period of TKA.

Together, these data suggest that knee OA results in the knee flexion while standing. With the progress of knee OA, hip is flexed, pelvis is posteriorly tilted, and the spine is bent forward. However, once the restriction of knee extension is corrected and lower extremity alignment is improved following TKA, lumbar and pelvic parameters are affected even in patients with normal SVA before surgery. Moreover, preoperative abnormal SVA tends to decrease with changes in knee flexion and lumbar parameters as knee–hip–spine syndrome (Figure 4). Therefore, TKA may help recovered knee function and correct lower extremity alignment in severe knee OA as well as improving posture to prevent falls.

13. Knee–Hip–Spine Syndrome

The current THA and TKA strategies have been developing since 1960s. At that time, the longevities of the artificial prostheses were much shorter than those in recent years. However, there were surgeries indicated for older patients and the mean lifespan was much shorter than the present years. Thus, the surgeons only needed a short observation period of the affected site.

Recently, the longevities of prostheses and surgical procedures have dramatically improved. These surgeries have also been performed in younger patients, and generally the mean lifespan has become longer than before. Therefore, long-term follow-up is indispensable after the primary surgery. During this longer period, additional concomitant symptoms may occur with age followed by the original pathology. In

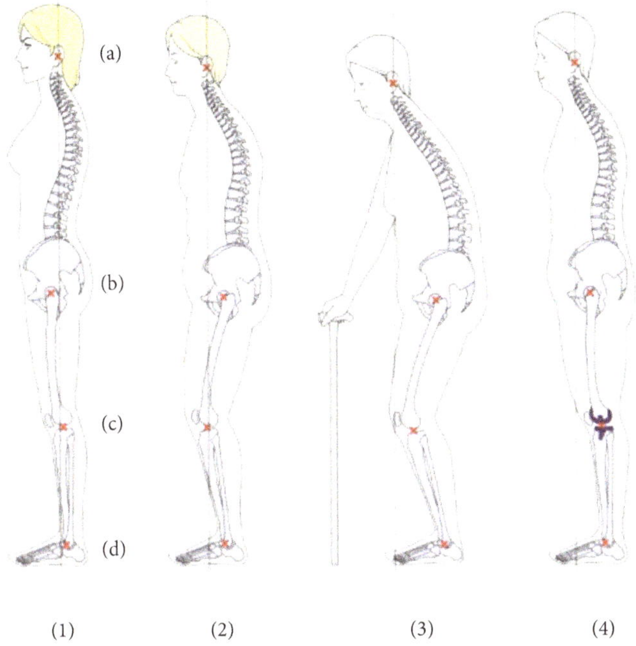

FIGURE 4: Age-related global postural changes. (a) The center of the acoustic meati, (b) the center of the hip, (c) the center of the knee, and (d) the center of the ankle. The vertical line shows the plumb line from the center of the acoustic meati. (1) The global alignment of the healthy subject. The plumb line from the center of the acoustic meati is close to the gravity line. The cervical and thoracic vertebrae are posterior to the gravity line. The lumbar vertebrae show lordosis, and L4 is anterior to the gravity line. The sacrum is posterior, and the hip center is anterior to the gravity line. The knee joint and ankle joint are posterior to the gravity line. (2) TK increases, LL decreases, and the pelvis tilts posteriorly while the hip, knee, and ankle flex. Consequently, the sagittal balance sifts anteriorly with age. (3) Older subjects show spinal kyphosis with the severe anterior shift of the sagittal balance. Consequently, the body balance is better maintained with support. (4) As the knee becomes extended and the lower extremity alignment is corrected with TKA, the global alignment and the sagittal balance can be improved.

addition to THA and TKA, reconstruction of the spinal alignment with the spinal long fusion has emerged as a new approach. Therefore, long-term follow-up after surgeries as well as additional treatments is essential for older patients with complex deformities of multiple structures to improve their QOL.

The spine, hip, and knee are anatomically connected, and all these structures undergo degenerative changes with age as ASD, hip OA, and knee OA. Clinically, pain and discomfort of the low back, hip, and knee are commonly occurring simultaneously, which are referred to as the knee–hip–spine syndrome. Occasionally, physicians misdiagnose and treat the wrong structures. The pendulum test is recommended to detect hip pathology from these symptoms to prevent misdiagnosis [43]. In addition, the abnormal posture occurs with ASD, hip OA, and knee OA. Treatments for the spine, hip, and knee are separated and specialized; however, physicians often carefully examine patients under the consideration with the knee–hip–spine syndrome as differential diagnosis.

At present, physicians often face new challenges of treating the complex multiple degenerative structures or additional degenerative changes following the changes to the primary affected structure. Thus, it is necessary to understand the knee–hip–spine syndrome and to elucidate the etiologies and compensatory mechanisms of the spine, hip, and knee, individually.

14. Conclusion

Musculoskeletal structures are interconnected, and pathologies of these structures are collectively referred to as the knee–hip–spine syndrome. Thus, when each structure is treated, its effect on the entire body must be considered. In this article, we reviewed the association between knee, hip, and spine, and our findings may be helpful for orthopaedic surgeons to bridge the gap between the treatments of these structures.

Abbreviations

QOL: Quality of life
ASD: Adult spinal deformity
hip OA: Osteoarthritis of the hip
THA: Total hip arthroplasty
knee OA: Osteoarthritis of the knee
TKA: Total knee arthroplasty
SVA: Sagittal vertical axis
TK: Thoracic kyphosis
LL: Lumbar lordosis
PI: Pelvic incidence
PT: Pelvic tilt
SS: Sacral slope.

References

[1] F. Schwab, V. Lafage, R. Boyce, W. Skalli, and J. Farcy, "Gravity line analysis in adult volunteers: age-related correlation with spinal parameters, pelvic parameters, and foot position," *The Spine Journal*, vol. 31, no. 25, pp. E959–E967, 2006.

[2] P. Roussouly and J. L. Pinheiro-Franco, "Biomechanical analysis of the spino-pelvic organization and adaptation in pathology," *European Spine Journal*, vol. 20, no. S5, pp. 609–618, 2011.

[3] R. P. Jackson and A. C. McManus, "Radiographic analysis of sagittal plane alignment and balance in standing volunteers and patients with low back pain matched for age, sex, and size: a prospective controlled clinical study," *The Spine Journal*, vol. 19, no. 14, pp. 1611–1618, 1994.

[4] K. Hasegawa, M. Okamoto, S. Hatsushikano et al., "Standing sagittal alignment of the whole axial skeleton with reference to the gravity line in humans," *Journal of Anatomy*, vol. 230, no. 5, pp. 619–630, 2017.

[5] J. Kim, J. Y. Hwang, J. K. Oh et al., "The association between whole body sagittal balance and risk of falls among elderly patients seeking treatment for back pain," *Bone & Joint Research* vol. 6, no. 5, pp. 337–344, 2017.

[6] S. Imagama, Z. Ito, N. Wakao et al., "Influence of spinal sagittal alignment, body balance, muscle strength, and physical ability on falling of middle-aged and elderly males," *European Spine Journal*, vol. 22, no. 6, pp. 1346–1353, 2013.

[7] K. Juhász, I. Boncz, B. Patczai, T. Mintál, and A. Sebestyén, "Risk factors for contralateral hip fractures following femoral neck fractures in elderly: Analysis of the Hungarian nationwide health insurance database," *Eklem Hastalıkları ve Cerrahisi*, vol. 27, no. 3, pp. 146–152, 2016.

[8] T. M. Lawrence, R. Wenn, C. T. Boulton, and C. G. Moran, "Age-specific incidence of first and second fractures of the hip," *The Journal of Bone & Joint Surgery (British Volume)*, vol. 92, no. 2, pp. 258–261, 2010.

[9] C. Jantzen, C. M. Madsen, J. B. Lauritzen, and H. L. Jørgensen, "Temporal trends in hip fracture incidence, mortality, and morbidity in Denmark from 1999 to 2012," *Acta Orthopaedica* vol. 89, no. 2, pp. 170–176, 2018.

[10] J. Herron, R. Hutchinson, F. Lecky et al., "The impact of age on major orthopaedic trauma: An analysis of the United Kingdom trauma audit research network database," *The Bone & Joint Journal*, vol. 99B, no. 12, pp. 1677–1680, 2017.

[11] S. Gawler, D. A. Skelton, S. Dinan-Young et al., "Reducing falls among older people in general practice: The ProAct65+ exercise intervention trial," *Archives of Gerontology and Geriatrics*, vol. 67, pp. 46–54, 2016.

[12] V. Lafage, F. Schwab, A. Patel, N. Hawkinson, and J.-P. Farcy, "Pelvic tilt and truncal inclination: two key radiographic parameters in the setting of adults with spinal deformity," *The Spine Journal*, vol. 34, no. 17, pp. E599–E606, 2009.

[13] R. Vedantam, L. G. Lenke, J. A. Keeney, and K. H. Bridwell, "Comparison of standing sagittal spinal alignment in asymptomatic adolescents and adults," *The Spine Journal*, vol. 23, no. 2, pp. 211–215, 1998.

[14] S. D. Glassman, S. Berven, K. Bridwell, W. Horton, and J. R. Dimar, "Correlation of radiographic parameters and clinical symptoms in adult scoliosis," *The Spine Journal*, vol. 30, no. 6, pp. 682–688, 2005.

[15] M. C. Marks, C. F. Stanford, A. T. Mahar, and P. O. Newton, "Standing lateral radiographic positioning does not represent customary standing balance," *The Spine Journal*, vol. 28, no. 11, pp. 1176–1182, 2003.

[16] Y. Shiba, H. Taneichi, S. Inami, H. Moridaira, D. Takeuchi, and Y. Nohara, "Dynamic global sagittal alignment evaluated by three-dimensional gait analysis in patients with degenerative lumbar kyphoscoliosis," *European Spine Journal*, vol. 25, no. 8, pp. 2572–2579, 2016.

[17] C. S. Lee, S. J. Park, S. S. Chung, and K. H. Lee, "The effect of simulated knee flexion on sagittal spinal alignment: Novel interpretation of spinopelvic alignment," *European Spine Journal*, vol. 22, no. 5, pp. 1059–1065, 2013.

[18] J. C. Le Huec, S. Aunoble, L. Philippe, and P. Nicolas, "Pelvic parameters: origin and significance," *European Spine Journal*, vol. 20, pp. 564–571, 2011.

[19] M. J. Lord, J. M. Small, J. M. Dinsay, and R. G. Watkins, "Lumbar lordosis: Effects of sitting and standing," *The Spine Journal*, vol. 22, no. 21, pp. 2571–2574, 1997.

[20] F. Schwab, B. Ungar, B. Blondel et al., "Scoliosis research society-schwab adult spinal deformity classification: a validation study," *The Spine Journal*, vol. 37, no. 12, pp. 1077–1082, 2012.

[21] S. Iyer, E. Sheha, M. C. Fu et al., "Sagittal spinal alignment in adult spinal deformity," *JBJS Reviews*, vol. 6, no. 5, article no e2, 2018.

[22] M. Cross, E. Smith, D. Hoy et al., "The global burden of hip and knee osteoarthritis: estimates from the global burden of disease 2010 study," *Annals of the Rheumatic Diseases*, vol. 73, no. 7, pp. 1323–1330, 2014.

[23] M. Tsubosaka, T. Matsumoto, K. Takayama, N. Nakano, and R. Kuroda, "Two cases of late medial instability of the knee due to hip disease after total knee arthroplasty," *International Journal of Surgery Case Reports*, vol. 37, pp. 200–204, 2017.

[24] C. M. Offierski and I. Macnab, "Hip-spine syndrome," *The Spine Journal*, vol. 8, no. 3, pp. 316–321, 1983.

[25] Y. Matsuyama, Y. Hasegawa, H. Yoshihara et al., "Hip-spine syndrome: Total sagittal alignment of the spine and clinical symptoms in patients with bilateral congenital hip dislocation," *The Spine Journal*, vol. 29, no. 21, pp. 2432–2437, 2004.

[26] P. Roussouly and C. Nnadi, "Sagittal plane deformity: an overview of interpretation and management," *European Spine Journal*, vol. 19, no. 11, pp. 1824–1836, 2010.

[27] H. Hirabayashi, J. Takahashi, H. Hashidate et al., "Characteristics of L3 nerve root radiculopathy," *World Neurosurgery*, vol. 72, no. 1, pp. 36–40, 2009.

[28] G. R. Fogel and S. I. Esses, "Hip spine syndrome: Management of coexisting radiculopathy and arthritis of the lower extremity," *The Spine Journal*, vol. 3, no. 3, pp. 238–241, 2003.

[29] W. J. Wang, F. Liu, Y. Zhu, M. Sun, Y. Qiu, and W. J. Weng, "Sagittal alignment of the spine-pelvis-lower extremity axis in patients with severe knee osteoarthritis," *Bone & Joint Research*, vol. 5, no. 5, pp. 198–205, 2016.

[30] T. Tsuji, Y. Matsuyama, M. Goto et al., "Knee-spine syndrome: Correlation between sacral inclination and patellofemoral joint pain," *Journal of Orthopaedic Science*, vol. 7, no. 5, pp. 519–523, 2002.

[31] Y. Murata, K. Takahashi, M. Yamagata, E. Hanaoka, and H. Moriya, "The knee-spine syndrome," *The Journal of Bone & Joint Surgery (British Volume)*, vol. 85, no. 1, pp. 95–99, 2003.

[32] K. Harato, T. Nagura, H. Matsumoto, T. Otani, Y. Toyama, and Y. Suda, "A gait analysis of simulated knee flexion contracture to elucidate knee-spine syndrome," *Gait & Posture*, vol. 28, no. 4, pp. 687–692, 2008.

[33] R. Tauchi, S. Imagama, A. Muramoto, M. Tsuboi, N. Ishiguro, and Y. Hasegawa, "Influence of spinal imbalance on knee osteoarthritis in community-living elderly adults," *Nagoya Journal of Medical Science*, vol. 77, no. 3, pp. 329–337, 2015.

[34] F. Schwab, A. Patel, B. Ungar, J.-P. Farcy, and V. Lafage, "Adult spinal deformity-postoperative standing imbalance: how much can you tolerate? An overview of key parameters in assessing alignment and planning corrective surgery," *The Spine Journal*, vol. 35, no. 25, pp. 2224–2231, 2010.

[35] A. A. Sultan, A. Khlopas, N. S. Piuzzi, M. Chughtai, N. Sodhi, and M. A. Mont, "The impact of spino-pelvic alignment on total hip arthroplasty outcomes: a critical analysis of current evidence," *The Journal of Arthroplasty*, vol. 33, no. 5, pp. 1606-1016, 2018.

[36] C. Rivière, J.-Y. Lazennec, C. Van Der Straeten, E. Auvinet, J. Cobb, and S. Muirhead-Allwood, "The influence of spine-hip relations on total hip replacement: A systematic review," *Orthopaedics & Traumatology: Surgery & Research*, vol. 103, no. 4, pp. 559–568, 2017.

[37] D. J. Blizzard, C. T. Penrose, C. Z. Sheets, T. M. Seyler, M. P. Bolognesi, and C. R. Brown, "Ankylosing spondylitis increases perioperative and postoperative complications after total hip arthroplasty," *The Journal of Arthroplasty*, vol. 32, no. 8, pp. 2474–2479, 2017.

[38] V. V. G. An, K. Phan, B. S. Sivakumar, R. J. Mobbs, and W. J. Bruce, "Prior lumbar spinal fusion is associated with an increased risk of dislocation and revision in total hip arthroplasty: a meta-analysis," *The Journal of Arthroplasty*, vol. 33, no. 1, pp. 297–300, 2018.

[39] H. Furuhashi, D. Togawa, H. Koyama, H. Hoshino, T. Yasuda, and Y. Matsuyama, "Repeated posterior dislocation of total hip arthroplasty after spinal corrective long fusion with pelvic fixation," *European Spine Journal*, vol. 26, pp. S100–S106, 2017.

[40] N. A. Bedard, C. T. Martin, S. E. Slaven, A. J. Pugely, S. A. Mendoza-Lattes, and J. J. Callaghan, "Abnormally high dislocation rates of total hip arthroplasty after spinal deformity surgery," *The Journal of Arthroplasty*, vol. 31, no. 12, pp. 2884-2885, 2016.

[41] S.-M. Lee, M. G. Yoon, M.-S. Moon, B.-J. Lee, S.-R. Lee, and Y. H. Seo, "Effect of correction of the contractured flexed osteoarthritic knee on the sagittal alignment by total replacement," *Asian Spine Journal*, vol. 7, no. 3, pp. 204–211, 2013.

[42] Y. Oshima, N. Watanabe, T. Takeoka et al., "Improvement in preoperative abnormal posture after total knee arthroplasty," in *Orthooaedic Research Society 2019 Annual Meeting*, 2019.

[43] Y. Oshima and J. Fetto, "Pendulum test: a highly accurate and simple physical examination maneuver to identify hip pathology," *Reconstructive Review*, vol. 5, no. 3, pp. 45–49, 2015.

14

The Impact of Preoperative Opioid Use Disorder on Complications and Costs following Primary Total Hip and Knee Arthroplasty

Jacob M. Wilson,[1] **Kevin X. Farley**,[1] **Matthew Aizpuru**,[2] **Eric R. Wagner**,[1] **Thomas L. Bradbury**,[1] **and George N. Guild**[1]

[1]*Department of Orthopaedic Surgery, Emory Orthopaedics & Spine Center, 59 S Executive Park NW, Atlanta, GA 30329, USA*
[2]*Emory School of Medicine, 201 Dowman Dr., Atlanta, GA 30322, USA*

Correspondence should be addressed to Jacob M. Wilson; jacobmwilson12@gmail.com

Academic Editor: Panagiotis Korovessis

Introduction. Multiple studies have demonstrated that patients taking opioids in the preoperative period are at elevated risk for complications following total hip (THA) and knee (TKA) arthroplasty. However, the incidence and impact of opioid use disorder (OUD) among these patients—both clinically and fiscally—remain unknown. The purpose of this study was to investigate this relationship. *Methods.* The Nationwide Readmission Database (NRD) was used to identify patients undergoing THA and TKA from 2011 to 2015. Coarsened exact matching was used to statistically match the OUD and non-OUD cohorts. Further analysis was then conducted on matched cohorts with multivariate analysis. The incidence of OUD was also determined, and the costs associated with this comorbidity were calculated. *Results.* The incidence of OUD in arthroplasty patients increased 80% over the study period. OUD patients had higher odds of prosthetic joint infection (OR 1.55, 95% CI 1.23–1.94), wound complication (OR 1.40, 95% CI 1.12–1.76), prosthetic complication (OR 1.37, 95% CI 1.10–1.70), and revision surgery (OR 1.47, 95% CI 1.19–1.81). OUD patients also had longer length of stays (TKA: +0.67 days; THA: +1.09 days), higher readmission (OR 1.60, 95% CI 1.43–1.79), and increased 90-day costs (TKA: +$3,602 [95% CI $3,138–4,065]; THA: +4,527 [95% CI $3,593–4,920). *Conclusion.* Opioid use disorder is becoming a more common comorbidity among THA and TKA patients. This is concerning as it represents a significant risk factor for postoperative complication. It additionally confers increased perioperative costs. Patients with OUD should be counseled on their elevated risk, and future work will be needed to determine if this is a modifiable risk factor.

1. Introduction

The opioid epidemic in the United States is well documented. The United States has experienced an alarming number of drug overdose deaths, and the majority (63% in 2015) involve opioids [1]. This epidemic, not surprisingly, has garnered attention from the media, government, and medical practitioners. In 2017, the White House declared the opioid crisis a public health emergency. While many of the aforementioned overdoses are a result of illicit drug use, prescription opioid use also contributes significantly [2]. Estimates are that patients treated with opioids for chronic pain misuse their narcotics 21–29% of the time, and 8–12% of these patients are addicted to the prescribed drug [3].

In the adult reconstruction realm, prior research has demonstrated that patients prescribed preoperative opioids are at higher risk for perioperative morbidity, revision, and less satisfactory outcomes [4–11]. Much attention has also been paid to postoperative opioid regimens, and there has been increasing recognition that conservative postoperative prescription patterns of opioids can be both safe and effective [12]. However, there has been a substantial increase in the number of patients being prescribed long-term opioids for chronic pain in the community (estimated at a 3-4% of those treated for chronic pain) [13, 14]. While the majority of these prescriptions are not written by orthopedists [15], surgical candidates taking opioids preoperatively are frequently encountered.

Less common is the patient with a diagnosed opioid use disorder (OUD). This diagnosis is defined by the Diagnostic and Statistical Manual of Mental Disorders 5 (DSM-5) as a problematic pattern of opioid use leading to clinically significant impairment or distress. DSM-IV had previously classified the same disorder as opioid abuse or dependence, and this diagnosis is made when 2 of 11 diagnostic criteria are present in a 12-month period [16]. Much less is known about this patient population, and how frequently these patients are receiving total joint arthroplasty is unknown. Defining risk in these patients is critical, and in value-based reimbursement models, understanding the economic impact of this diagnosis is important.

Therefore, the purpose of this investigation was threefold: (1) we sought to determine the incidence of opioid dependence or abuse in the total hip and knee arthroplasty population, (2) to determine if those with opioid dependence are at higher risk for postoperative complication, and (3) to determine the economic burden associated with this diagnosis. We hypothesized that the incidence of opioid dependence among total joint arthroplasty patients is increasing and that these patients would have higher complication rates and increased resource utilization.

2. Materials and Methods

2.1. Data Acquisition. Patients included in this study were selected from the Nationwide Readmission Database (NRD), a publicly available administrative database maintained by the Agency for Healthcare Research and Quality (AHRQ), a part of the Healthcare Cost and Utilization Project (HCUP). Information regarding this database can be found at https://www.hcup-us.ahrq.gov/tech_assist/centdist.jsp. The NRD includes information on patients of all payer types, including the uninsured. The database provides a nationally representative sample and is able to capture all readmissions occurring in the same state, including readmissions to hospitals different from where the index admission took place. The database contains data on the patient's initial inpatient stay, as well as all subsequent inpatient admissions occurring in the same calendar year. It can thus be queried for postoperative inpatient complication data, as well as diagnoses leading to readmission. This allows for the capture of major complications requiring readmission out to 90 days postoperatively.

Patients were identified using the International Classification of Disease, Ninth Revision, Clinical Modification (ICD-9-CM) procedural codes (total hip arthroplasty 81.51; total knee arthroplasty 81.54). The database was queried from 2011 to 2015 quarter 3 (Q3). This was chosen as the end date for this study as this was when the database switched to ICD-10 codes, and exclusion of this transition allowed for equal comparisons. The NRD cannot track patients from year to year, and therefore, we excluded all patients undergoing primary hip or knee arthroplasty in quarter 4 (Q4) of each year as complete 90-day follow-up could not be obtained in these Q4 patients.

ICD-9 diagnosis codes were used to identify patients with opioid use disorders (OUD; abuse or dependence), and the following codes were used: 304.00–304.03, 304.70–304.73, and 305.50–305.53. Similarly, postoperative complications were identified using ICD-9 codes. Hospital costs were calculated using NRD cost-to-charge ratios and were inflation adjusted to the year 2015 using the Consumer Price Index from the Federal Reserve Bank [17].

2.2. Baseline Patient Information. Baseline patient data were collected including the following variables: age, sex, surgery type (THA or TKA), insurance status, zip code income quartile, hospital size, comorbidities, and the presence or not of perioperative transfusion. The included comorbidities were obtained from the Elixhauser Comorbidity Measure [18] and included obesity, diabetes mellitus (DM), preoperative anemia, congestive heart failure (CHF), chronic kidney disease (CKD), chronic obstructive pulmonary disease (COPD), psychiatric illness, and tobacco use. Perioperative transfusion was included in this category as it is well established as a risk factor for postoperative infection [19].

2.3. Outcomes. The incidence of opioid use disorders among total hip and knee arthroplasty patients was calculated on an annual basis by dividing the number of patients with opioid use disorder by the total number of patients undergoing the procedure (with or without OUDs) annually. This was then compared between years. Additionally, we collected information on the following postoperative complications: prosthetic joint infection (PJI), superficial surgical site infection, other wound complications, prosthetic complications (including mechanical complication, loosening, dislocation, prosthetic fracture, and periprosthetic fracture), revision surgery, and postoperative pain (ICD-9 codes 338.18 and 338.19; acute postoperative pain). Complications were included in this study if they occurred on the initial inpatient stay or if they were the cause of readmission. We additionally collected length of stay, readmission, inpatient hospital costs, and 90-day episode costs for all included patients.

2.4. Statistical Analysis. After identification of all patients undergoing THA or TKA, the patients were then divided into two cohorts: patients with and without OUD. HCUP-provided weights were then used to create nationally representative estimates, and further analysis was then conducted. Ultimately, 3,438,105 patients were identified, and of these, 9,832 (0.29%) were found to have a concomitant diagnosis of OUD. First, analysis was conducted comparing baseline patient information between groups using chi-square analysis for categorical values and *t*-tests for continuous variables.

Given the differences identified between nonopioid dependent and OUD patients, statistical matching was performed using coarsened exact matching (CEM) to match patients based on a number of baseline factors. In short, CEM is a validated method of matching [20, 21] that temporarily coarsens data which then allows for exact matching. After matching is performed, typical multivariate analysis can then be conducted on matched cohorts. Patients were matched on all of the variables given in Table 1. While many were significantly different prior to matching, after matching was performed, no differences remained ($p \geq 0.997$). Further analysis was then conducted on these matched cohorts.

Binomial logistic regression, controlling for the variables listed in Table 1, was conducted on matched cohorts to determine if a diagnosis of OUD was an independent predictor of postoperative complications, readmission, or nonhome discharge. Furthermore, cost and LOS were analyzed with linear regression. Additionally, linear regression was used to analyze the trend of incidence of OUD over time. A p value of <0.05 was considered significant. All statistics were performed using SPSS Statistics (IBM Corporation, Version 25, Armonk, NY).

3. Results

3.1. Baseline Patient Information and the Incidence of Opioid Use Disorder. Ultimately, 3,438,105 (THA: 35%, and TKA: 65%) patients were identified for inclusion in this study. 9,982 (0.29%) patients were identified as having a preexisting OUD (opioid abuse or dependency). Analysis comparing baseline patient information between patients with and without OUD was conducted prior to matching. This analysis revealed that opioid dependent patients included significantly more males, significantly more patients with Medicaid (and less with Medicare or private insurance), significantly younger patients, a higher rate of perioperative transfusion, a higher number of patients in lower income quartile zip codes, and a higher number of patients treated at high-volume centers, as well as significantly different comorbidity profiles ($p < 0.001$ for all comparisons) (Table 1).

The incidence of opioid use disorder among those undergoing total hip or knee arthroplasty in the United States was determined by dividing the number of those with OUD each year by the total number of patients undergoing THA or TKA in the corresponding year. We found that the incidence of OUD in arthroplasty patients is increasing significantly, and from 2011 to 2015, the incidence nearly doubled from 0.2% to 0.36% (80% increase, $p < 0.001$) Figure 1.

3.2. Opioid Use Disorder and Postoperative Complications. Multivariate analysis conducted on matched cohorts found significant differences in the odds of multiple postoperative complications. These included prosthetic joint infection (OR 1.55, 95% CI 1.23–1.94, $p < 0.001$), superficial surgical site infection (OR 1.66, 95% CI 1.34–2.05, $p < 0.001$), noninfectious wound complication (OR 1.40, 95% CI 1.12–1.76, $p = 0.003$), prosthetic complication (OR 1.37, 95% CI 1.10–1.70, $p = 0.005$), need for early revision surgery (all cause revision; OR 1.47, 95% CI 1.19–1.81, $p < 0.001$), and for clinically important acute postoperative pain (OR 2.97, 95% CI 2.72–3.23, $p < 0.001$) (Table 2).

3.3. Length of Stay, Nonhome Discharge, 90-Day Readmission, and Economic Burden of Opioid Use Disorder. Multivariate analysis, again controlling for patient characteristics, was conducted to examine postoperative length of stay, nonhome discharge, and 90-day readmission. This analysis revealed that patients with OUD undergoing TKA and THA have significantly longer length of stays (TKA: +0.67 days; THA: +1.09 days, $p < 0.001$) as well as significantly higher odds of nonhome discharge (TKA: OR 1.47, 95% CI 1.30–1.64, $p < 0.001$; THA: OR 1.40, 95% CI 1.28–1.53, $p < 0.001$) and 90-day readmission (TKA: OR 1.60, 95% CI 1.43–1.79, $p < 0.001$; THA: OR 1.53, 95% CI 1.43–1.79, $p < 0.001$). We additionally compared both inpatient and 90-day costs between patients with and without OUD. This analysis revealed that OUD was associated with significantly increased inpatient (TKA: +$2,522 [95% CI $2,170–2,874]; THA: +2,924 [95% CI $2,496–3,353], $p < 0.001$) and total 90-day costs (TKA: +$3,602 [95% CI $3,138–4,065]; THA: +4,527 [95% CI $3,593–4,920], $p < 0.001$) in both TKA and THA (Table 3).

4. Discussion

The current investigation identifies a clear and concerning increase in the incidence of total hip and knee arthroplasty patients with concomitant opioid use disorders. This is troubling given that our study also demonstrates that this cohort of patients is at elevated perioperative risk for complications, increased length of stay, readmission, and resource utilization.

Our results demonstrated that the incidence of opioid use disorder among total hip and knee arthroplasty patients is increasing on an annual basis. This may be expected given the well-established opioid epidemic [13] along with chronic pain prescribing patterns [14]. A similar analysis conducted on pregnant women demonstrated similar findings with significantly increased rates of opioid use disorders over time [22]. The incidence of OUDs in patients undergoing lumbar fusion was found to be 0.91%, which is higher than our identified rate of 0.36% in 2015 [23]. This is also lower than the rate that was found in a similar study performed on patients undergoing lower extremity bypass (0.63%) [24] and lower than the 0.81% that has been reported for the general population [24, 25]. The lower rate observed in our cohort likely reflects the fact that patients undergoing total joint arthroplasty are typically older than the general population, and while substance abuse is becoming more common in a geriatric population [26], it remains much more commonly encountered in younger populations. This is also reflected in our two cohorts. Opioid dependent patients were, on average, younger than those without OUD. We controlled for this fact by matching patients on age and subsequently controlling for age in our multivariate regression.

Though novel, our finding that patients with OUD sustain high postoperative morbidity is consistent with prior literature. Similar analyses conducted on patients undergoing lumbar fusion [23] and lower extremity bypass [24] procedures demonstrated similar results, findings that

TABLE 1: Patient demographics and comorbidities.

Characteristic		Nonopioid dependent (*n* (%))	Opioid dependent (*n* (%))	*p* value Before matching	*p* value After matching
Total patients		3,428,273 (99.7)	9,832 (0.3)		
Surgery type	THA	1,198,470 (35)	4,258 (43.3)	<0.001	0.999
	TKA	2,229,803 (65)	5,574 (56.7)		
Sex	Male	1,347,632 (39.3)	4,693 (47.7)	<0.001	0.999
	Female	2,080,641 (60.7)	5,140 (52.3)		
Insurance	Medicare	1,941,276 (56.7)	4,576 (46.6)	<0.001	0.998
	Private	1,226,412 (35.8)	2,828 (28.8)		
	Medicaid	118,405 (3.5)	1,869 (19.0)		
	Other	137,350 (4.0)	552 (5.6)		
Age category	<55	486,664 (14.2)	3,550 (36.1)	<0.001	0.998
	55–64	984,362 (28.7)	3,852 (39.2)		
	65–74	1,191,172 (34.7)	1,810 (18.4)		
	75–84	653,333 (19.1)	540 (5.5)		
	85+	112,742 (3.3)	81 (0.8)		
Perioperative transfusion		374,279 (10.9)	1,463 (14.9)	<0.001	0.998
Zip code income quartile	1	728,949 (21.6)	2,348 (24.3)	<0.001	0.997
	2	861,933 (25.5)	2,602 (26.9)		
	3	900,568 (26.7)	2,523 (26.1)		
	4	886,595 (26.2)	2,189 (22.7)		
Hospital size	Low	741,092 (21.6)	1,278 (13.0)	<0.001	0.999
	Medium	866,705 (25.3)	2,596 (26.4)		
	High	1,820,476 (53.1)	5,958 (60.6)		
Comorbidity	Obesity	737,221 (21.5)	2,920 (29.7)	<0.001	0.999
	Diabetes	660,785 (19.3)	1,626 (16.5)	<0.001	0.999
	Psychiatric disorder	524,428 (15.3)	3,961 (40.3)	<0.001	0.998
	Anemia	490,946 (14.3)	2,046 (20.8)	<0.001	0.999
	CHF	87,133 (2.5)	335 (3.4)	<0.001	0.998
	Renal failure	165,033 (4.8)	562 (5.7)	<0.001	0.999
	COPD	507,748 (14.8)	2,655 (27.0)	<0.001	0.999
	Tobacco use	268,528 (7.8)	3,028 (30.8)	<0.001	0.998

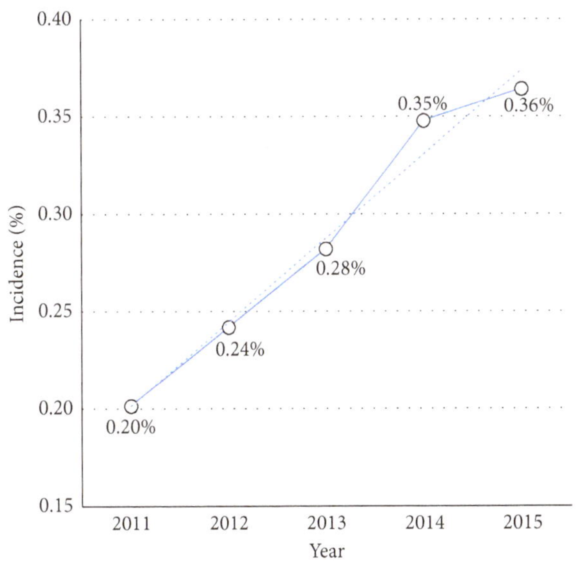

FIGURE 1: The annual incidence of opioid use disorder among patients undergoing total hip or knee arthroplasty in the United States from 2011 to 2015.

patients with OUDs had higher rates of complications and nonhome discharge, as well as increased length of stay and total charges. Additionally, patients who are prescribed preoperative opioids before undergoing a THA or TKA are known to be at higher risk for postoperative complications and increased postoperative opioid consumption [4–7, 9–11, 27]. However, until now, analysis of patients with OUD has been limited to small series [28–30]. This population is likely very different than patients simply receiving opioids preoperatively for pain. In fact, the current study found that patients with opioid use disorder who undergo THA or TKA are on average, younger, from lower income zip codes, more likely to be smokers, and have higher comorbid burdens. These are important differences to consider given their impact on postoperative outcomes. While we took multiple steps (statistical matching and subsequently controlling for these differences in our statistical model) to control for these differences in our analysis, it should be recognized that patients with OUD are likely fundamentally different than those without OUD and the entirety of this difference may be difficult to fully account for. However, even when controlling for these differences

Table 2: Multivariate-adjusted analysis of complications in patients with and without opioid use disorder.

Complication	Nonopioid dependent	Opioid dependent	Odds ratio[a]	p value (multivariate)
Prosthetic joint infection	22,702 (0.7%)	190 (1.9%)	1.55 (1.23–1.94)	<0.001
Superficial surgical site infection	24,020 (0.7%)	216 (2.2%)	1.66 (1.34–2.05)	<0.001
Noninfectious wound complication	30,492 (0.9%)	209 (2.1%)	1.40 (1.12–1.76)	0.003
Prosthetic complication	36,874 (1.1%)	217 (2.2%)	1.37 (1.10–1.70)	0.005
Revision	33,965 (1.0%)	238 (2.4%)	1.47 (1.19–1.81)	<0.001
Postoperative pain	135,788 (4.0%)	1,405 (14.3%)	2.97 (2.72–3.23)	<0.001

[a]Odds ratio with 95% confidence interval obtained through multivariate regression on matched cohorts while controlling for patient and operative characteristics.

Table 3: Multivariate analysis of healthcare utilization-associated factors.

Complication		Nonopioid dependent[a]	Opioid dependent[a]	Beta coefficient or odds ratio[b]	p value (multivariate)
	Nonhome discharge	621,157 (27.9%)	1,729 (31.0%)	1.47 (1.30–1.64)	<0.001
	90-day readmission	190,769 (8.6%)	823 (14.8%)	1.60 (1.43–1.79)	<0.001
TKA	Length of stay (days)	3.43 ± 2.74	4.39 ± 4.22	+0.67 days (0.56–0.78)	<0.001
	Inpatient cost (USD)	$17,013 ± 8,923	$20,394 ± 11,067	+$2,522 (2,170–2,874)	<0.001
	Total 90-day cost (USD)	$18,250 ± 11,575	$22,873 ± 15,793	+$3,602 (3,138–4,065)	<0.001
	Nonhome discharge	327,408 (27.3%)	1,357 (31.9%)	1.40 (1.28–1.53)	<0.001
	90-day readmission	112,624 (9.4%)	777 (18.2%)	1.53 (1.43–1.79)	<0.001
THA	Length of stay (days)	3.48 ± 3.59	5.26 ± 9.40	+1.09 days (0.95–1.24)	<0.001
	Inpatient cost (USD)	$17,943 ± 9,799	$22,307 ± 15,385	+$2,924 (2,496–3,353)	<0.001
	Total 90-day cost (USD)	$19,603 ± 13,252	$26,198 ± 21,360	+$4,257 (3,593–4,920)	<0.001

[a]Presented as mean ± standard deviation for continuous variables or n (%) for categorical variables, and univariate values represent unmatched cohorts.
[b]Odds ratio or beta coefficient with 95% confidence interval obtained through multivariate regression on matched cohorts while controlling for patient and operative characteristics; beta represents an increase in days and dollars associated with an opioid use disorder.

and performing analysis on matched cohorts, rates of complication were significantly higher in the OUD cohort.

Infectious complications have previously been associated with substance abuse, as Bauer et al. found nearly a 40% infection rate in patients who illicitly use intravenous drugs after TKA [31]. Preoperative opioid use has been repeatedly associated with surgical site infections in arthroplasty [9, 11, 27] as well as other general surgery procedures [32, 33]. Why this may be the case is likely multifactorial and could include patient and socioeconomic factors. Nonetheless, some limited evidence exists to suggest that opioids are associated with delayed wound healing which could be partially responsible for some of our observed associations [34]. This is further supported by the finding that OUD patients had significantly higher rates of wound healing issues—both infectious and noninfectious. Direct impairment of immune cells by opioids has also been demonstrated in vitro and in animal models [35].

A significant finding of this investigation is that OUD represents an expensive comorbidity. As value-based models emerge, this is an important consideration and adjustments will need to be made for patients with OUD as they are at increased risk for readmission, complications, and subsequent increased costs. In this study, patients with OUD were significantly more costly. This was by over $2500 + for inpatient costs and $3600 + for total 90-day costs in both THA and TKA. These differences persisted, even when controlling for demographic, procedural, and comorbid data. Alternatively, we do not suggest that prior OUD is a contraindication to arthroplasty as prior studies demonstrate these patients do improve [6]. However, these patients must be recognized and counseled that they are at high risk, and when possible, should be weaned from narcotics preoperatively to reduce their risk of complications [9, 29].

There are multiple limitations to this investigation, most of which are inherent to analysis of large administrative databases. First, our analysis is reliant on accurate coding. It is possible that some patients with opioid abuse or dependence were not coded as such and were therefore included in the incorrect cohort. The same is true of the preoperative comorbidities included in our match and as controls in our multivariate model as well as our examined outcomes. On the same note, we assumed in our analysis that coding frequency stayed the same over time. Our observed increase in incidence, therefore, could be partially accounted for by an increased awareness of the opioid epidemic and increased coding for OUD over time. Similarly, the NRD reports only on patients who were treated as inpatients. Given the movement to outpatient total joint arthroplasty, this likely means that many patients were not captured. However, inclusion of patients treated as outpatients may have actually increased our observed differences between cohorts as these are generally healthy patients with low-risk profiles. Generally, opioid use disorder would be considered a contraindication to outpatient arthroplasty [36] and it, therefore, is likely that the vast majority of these patients have been captured in this investigation. Additionally, using the NRD, only inpatient complications are captured unless the complication leads to readmission and even readmissions are tracked only to 90 days. This could mean that our complication rates are underestimated. Last, it is true that complete isolation of OUD may be difficult. Still, this analysis was performed on matched cohorts and controlling for available comorbid, socioeconomic, and procedural data, likely providing the best analysis possible.

Despite its limitations, the use of the Nationwide Readmission Database is a strength of this study as it allows for national estimates and provides a very large, all-payer sample. It additionally allows for controlling of socioeconomic factors by reporting insurance status as well as zip code income quartile. Both factors that have been associated with outcomes [37–39], and the ability to control for these represents an important strength compared to other database studies. Also, readmissions can be tracked even if the readmission occurs at a different institution, therefore providing a higher capture rate for outcomes. Additionally, trends in incidence of OUD in the arthroplasty population could not confidently be reported without the use of a large administrative database, representing an advantage over single-institution studies. Finally, the NRD provides charge-cost ratios and reports economic data allowing for quantification of the additional cost conferred by OUD as a comorbid condition. As value-based reimbursement models emerge and evolve, this information is invaluable.

In conclusion, opioid use disorder as a preoperative comorbid condition is becoming increasingly common in the primary total hip and total knee arthroplasty patients. This is an important finding as this patient cohort has elevated risk for multiple important complications, readmission, extended length of stay, and increased economic burden in the early postoperative period. This patient population must be counseled on their elevated risks. Furthermore, this study adds to the evidence suggesting these patients should be weaned from preoperative narcotics, as opioid freedom prior to surgery, even after long-term use, confers a risk reduction [6, 7, 9, 27]. Future research may be directed at evaluating preoperative opioid use in morphine equivalents to determine cutoff values for safe surgery.

References

[1] P. Seth, L. Scholl, R. A. Rudd, and S. Bacon, "Overdose deaths involving opioids, cocaine, and psychostimulants—United States, 2015-2016," *MMWR. Morbidity and Mortality Weekly Report*, vol. 67, no. 12, pp. 349–358, 2018.

[2] A. D. Kaye, M. R. Jones, A. M. Kaye et al., "Prescription opioid abuse in chronic pain: an updated review of opioid abuse predictors and strategies to curb opioid abuse: Part 1," *Pain Physician*, vol. 20, no. 2S, pp. S93–S109, 2017.

[3] K. E. Vowles, M. L. McEntee, P. S. Julnes, T. Frohe, J. P. Ney, and D. N. van der Goes, "Rates of opioid misuse, abuse, and addiction in chronic pain," *Pain*, vol. 156, no. 4, pp. 569–576, 2015.

[4] J. C. Rozell, P. M. Courtney, J. R. Dattilo, C. H. Wu, and G.-C. Lee, "Preoperative opiate use independently predicts narcotic consumption and complications after total joint arthroplasty," *The Journal of Arthroplasty*, vol. 32, no. 9, pp. 2658–2662, 2017.

[5] S. R. Smith, J. Bido, J. E. Collins, H. Yang, J. N. Katz, and E. Losina, "Impact of preoperative opioid use on total knee arthroplasty outcomes," *The Journal of Bone and Joint Surgery*, vol. 99, no. 10, pp. 803–808, 2017.

[6] C. M. Goplen, W. Verbeek, S. H. Kang et al., "Preoperative opioid use is associated with worse patient outcomes after total joint arthroplasty: a systematic review and meta-analysis," *BMC Musculoskelet Disord*, vol. 20, no. 1, p. 234, 2019.

[7] A. Ben-Ari, H. Chansky, and I. Rozet, "Preoperative opioid use is associated with early revision after total knee arthroplasty," *The Journal of Bone and Joint Surgery*, vol. 99, no. 1, pp. 1–9, 2017.

[8] J. Starr, I. Rozet, and A. Ben-Ari, "A risk calculator using preoperative opioids for prediction of total knee revision arthroplasty," *The Clinical Journal of Pain*, vol. 34, no. 4, pp. 328–331, 2018.

[9] N. Jain, J. L. Brock, A. T. Malik, F. M. Phillips, and S. N. Khan, "Prediction of complications, readmission, and revision surgery based on duration of preoperative opioid use," *The Journal of Bone and Joint Surgery*, vol. 101, no. 5, pp. 384–391, 2019.

[10] J. Weick, H. Bawa, D. R. Dirschl, and H. H. Luu, "Preoperative opioid use is associated with higher readmission and revision rates in total knee and total hip arthroplasty," *The Journal of Bone and Joint Surgery*, vol. 100, no. 14, pp. 1171–1176, 2018.

[11] K. L. Bell, N. Shohat, K. Goswami, T. L. Tan, I. Kalbian, and J. Parvizi, "Preoperative opioids increase the risk of periprosthetic joint infection after total joint arthroplasty," *The Journal of Arthroplasty*, vol. 33, no. 10, pp. 3246–3251.e1, 2018.

[12] A. J. Holte, C. N. Carender, N. O. Noiseux, J. E. Otero, and T. S. Brown, "Restrictive opioid prescribing protocols following total hip arthroplasty and total knee arthroplasty are safe and effective," *The Journal of Arthroplasty*, vol. 34, no. 7, pp. S135–S139, 2019.

[13] N. D. Volkow and A. T. McLellan, "Opioid abuse in chronic pain—misconceptions and mitigation strategies," *New England Journal of Medicine*, vol. 374, no. 13, pp. 1253–1263, 2016.

[14] D. Boudreau, M. Von Korff, C. M. Rutter et al., "Trends in long-term opioid therapy for chronic non-cancer pain," *Pharmacoepidemiology and Drug Safety*, vol. 18, no. 12, pp. 1166–1175, 2009.

[15] R. S. Namba, E. W. Paxton, and M. C. Inacio, "Opioid prescribers to total joint arthroplasty patients before and after surgery: the majority are not orthopedists," *The Journal of Arthroplasty*, vol. 33, no. 10, pp. 3118–3124.e3, 2018.

[16] American Psychiatric Association, *Diagnostic and Statistical Manual of Mental Disoders: DSM-5*, American Psychiatric Association Publishing, Washington, DC, USA, 2013.

[17] S. L. Fed, "Economic research: consumer price indexes (CPI and PCE)," https://fred.stlouisfed.org/categories/9.

[18] A. Elixhauser, C. Steiner, D. R. Harris, and R. M. Coffey, "Comorbidity measures for use with administrative data," *Medical Care*, vol. 36, no. 1, pp. 8–27, 1998.

[19] J. L. Kim, J.-H. Park, S.-B. Han, I. Y. Cho, and K.-M. Jang, "Allogeneic blood transfusion is a significant risk factor for surgical-site infection following total hip and knee arthroplasty: a meta-analysis," *The Journal of Arthroplasty*, vol. 32, no. 1, pp. 320–325, 2017.

[20] S. M. Iacus, G. King, and G. Porro, "Causal inference without balance checking: coarsened exact matching," *Political Analysis*, vol. 20, no. 1, pp. 1–24, 2012.

[21] S. M. Iacus, G. King, and G. Porro, "Multivariate matching methods that are monotonic imbalance bounding," *Journal of the American Statistical Association*, vol. 106, no. 493, pp. 345–361, 2011.

[22] S. C. Haight, J. Y. Ko, V. T. Tong, M. K. Bohm, and W. M. Callaghan, "Opioid use disorder documented at delivery hospitalization—United States, 1999-2014," *MMWR. Morbidity and Mortality Weekly Report*, vol. 67, no. 31, pp. 845–849, 2018.

[23] M. L. Martini, D. A. Nistal, B. C. Deutsch, and J. M. Caridi, "Characterizing the risk and outcome profiles of lumbar fusion procedures in patients with opioid use disorders: a step toward improving enhanced recovery protocols for a unique patient population," *Neurosurgical Focus*, vol. 46, no. 4, p. E12, 2019.

[24] M. Aizpuru, L. K. Gallo, K. X. Farley et al., "Economic burden and clinical impact of pre-operative opioid dependence for patients undergoing lower extremity bypass surgery," *Journal of Vascular Surgery*, 2019, in Press.

[25] Medicine ASoA, "Opioid addiction: 2016 facts and figures," 2016, https://www.asam.org/docs/default-source/advocacy/opioid-addiction-disease-facts-figures.pdf.

[26] S. Yarnell, L. Li, B. MacGrory, L. Trevisan, and P. Kirwin, "Substance use disorders in later life: a review and synthesis of the literature of an emerging public health concern," *The American Journal of Geriatric Psychiatry*, 2019, in Press.

[27] M. Blevins Peratikos, H. L. Weeks, A. J. B. Pisansky, R. J. Yong, and E. A. Stringer, "Effect of preoperative opioid use on adverse outcomes, medical spending, and persistent opioid use following elective total joint arthroplasty in the United States: a large retrospective cohort study of administrative claims data," *Pain Medicine*, 2019.

[28] C. R. Lehman, M. D. Ries, G. D. Paiement, and A. B. Davidson, "Infection after total joint arthroplasty in patients with human immunodeficiency virus or intravenous drug use," *The Journal of Arthroplasty*, vol. 16, no. 3, pp. 330–335, 2001.

[29] L.-C. L. Nguyen, D. C. Sing, and K. J. Bozic, "Preoperative reduction of opioid use before total joint arthroplasty," *The Journal of Arthroplasty*, vol. 31, no. 9, pp. 282–287, 2016.

[30] K. Wieser, P. O. Zingg, M. Betz, G. Neubauer, and C. Dora, "Total hip replacement in patients with history of illicit injecting drug use," *Archives of Orthopaedic and Trauma Surgery*, vol. 132, no. 7, pp. 1037–1044, 2012.

[31] D. E. Bauer, A. Hingsammer, L. Ernstbrunner et al., "Total knee arthroplasty in patients with a history of illicit intravenous drug abuse," *International Orthopaedics*, vol. 42, no. 1, pp. 101–107, 2018.

[32] D. C. Cron, M. J. Englesbe, C. J. Bolton et al., "Preoperative opioid use is independently associated with increased costs and worse outcomes after major abdominal surgery," *Annals of Surgery*, vol. 265, no. 4, pp. 695–701, 2017.

[33] A. D. Harris, B. Fleming, J. S. Bromberg et al., "Surgical site infection after renal transplantation," *Infection Control & Hospital Epidemiology*, vol. 36, no. 4, pp. 417–423, 2015.

[34] V. K. Shanmugam, K. S. Couch, S. McNish, and R. L. Amdur, "Relationship between opioid treatment and rate of healing in chronic wounds," *Wound Repair and Regeneration*, vol. 25, no. 1, pp. 120–130, 2017.

[35] L. M. Plein and H. L. Rittner, "Opioids and the immune system—friend or foe," *British Journal of Pharmacology*, vol. 175, no. 14, pp. 2717–2725, 2018.

[36] R. M. Meneghini, M. Ziemba-Davis, M. K. Ishmael, A. L. Kuzma, and P. Caccavallo, "Safe selection of outpatient joint arthroplasty patients with medical risk stratification: the "outpatient arthroplasty risk assessment score"," *The Journal of Arthroplasty*, vol. 32, no. 8, pp. 2325–2331, 2017.

[37] D. Shau, N. Shenvi, K. Easley, M. Smith, T. Bradbury, and G. Guild III, "Medicaid payer status is associated with increased 90-day morbidity and resource utilization following primary total hip arthroplasty," *The Journal of Bone and Joint Surgery*, vol. 100, no. 23, pp. 2041–2049, 2018.

[38] D. Shau, N. Shenvi, K. Easley, M. Smith, and G. Guild III, "Medicaid is associated with increased readmission and resource utilization after primary total knee arthroplasty: a propensity score-matched analysis," *Arthroplasty Today*, vol. 4, no. 3, pp. 354–358, 2018.

[39] P. M. Courtney, J. I. Huddleston, R. Iorio, and D. C. Markel, "Socioeconomic risk adjustment models for reimbursement are necessary in primary total joint arthroplasty," *The Journal of Arthroplasty*, vol. 32, no. 1, pp. 1–5, 2017.

15

Health-Related Quality of Life and Outcome after Total Knee Replacement: Results from a Cross-Sectional Survey in Jordan

Yazan Al Thaher[1] **Othman A. Alfuqaha**[2] **and Ahmed Dweidari**[3]

[1]*Faculty of Pharmacy, Philadelphia University, Amman 19392, Jordan*
[2]*Scientific Research Office, Jordan University Hospital, The University of Jordan, Amman 11942, Jordan*
[3]*Department of Special Procedure, Division of Orthopedics, School of Medicine, The University of Jordan, Amman 11942, Jordan*

Correspondence should be addressed to Othman A. Alfuqaha; othman_alfoqaha@yahoo.com

Academic Editor: Francesco Liuzza

Total knee replacement (TKR) is a common procedure that is considered cost-effective with excellent long-term survivorship. This cross-sectional study, which includes 118 selected patients in Jordan from January 2020 to January 2021, aims to assess health-related quality of life (HQOL), functional status, and associated factors before and after 3 to 12 months of TKR. Furthermore, several demographical factors were included in this study to evaluate the potential association with the procedure's outcome. Western Ontario and McMaster Universities Osteoarthritis Index scale (WOMAC) and Short Form-36 (SF-36) scale were used in this study. It was found that the main change occurred 6–12 months after the procedure. Gender and age were found to be the primary predictor of quality of life among TKR patients. Patients before the TKR procedure experienced severe pain, joint stiffness, physical impairment, and psychological demand issues. After the TKR procedure, all symptoms were improved significantly. The TKR procedure can improve the quality of life for patients, which can be detected for several months after the procedure. Function and pain are the most critical indicators of improvement in quality of life. Assessing the quality of life is a key indicator for identifying patients without improvement, as well as improving the health care process and comparing other alternative interventions.

1. Introduction

Osteoarthritis of the knee is a prevalent problem that causes pain and functional limitations, especially in the elderly population (>80% in population above 65 years) [1]. Common treatments for osteoarthritis involve the use of medications (e.g., nonsteroidal anti-inflammatory drugs) [2]. Other treatment approaches involve physical therapy, for example, backward walking on static stability [3], topical sesame oil [4], and topical *Linum usitatissimum* L. (flaxseed) oil [5]. End-stage osteoarthritis, disability, and loss of HQOL all necessitate TKR, which relieves pain, improves long-term function, and restores mobility. The TKR is one of the common procedures performed globally and is considered cost-effective with excellent long-term survivorship, with substantial variations in rates across different countries [6, 7].

Although most patients have a favorable clinical outcome after TKR, several studies have reported that more than 20% of patients are dissatisfied with the outcome after procedure [8–10]. This deficiency in patient satisfaction drives research and development in this field. Improving outcomes can be done by changing implant design, implantation methods, improving preoperative care for patients, etc. Therefore, measuring patients' quality of life and their perception of the procedure is of paramount value to improve this procedure and increase the proportion of patients who have successful outcomes and improved quality of life [10].

A highly effective evaluation for the outcome after TKR is essential for making patient-reported outcome measures. The outcome evaluation should account for different aspects of the patient's life, including activity and functional aspects, social aspects, as well as psychological or emotional aspects [9]. Several scores are developed for this purpose, which features the patient in the assessment of the TKR outcome. These scores can be divided into two types: those measuring HQOL for aspects that can be influenced by feelings of physical well-being or mental state and those evaluating the knee function and pain. Examples of the former are the 36-Item Short Form (SF-36) and 12-Item Short Form (SF-12) that are not specific for the outcome after TKR. However, more specific scores are available, such as the Osteo Arthritis Knee and Hip Quality of Life (OAKHQOL) and the Knee Quality of Life-26 (KQOL-26). The second type of score is called functional scores, which evaluate the knee function and pain, such as the Knee Society Score, WOMAC, and Oxford Knee Score. A combination of these two types of scores is mostly used to evaluate the outcome after TKR [11, 12].

Most studies in the literature use one generic score from the first type previously mentioned and one specific score from the second type [9, 13]. The two questionnaires complement each other and measure different aspects of patient outcomes. The SF-36 and WOMAC scores are the most commonly used combination in literature [14]. While the WOMAC score measures the joint's stiffness, pain, and physical functioning, the SF-36 measures HQOL for the patient.

This study aims to assess HQOL, functional status, and associated factors before and after TKR, consequently, measuring the clinical effectiveness or outcome of the TKR. There was no recent multicenter data regarding preoperative or postoperative measurement for HQOL or patient outcomes in Jordan. This helps identify patient satisfaction deficiencies to make future patient-informed measures to this procedure and improve current clinical practice. The results will be important for orthopedics and physicians who treat TKR patients. Herein, HQOL was evaluated before and after TKR. Moreover, patients' HQOL was evaluated in patients after 3 to 12 months after TKR. Several demographical factors were included in this study to assess any potential association with the procedure's outcome.

2. Materials and Methods

2.1. Design. This cross-sectional study evaluates the HQOL, outcome, and functional status before and after TKR among patients in Jordan. The authors adhered to STROBE guidelines.

2.2. Settings and Participants. The population of this study comprises all patients on the waiting list for TKR who have been diagnosed with knee osteoarthritis and patients who have had TKR. This study was conducted in a tertiary hospital in Amman (the capital of Jordan) since they had the largest number of TKR patients in Jordan, among other Jordanian cities. All patients admitted to the hospital for TKR in 2020 were invited to participate in this study. According to a previous study [15], a total of 100–300 samples will have a confidence interval of 95% and an error estimation of 5%. Exclusion criteria were patients with a road traffic accident that caused TKR, malignant tumors, and psychiatric disorders. Consecutive patients with primary TKR in the selected hospital were eligible to participate in this study. In the selected hospital, a total of 200 TKR patients had the procedure in 2020 in the selected hospital. A convenient sampling process was selected to collect the data over one year (from January 2020 to January 2021). A total of 118 patients were followed up and completed an envelope survey, with a response rate of 59%. All patients received a letter informing them about the study and asking for voluntary participation. Patients were followed before TKR and up to a year after procedure.

Patients visited the orthopedic clinic within the first 3 months and 3 to 6 months after having a TKR procedure. During their visit, data were collected through an interview. Patients were contacted 6 months to 12 months after TKR procedure by phone for data collection because they usually do not come to the clinic unless serious complications happen. However, all participants completed the SF-36 and WOMAC scores, as well as additional questions about the clinical disease aspects and sociodemographic information. The data were collected from participants before and after the procedure within one year after the procedure. After the procedure, patients who did not come to the clinic were contacted via phone call. The ethical guidelines of scientific research were followed during the interview and phone call.

2.3. Data Measurement. Patients were asked to complete the following scales.

2.3.1. Part One. Sociodemographic characteristics of patients included gender, age, marital status, educational level, weight, height, body mass index (BMI), location, site of knee procedure, previous TKR procedure, and comorbidities.

2.3.2. Part Two. WOMAC scale was used in this study. This scale consisted of 24 items divided into three dimensions: pain severity (5 items), joint stiffness (2 items), and daily physical daily functioning of the joint (17 items). A five-point Likert type scale was used to answer the items of WOMAC scale from 1 "None" to 5 "Extremely." It is widely recognized that the WOMAC scale has reliable psychometric properties [16]. Alfatafta [17] recently found that the Arabic WOMAC scale is an effective tool to evaluate the quality of life among Jordanian patients after a TKR. Therefore, the Arabic version of the WOMAC scale was used, and its validity and reliability were checked. The five-point Likert mean score has a mild mean score from 1 to 2.33, a moderate mean score from 2.34 to 3.67, and a high mean score from 3.68 to 5. A high mean score represents severe pain, stiffness, and difficulties in performing daily activities.

2.3.3. Part Three. SF-36 was used in this study. It consists of 36 items divided into two main dimensions: physical demand (22 items) and psychological demand HQOL (14 items). Since the WOMAC scale measures the physical

Table 1: Correlation coefficients and Cronbach's alpha for the scales used in this study.

#	Factor	1	2	3	4	5	Cronbach's alpha
1	Total WOMAC scale	—					0.84
2	Pain severity	0.62**	—				0.76
3	Joint stiffness	0.31**	0.37**	—			0.62
4	Physical functioning impairment	0.71**	0.30**	0.46**	—		0.79
5	Psychological demand (SF-36)	0.28**	0.21**	0.01	0.22**	—	0.76

** *P* value: <0.001.

demand, the psychological demand section was only taken from SF-36 to measure different aspects of psychological issues such as emotional problems, depression, worn out, downheartedness, and lack of accomplishment. The Arabic version of SF-36 was used after obtaining the necessary permissions [18], and this scale's validity and reliability were checked. A five-point Likert type scale was used to answer the 14 items of the SF-36 scale from 1 "None" to 5 "Extremely." The cut-off point for this scale was measured the same as for the WOMAC scale. A high mean score represents severe emotional problems, downheartedness, blue, and lack of accomplishment.

2.4. Validity and Reliability. Validity and reliability were assessed for the Arabic scales used in this study. Cronbach's alpha, correlation coefficient, Kaiser–Meyer–Olkin (KMO) test, and Bartlett's test of sphericity were calculated (presented in Table 1).

As shown in Table 1, Cronbach's alpha for the WOMAC scale and SF-36 were considered applicable. Pearson correlation coefficient ranged between 0.31 and 0.71 for the Arabic WOMAC scale, and its dimension indicated a discriminant validity due to moderate correlation. A positive correlation coefficient was found between the total WOMAC scale and (SF-36) psychological demand. The KMO test was 0.75 for the Arabic WOMAC scale, which is considered adequate (>0.70) [19]. Bartlett's test of sphericity $p < 0.05$ was deemed significant [19]. Regarding (SF-36) psychological demand dimension, the KMO test was 0.76 and Bartlett's test of sphericity was significant. These results suggested that the Arabic WOMAC scale and Arabic SF-36 were valid and reliable for this study.

2.5. Statistical Analysis. The Statistical Package for the Social Sciences (SPSS) version 22 was used to analyze the study results. Descriptive statistics, multiple linear regression analysis (stepwise method), Pearson correlation coefficients, and *t*-test were used in this study.

2.6. Ethical Considerations. Ethical approval was obtained from the institutional review boards in the selected hospital (No. 10/2020/21599) before collecting the information for this study. The study's primary aim was explained to all patients, and they were informed about their right to refuse or withdraw from the study. Moreover, patients were informed about confidentiality and anonymity during data analysis.

3. Results

One hundred eighteen patients participated in this study, with a total response rate of 59% of the total number of participants (200 patients). Females represented 53.8% of the sample. All participants were married and had a mean age of 66 years, and the majority lived at central of Jordan (Table 2).

The educational level for most of the participants was high school or less, while participants' average BMI was found to be overweight (26.17 ± 3.32). The location of the knee procedure was almost equal between the right and left sides. Diabetes mellitus and hypertension were found to be the most common comorbidities among participants in this study.

The differences in quality of life among participants are shown in Table 3, where the quality of life was calculated before and after TKR and means, standard deviations, percentages, *t*-test, and *p* value.

Before the TKR procedure, patients experienced severe pain, joint stiffness, physical impairment, and psychological demand issues. Physical functioning impairment before TKR procedure exhibited the highest mean score on the WOMAC scale. On the other hand, psychological demand (SF-36) in patients before TKR reported severe anxiety levels, downheartedness, emotional problems, and lack of accomplishment. After TKR procedure, there was a significant improvement in all dimensions of the WOMAC scale, with an overall mild level. Physical functioning impairment was decreased significantly after the TKR procedure. Psychological demand in SF-36 decreased significantly to a moderate level. Furthermore, the quality of life after TKR procedure was improved significantly, as expressed by the total WOMAC scale.

During the data collection period, participants were added into 3 major groups according to the date of follow-up after a TKR procedure. A total of 38 participants were seen in orthopedic clinics within the first 3 months of the TKR procedure (group 1), 48 participants were seen between 3 and 6 months after the TKR (group 2), and a total of 32 participants were contacted by phone from 6 months to 12 months after the TKR (group 3). The demographic factors of these three groups are shown in Table 4.

Moreover, means, standard deviations, and overall level were calculated to measure the quality of life among these groups, as shown in Table 5.

Regarding the psychological demand, a *t*-test was performed between groups 1, 2, and 3 and the results showed no significant association between all three groups ($p > 0.05$). Regarding the total quality of life, there was a significant

Table 2: Patients' demographics ($N = 118$).

Variables	Descriptive	Frequency (%)
Gender	Male	54 (45.4)
	Female	64 (53.8)
Marital status	Single	0
	Married	103 (87.3)
	Divorced/widow	15 (12.7)
Age (years)	M ± SD	66.06 ± 6.83
Body mass index	Weight/(height^2)	26.17 ± 3.32
Location	Middle	87 (73.7)
	South	23 (19.5)
	North	8 (6.8)
Educational level	High school or less	66 (55.9)
	Diploma degree	28 (23.7)
	Bachelor's degree	24 (20.3)
	Postgraduate degree	0
Site of knee procedure	Right knee	56 (47.5)
	Left knee	49 (41.5)
	Both knees	13 (11)
Previous TKR procedure	No	101 (85.6)
	Once	14 (11.9)
	More than once	3 (2.5)
Comorbidities	Not applicable	13 (11.1)
	Diabetes mellitus	17 (14.4)
	Hypertension	19 (8.5)
	Diabetes mellitus + hypertension	59 (50)
	Arthritis	10 (8.5)

M ± SD: mean ± standard deviation.

Table 3: The quality-of-life differences among patients before and after TKR ($N = 118$).

Variables		Before TKR, M ± SD	Status level	After TKR, M ± SD	Status level	t-test	p value
Psychological demand (SF-36)		3.88 ± 0.37	Severe	2.36 ± 0.21	Moderate	19.13	<0.001**
Quality of life (WOMAC scale)	Pain severity	3.95 ± 0.46	Severe	1.86 ± 0.31	Mild	13.45	<0.001**
	Joint stiffness	3.91 ± 0.67	Severe	1.79 ± 0.50	Mild	12.43	<0.001**
	Physical functioning impairment	4.03 ± 0.30	Severe	1.96 ± 0.26	Mild	14.69	<0.001**
	Total WOMAC scale	4.00 ± 0.31	Severe	1.92 ± 0.21	Mild	14.36	<0.001**

M ± SD: mean ± standard deviation; TKR: total knee replacement. **p value: <0.001.

difference between groups 1 and 2 ($t = 4.99$, $p < 0.001$) and between groups 1 and 3 ($t =$, $p < 0.001$). However, there was no significant difference between groups 2 and 3 ($t = 0.23$, $p < 0.82$). Group 3 had the lowest mean score among other groups, with an improved quality of life status. In the current study, the best improvement in the quality of life was from 6 to 12 months after TKR. Overall, patients presented lower levels of pain, stiffness, and psychological issues.

Finally, linear regression analysis (stepwise method) was conducted (as shown in Table 6) to study the contribution of many demographic factors such as gender, age, marital status, educational level, BMI, location, qualification, and site of the knee procedure in predicting quality of life outcome.

Gender and age are the main predictors of quality of life among TKR patients, with a total variation of 39.4%. While gender was found to account for 37.1% of the variances in quality of life ($R^2 = 0.371$, $p < 0.001$), age was a significant predictor of quality of life with a total variation of 2.3% ($R^2 = 0.023$, $p < 0.05$). Descriptive statistics were performed to determine which gender type and age categories had more levels of quality of life after TKR procedure. The results showed that male patients had higher levels of quality of life than female patients ($\text{mean}_{\text{male}} = 2.06$, $\text{mean}_{\text{female}} = 1.80$). Based on age categories, mean ages below 65 years are associated with a higher quality of life after TKR. However, other factors such as marital status, educational level, BMI, location, qualification, and site of knee procedure were excluded as predictors in this study.

4. Discussion

The results of this study provided information about the quality of life and outcome of TKR patients. This study provides information about pain, stiffness, physical impairment, and psychological demand issues before TKR and

Table 4: Participants' demographics based on groups.

Variables	Descriptive	Group 1, $n = 38$, frequency (%)	Group 2, $n = 48$, frequency (%)	Group 3, $n = 32$, frequency (%)
Gender	Male	25 (21.2)	18 (15.3)	11 (9.3)
	Female	13 (11)	30 (25.4)	21 (17.8)
Marital status	Single	0	0	0
	Married	34 (28.8)	42 (35.6)	27 (22.9)
	Divorced/widow	4 (3.4)	6 (5.1)	5 (4.2)
Age (Years)	M ± SD	66.76 ± 7.05	66.04 ± 6.51	66.25 ± 7.14
Body Mass index	Weight/(height^2)	25.71 ± 3.34	26.37 ± 3.40	26.41 ± 3.23
Location	Middle	30 (25.4)	37 (31.4)	20 (16.9)
	South	7 (5.9)	9 (7.6)	7 (5.9)
	North	1 (0.8)	2 (1.7)	5 (4.2)
Educational level	High school or less	21 (17.8)	25 (21.2)	20 (16.9)
	Diploma degree	9 (7.6)	13 (11)	6 (5.1)
	Bachelor's degree	8 (6.8)	10 (8.5)	6 (5.1)
	Postgraduate degree	0	0	0
Site of knee procedure	Right knee	16 (13.6)	27 (22.9)	13 (11)
	Left knee	18 (15.3)	16 (13.6)	15 (12.7)
	Both knees	4 (3.4)	5 (4.2)	4 (3.4)
Previous TKR procedure	No	31 (26.3)	42 (35.6)	28 (23.7)
	Once	6 (5.1)	5 (4.2)	3 (2.5)
	More than once	1 (0.8)	1 (0.8)	1 (0.8)
Comorbidities	Not applicable	3 (2.5)	9 (7.6)	4 (3.4)
	Diabetes mellitus	5 (4.2)	9 (7.6)	6 (5.1)
	Hypertension	8 (6.8)	9 (7.6)	4 (8.5)
	Diabetes Mellitus + hypertension	21 (17.8)	16 (13.5)	17 (14.4)
	Arthritis	1 (0.8)	5 (4.2)	1 (0.8)

%: percentage of total. M ± SD: mean ± standard deviation.

Table 5: The duration differences of quality of life among patients after TKR ($N = 118$).

Variables		Group 1, M ± SD	Status level	Group 2, M ± SD	Status level	Group 3, M ± SD	Status level
Psychological demand (SF-36)		2.41 ± 0.21	Moderate	2.33 ± 0.20	Moderate	2.32 ± 0.22	Moderate
Quality of life (WOMAC)	Pain severity	1.97 ± 0.30	Mild	1.84 ± 0.30	Mild	1.74 ± 0.28	Mild
	Joint stiffness	1.95 ± 0.50	Mild	1.73 ± 0.53	Mild	1.70 ± 0.42	Mild
	Physical functioning impairment	2.11 ± 0.20	Mild	1.88 ± 0.22	Mild	1.89 ± 0.25	Mild
	Total WOMAC scale	2.06 ± 0.19	Mild	1.86 ± 0.18	Mild	1.85 ± 0.20	Mild

M ± SD: mean ± standard deviation; TKR: total knee replacement; Group 1: the first 3 months after TKR ($n = 38$); Group 2: between 3 and 6 months ($n = 48$); Group 3: between 6 and 12 months ($n = 32$). $^{**}p$ value: <0.001.

Table 6: Results of linear regression analysis (stepwise regression) for quality-of-life predictors ($N = 118$).

Factor	Model	R	R^2	R change	Unstandardized coefficient B	Std. error	t-test	Sig.
Quality of life (WOMAC)							46.021	<0.001**
	1[a]	0.609	0.365	0.371	2.321	0.050		
					0.257	0.031	8.270	<0.001**
					2.641	0.161	16.393	<0.001**
	2[b]	0.628	0.394	0.023	0.263	0.031	8.543	<0.001**
					0.005	0.002	2.093	0.039*

[a]Predictors: constant and gender. [b]Predictors: constant, gender, and age. p value significant at **<0.01 and *<0.05.

12 months after the intervention. The main change was found to occur 3–6 months after the procedure. The WOMAC progress score decreased from severe to mild before and after the TKR procedure. Moreover, the psychological demand (SF-36) scale was changed from severe to moderate after the TKR procedure. Following the intervention, patients' physical and psychological assessments changed significantly.

Elderly patients had longer hospital stays and higher mortality and morbidity compared to younger patients. However, no significant differences in functional performance and pain were found between elderly (>65 years) and younger patients (<65 years) [20]. In another study, elderly patients' differences in everyday comfort and pain-related scores were significant between preoperative and postoperative evaluations [21]. In a study including 661 young patients with an average age of 54 years, it was found that 33% had swelling, 33% had residual pain, and 41% had stiffness after TKR [22]. In contrast, another study highlighted that advanced age and complications such as pulmonary disease limited the gains in scoring and reaching a satisfactory quality of life [23]. In this study, younger patients had a better quality of life compared to elderly patients. It was found that the lower the age of TKR patients, the more improved the quality of life or procedure outcome.

There is evidence that men's activity levels and functional scores after TKR are higher than in women [24]. The negative result of the female gender, especially on stiffness and residual pain after TKR, has been established by others [9]. Moreover, females with low social support and primary educational level, and patients with worse mental health before procedure, presented a poorer HQOL after TKR [13]. Our results agree with previous studies, where male patients are associated with better outcomes after TKR compared to female patients.

Obesity had been associated with worse scores in all dimensions of the WOMAC score. It negatively affected the initial and long-term assessment results and predicted poorer patients' quality of life [12]. Dietary and lifestyle modifications aiming at obesity improve patients' overall quality of life. In addition, TKR had a positive outcome on BMI and functional outcomes over the long term, with weight loss observed in 31% of cases obviously because of retrieving mobility after procedure [25]. In this study, no association was found between obesity and quality of life in the study participants.

Patients with comorbidities such as arthritis, lupus, and multijoint disease have the most significant functional improvement, especially in most severe cases [9]. However, it has been reported that WOMAC and SF-36 predictors of function and pain scores are increased with increasing comorbidities and low preoperative SF-36 mental health scores [26]. Patients with poor psychological status, for example, anxiety and depression, had a high dissatisfaction rate despite having functional improvements after TKR [9]. Other demographic factors, such as educational level and housing location, had no effect on the outcome after TKR, and they were not good predictors of quality of life after TKR [26]. In our study, no association was found between comorbidities and quality of life.

Improvement in functional aspects after the initial assessment was reported in several studies. Kilic et al. [27] used the SF-36 and Knee Society Clinical Rating System (KSCRS) to evaluate patients after 6 weeks and 6 months; significant improvements were observed in all scales after 6 months. Nevertheless, the physical dimension continued to improve significantly till 6 months. Bruyère et al. [28] maintained the observed improvements in emotional and functional state dimensions in WOMAC and SF-36 until the follow-up ended after 7 years.

Fernandes et al. [29] observed excellent improvement in 28 patients who performed TKR after 6 months. The balance and quality of life were assessed using WOMAC, Short Form Health Survey, and McMaster Universities Osteoarthritis Index questionnaire. However, despite the improvement, the level of physical activity did not reach the level expected for healthy individuals. Furthermore, the habit of practicing physical activity seems to influence the level of activity more than the treatment itself.

Many studies have found that pain levels improve in the first few weeks and even several years after procedure [26]. The improvement of pain is strongly correlated with improving the scores in different scales and the patient's quality of life after the procedure. Therefore, persistent pain in the assessments after procedure is negatively correlated with the possibility of attaining a good outcome. Moreover, pain and joint function improvements are closely associated with physical activity and social support before the procedure [30].

It is essential to mention some limitations of this cross-sectional study. The SF-36 and WOMAC scores were answered using a five-point Likert scale. Some other authors have employed a seven-point Likert scale or have more options answer scale [14]. In this study, the high mean age of the population and level of education made it difficult to have a more complicated answering system. In addition, another inherent problem was the percentage of missing or nonresponding patients and could be attributed to patients with worse health conditions. In this study, 118 patients completed the study out of 200 patients, which is considered satisfactory compared to the length of follow-up after procedure. Although the losses of the volunteers could affect the validity of the sample size, the effect is probably minimal, and the results can be generalized for the whole sample, as seen in other studies [17].

In terms of sample size and representativeness, recruited patients were fewer than expected, especially in the frequency of TKR indications. Another limitation of this study could be that it did not measure patients' expectations before the procedure. Attainment of expectations was highly linked with the level of satisfaction. Patients who stated that their prospects had been met after procedure reported better quality of life [27]. Meanwhile, another study emphasized the importance of developing realistic expectations regarding TKR to avoid dissatisfaction with the surgical outcome [31].

5. Conclusion

A TKR procedure can provide an overall improvement in patients' quality of life. These improvements can be detected for several months after the procedure. Function and pain are the most critical indicators of improvement in quality of life. After a TKR procedure, psychological demand decreased significantly to a moderate level. The physical functioning and pain after the TKR procedure was improved significantly, as expressed by the total WOMAC scale. Among the studied demographic factors, gender and age are the main predictors of quality of life among TKR patients. However, other factors such as marital status, educational level, BMI, location, qualification, and site of knee procedure were excluded as predictors in this study. Future studies should consider other patients' groups (e.g., patients with partial knee replacement) and control groups. In addition, other factors should be taken into consideration, such as implant type, patient characteristics, previous health status, and a bigger sample size. Moreover, it is advisable to consider other additional interventions that can help improve the procedure's outcome. The planning for health care resources and the perception of mental and physical activity should be considered, especially in elderly female patients. The application of scales (e.g., WOMAC and SF-36) will give us valuable tools for gathering information before decision-making in health care systems.

Acknowledgments

The authors would like to thank all patients for their time to complete the selected scales in this study as well as Jordan University Hospital for their kindness and their collaboration. The authors would like to thank Philadelphia University for their support.

References

[1] K. Shriram, A. B. Govindaraj, A. N. Vivek, S. VijayKumar, and M. Anand, "Functional outcome of single stage bilateral total knee replacement measured using oxford knee score," *Journal of Arthroscopy and Joint Surgery*, vol. 6, no. 2, pp. 94–97, 2019.

[2] C. Ding, "Do NSAIDs affect the progression of osteoarthritis?" *Inflammation*, vol. 26, no. 3, pp. 139–142, 2002.

[3] Z. Chen, X. Ye, Y. Wang et al., "The efficacy of backward walking on static stability, proprioception, pain, and physical function of patients with knee osteoarthritis: a randomized controlled trial," *Evidence Based Complementary and Alternative Medicine*, vol. 11, Article ID 5574966, 2021.

[4] A. Askari, S. A. Ravansalar, M. M. Naghizadeh et al., "The efficacy of topical sesame oil in patients with knee osteoarthritis: a randomized double-blinded active-controlled non-inferiority clinical trial," *Complementary Therapies in Medicine*, vol. 47, Article ID 102183, 2019.

[5] S. H. Mosavat, N. Masoudi, H. Hajimehdipoor et al., "Efficacy of topical Linum usitatissimum L. (flaxseed) oil in knee osteoarthritis: a double-blind, randomized, placebo-controlled clinical trial," *Complementary Therapies in Clinical Practice*, vol. 31, pp. 302–307, 2018.

[6] M. Collins, M. Lavigne, J. Girard, and P.-A. Vendittoli, "Joint perception after hip or knee replacement procedure," *Orthopaedics & Traumatology: Surgery & Research*, vol. 98, pp. 275–280, 2021.

[7] M. Romeo, G. Rovere, L. Stramazzo et al., "Single use instruments for total knee arthroplasty," *Medical Association of Zenica-Doboj Canton, Bosnia and Herzegovina*, vol. 18, no. 1, pp. 247–251, 2021.

[8] H. D. E. Atkinson, "The negatives of knee replacement surgery: complications and the dissatisfied patient," *Orthopaedics and Traumatology*, vol. 31, no. 1, pp. 25–33, 2017.

[9] F. Canovas and L. Dagneaux, "Quality of life after total knee arthroplasty," *Orthopaedics & Traumatology: Surgery & Research*, vol. 104, no. 1, pp. S41–S46, 2018.

[10] A. J. Price, A. Alvand, A. Troelsen et al., "Knee replacement," *The Lancet*, vol. 392, pp. 1672–1682, Article ID 10158, 2018.

[11] Y. Ko, S. Narayanasamy, H.-L. Wee et al., "Health-related quality of life after total knee replacement or unicompartmental knee arthroplasty in an urban asian population," *Value in Health*, vol. 14, no. 2, pp. 322–328, 2011.

[12] M. Núñez, E. Núñez, J. L. del Val et al., "Health-related quality of life in patients with osteoarthritis after total knee replacement: factors influencing outcomes at 36 months of follow-up," *Osteoarthritis and Cartilage*, vol. 15, pp. 1001–1007, 2007.

[13] V. Serra-Sutton, A. Allepuz, O. Martínez, and M. Espallargues, "En nombre del Grupo de Trabajo de Evaluación de las Artroplastias en Cataluña (2013) [Quality of life-associated factors at one year after total hip and knee replacement: a multicentre study in Catalonia]," *Revista Española de Cirugía Ortopédica y Traumatología*, vol. 57, pp. 254–262, 2013.

[14] A. Escobar, J. M. Quintana, A. Bilbao, I. Aróstegui, I. Lafuente, and I. Vidaurreta, "Responsiveness and clinically important differences for the WOMAC and SF-36 after total knee replacement," *Osteoarthritis and Cartilage*, vol. 15, no. 3, pp. 273–280, 2007.

[15] J. F. Hair, W. C. Black, B. J. Babin, and R. E. Anderson, *Multivariate Data Analysis*, Pearson Education, Upper Saddle River, 7th edition, 2014.

[16] P. T. S. Lage, L. A. C. Machado, S. M. Barreto, R. C. de Figueiredo, and R. W. Telles, "Measurement properties of Portuguese-Brazil Western Ontario and McMaster Universities osteoarthritis index (WOMAC) for the assessment of knee complaints in Brazilian adults: ELSA-Brasil Musculoskeletal cohort," *Rheumatology International*, vol. 40, no. 2, pp. 233–242, 2020.

[17] H. Alfatafta, "Evaluation the impacts of knee osteoarthritis on quality of life among Jordanian patients using the Arabic version of the western Ontario and MCmaster Universities arthritis index (WOMAC)," *Progress in Orthopedics and Rheumatology Open access Journal*, vol. 2, no. 1, pp. 1–4, 2018.

[18] K. A. Sheikh, U. Yagoub, M. Elsatouhy, R. Al Sanosi, and S. A. Mohamud, "Reliability and validity of the Arabic version of the SF-36 health survey questionnaire in population of Khat chewers-Jazan region-kingdom of Saudi Arabia," *Applied Research in Quality of Life*, vol. 10, no. 1, pp. 1–13, 2015.

[19] N. Shrestha, "Factor Analysis as a tool for survey analysis," *American Journal of Applied Mathematics and Statistics, Science and Education Publishing*, vol. 9, pp. 4–11, 2021.

[20] E. F. Kuperman, M. Schweizer, P. Joy, X. Gu, and M. M. Fang, "The effects of advanced age on primary total knee arthroplasty: a meta-analysis and systematic review," *BMC Geriatrics*, vol. 16, no. 1, p. 41, 2016.

[21] J. F. Maempel, F. Riddoch, N. Calleja, and I. J. Brenkel, "Longer hospital stay, more complications, and increased mortality but substantially improved function after knee replacement in older patients," *Acta Orthopaedica*, vol. 86, no. 4, pp. 451–456, 2015.

[22] J. Parvizi, R. M. Nunley, K. R. Berend et al., "High level of residual symptoms in young patients after total knee arthroplasty," *Clinical Orthopaedics & Related Research*, vol. 472, no. 1, pp. 133–137, 2014.

[23] P. Rissanen, S. Aro, H. Sintonen, P. Slatis, and P. Paavolainen, "Quality of life and functional ability in hip and knee replacements: a prospective study," *Quality of Life Research*,

vol. 5, no. 1, pp. 56–64, 1996.

[24] J. J. Cherian, M. I. O'Connor, K. Robinson, J. J. Jauregui, J. Adleberg, and M. A. Mont, "A prospective, longitudinal study of outcomes following total knee arthroplasty stratified by gender," *The Journal of Arthroplasty*, vol. 30, no. 8, pp. 1372–1377, 2015.

[25] M. P. Ast, M. P. Abdel, Y.-Y. Lee, S. Lyman, A. V. Ruel, and G. H. Westrich, "Weight changes after total hip or knee arthroplasty," *Journal of Bone and Joint Surgery*, vol. 97, no. 11, pp. 911–919, 2015.

[26] R. R. Da Silva, A. A. M. Santos, J. De Sampaio Carvalho Júnior, and M. A. Matos, "Quality of life after total knee arthroplasty: systematic review," *Revista Brasileira de Ortopedia (English Edition)*, vol. 49, no. 5, pp. 520–527, 2014.

[27] E. Kilic, E. Sinici, V. Tunay, D. Hasta, S. Tunay, and M. Basbozkurt, "Evaluation of quality of life of female patients after bilateral total knee arthroplasty," *Acta Orthopaedica et Traumatologica Turcica*, vol. 43, no. 3, pp. 248–253, 2009.

[28] O. Bruyère, O. Ethgen, A. Neuprez et al., "Health-related quality of life after total knee or hip replacement for osteoarthritis: a 7-year prospective study," *Archives of Orthopaedic and Trauma Surgery*, vol. 132, pp. 1583–1587, 2012.

[29] D. A. Fernandes, L. S. Martins, C. A. D. Q. Lima, F. D. Rosa Neto, and F. Au, "Balance and quality of life after total knee arthroplasty," *Revista Brasileira de Ortopedia (English Edition)*, vol. 53, no. 6, pp. 747–753, 2018.

[30] M. Brandes, M. Ringling, C. Winter, A. Hillmann, and D. Rosenbaum, "Changes in physical activity and health-related quality of life during the first year after total knee arthroplasty," *Arthritis Care & Research*, vol. 63, pp. 328–334, 2011.

[31] M. Gonzalez Sáenz de Tejada, A. Escobar, C. Herrera, L. García, F. Aizpuru, and C. Sarasqueta, "Patient expectations and health-related quality of life outcomes following total joint replacement," *Value in Health*, vol. 13, pp. 447–454, 2010.

16

A Comparison of the Incidences of Venous Thromboembolism after Total Hip Arthroplasty between the Direct Anterior Approach and the Direct Lateral Approach, Especially in the Early Period after Introduction of the Direct Anterior Approach

Tetsuya Kawano,[1,2] Hiroaki Kijima,[1,2] Shin Yamada,[2] Natsuo Konishi,[2] Hitoshi Kubota,[2] Hiroshi Tazawa,[2] Takayuki Tani,[2] Norio Suzuki,[2] Keiji Kamo,[2] Yoshihiko Okudera,[2] Masashi Fujii,[1,2] Ken Sasaki,[2] Yosuke Iwamoto,[2] Itsuki Nagahata,[2] Takanori Miura,[1,2] Naohisa Miyakoshi,[1] and Yoichi Shimada[1]

[1]*Department of Orthopedic Surgery, Akita University Graduate School of Medicine, Akita, Japan*
[2]*Akita Hip Research Group (AHRG), Akita, Japan*

Correspondence should be addressed to Tetsuya Kawano; iwtbagdtk@gmail.com

Academic Editor: Benjamin Blondel

Objective. To compare the incidence of venous thromboembolism (VTE) after total hip arthroplasty (THA) using the direct anterior approach (DAA) with that using the direct lateral approach (DLA). In addition, patient background characteristics and the incidence of VTE were compared between the first half and the latter half of the period after introducing DAA and against DLA. *Method.* This was a retrospective, multicenter study involving 109 patients (116 hips) who had undergone primary unilateral THA. Thirty-six hips underwent THA using DAA and 80 hips underwent THA using DLA. Patient information including sex, age, and preoperative diagnosis was collected. The incidence of VTE was compared between DAA and DLA. Moreover, the patients who underwent THA using DAA were divided into 2 groups (first half and latter half groups), and sex, age, body mass index (BMI), and surgical time were compared between the 2 groups. Moreover, the incidence of VTE was compared among the 3 groups (first half of DAA, latter half of DAA, and DLA). *Results.* The incidence of VTE in the DAA group was significantly higher than that in the DLA group ($p = 0.014$). The incidence of VTE in the first half group was significantly higher than in the latter half group and the DLA group ($p = 0.035$ and $p = 0.001$, respectively), and there was no difference in the incidence of VTE between the latter half group and the DLA group ($p = 0.923$). Surgical time was significantly longer in the first half group than in the latter half group ($p = 0.046$). *Conclusions.* In the first half of the period after introducing the DAA, more VTEs occurred than in the DLA. It may be important to shorten the surgical time in the early stage of introducing the DAA, and aggressive anticoagulation therapy may be required until the surgeon becomes familiar with the procedure.

1. Introduction

Venous thromboembolism (VTE) is a generic term for pulmonary embolism (PE) and deep venous thrombosis (DVT), and it is a serious complication that can occur after total hip arthroplasty (THA). Because the mortality rate of symptomatic PE is high, the prevention of VTE is very important. This includes anticoagulation therapy and physical prevention; however, when anticoagulation therapy is given to the patients with a risk of hemorrhage, aged patients, and those with impaired renal function, attention must be paid to the occurrence of hemorrhagic complications [1]. On the other hand, physical methods of prevention, such as early postoperative mobilization, have a low cost and a low risk of complications. Therefore, the American Academy of Orthopaedic Surgeons (AAOS) guidelines recommended physical prevention for preventing VTE [2].

There are several approaches to THA. The direct anterior approach (DAA) uses a natural intramuscular and intranerve interval [3]. This approach can lead to more rapid recovery after surgery because it is less invasive. From August 2015, we changed the standard approach for THA from a direct lateral approach (DLA), including the Dall and Hardinge approach, to DAA. However, we had many cases of VTE immediately after introduction of DAA, in contrary to our expectations. Thus, the aim of this study was to compare the incidence of VTE after THA using DAA with that using DLA. In addition, the incidence of VTE in two time periods after introducing the DAA was investigated.

2. Materials and Methods

This was a retrospective, multicenter study. Patients were recruited from January 2014 to November 2017. Of these cases, patients who underwent bilateral THAs on the same day, underwent revision THA, underwent THA after osteotomy, or underwent THA due to fracture were excluded. A total of 109 patients (116 hips) who had undergone primary unilateral THA were included. One surgeon performed THA using DAA (36 hips), and 3 experienced surgeons performed THA using DLA (Dall approach, 62 hips; Hardinge approach, 18 hips). THAs using DAA and DLA were performed with the patient placed in the supine position and in the lateral decubitus position, respectively, on a regular table under general anesthesia. All THAs were performed with cementless stems and cups. All patients undergoing both DAA and Hardinge approaches could leave their beds and were permitted full weight-bearing after drain removal. Patients who underwent THAs using the Dall approach required restricted weight-bearing for 3 weeks to avoid detaching the greater trochanter. Patient information including sex, age, and preoperative diagnosis was collected. The incidence of VTE was compared between DAA and DLA. The patients who underwent THA using DAA were divided into 2 groups (first half and latter half of the period after introduction of DAA), and sex, age, body mass index (BMI), and surgical time were compared between the 2 groups. Additionally, the incidence of VTE was compared among 3 groups: the first half and latter half of DAA, and DLA. Enhanced computed tomography (CT) or lower extremity ultrasound (US) was performed to investigate for VTE at 2 weeks after THA. The sensitivity and specificity of enhanced CT for VTE were reported to be 89–100% and 94–100%, respectively [4–6]. The sensitivity and specificity of lower extremity US for VTE were reported to be 90.1–94% and 98.5–97.3%, respectively [7].

Manual calf massage was performed to maintain venous circulation and increase the blood flow velocity and muscular pumping of the calf by passive ankle motion after THA for VTE prevention according to the method reported by Funayama et al. and Imai et al. [8, 9].

2.1. Statistical Analysis. Comparisons between groups were performed using the Mann–Whitney U test. Proportions were analyzed using the chi-squared test. All statistical analyses were performed using Statistical Package for the Biosciences software (SPBS version 9.68) [10]. This study was performed with the approval of our institutional ethics committee. The patients and/or their families were informed that their data would be submitted for publication, and they gave their consent.

3. Results

Preoperative diagnoses in the DAA group were osteoarthritis (OA; 29 hips), rapid destructive coxarthropathy (RDC; 5 hips), and idiopathic osteonecrosis of the femoral head (ION; 2 hips). Preoperative diagnoses in the DLA group were OA (74 hips), RDC (1 hips), ION (4 hips), and rheumatoid arthritis (RA; 1 hip). The DAA group had a significantly higher percentage of female patients ($p = 0.009$). The incidence of VTE was significantly higher in the DAA group ($p = 0.014$). The mean surgical time was significantly longer in the DLA group ($p < 0.001$) (Table 1).

There was no significant difference in the sex, age, and BMI between the first half and latter half groups. Surgical time was significantly longer in the first half group than in the latter half group ($p = 0.046$) (Table 2). The incidence of VTE in the first half group was higher than in the latter half group and the DLA group ($p = 0.035$ and $p = 0.001$, respectively). However, there was no difference in the incidence of VTE between the latter half group and the DLA group ($p = 0.923$).

4. Discussion

This study compared the incidence of VTE after THA using DAA and using DLA. The incidence of VTE after THA was significantly higher after DAA than after DLA. In particular, the incidence of VTE was higher during the first half of the period following introduction of DAA.

The cause of VTE has been described as Virchow's triad: venous stasis, endothelial insult, and hypercoagulability. The surgical approach was one of the causes of venous stasis and endothelial insult. In both posterior and lateral approaches, the combination of femoral flexion, adduction, and internal rotation required for canal preparation causes obstruction of the femoral vein in both the posterior and lateral approaches [11]. On the other hand, the combination of femoral extension, adduction, and external rotation required for canal preparation in the DAA does not cause femoral vein obstruction [12–14]. Therefore, the position for canal preparation during THA using DAA may not be the cause of VTE. However, in the present study, the prevalence of VTE was higher in the DAA group, especially during the first half of the period after introduction of DAA, than in the DLA group. A previous study reported that the femoral venous cross-sectional area and peak flow were significantly

TABLE 1: Patients' characteristics and VTE incidence in the DAA and DLA groups.

	DAA ($n = 36$)	DLA ($n = 80$)	p value
Female, n (%)	34 (94.4)	59 (73.8)	0.009
Age (years)	65.1 ± 10.8	62.4 ± 11.2	0.265
Preoperative diagnosis			
OA	29	74	
RDC	5	1	
ION	2	4	
RA	0	1	
Surgical time (minutes)	140.1 ± 18.1	169.2 ± 47.6	0.001
The incidence of VTE, n (%)	7 (19.4)	4 (5.0)	0.014

VTE: venous thromboembolism, DAA: direct anterior approach, DLA: direct lateral approach, OA: osteoarthritis, RDC: rapid destructive coxarthropathy, ION: idiopathic osteonecrosis of femoral head, RA: rheumatoid arthritis. Data represent mean ± SD or number of patients.

TABLE 2: Comparison of patients' and surgical characteristics according to the period after introducing DAA.

	First half ($n = 18$)	Latter half ($n = 18$)	p value
Female, n (%)	16 (88.9)	18 (100)	0.146
Age (years)	65.8 ± 10.8	64.4 ± 11.0	0.635
BMI (kg/m^2)	24.2 ± 2.7	23.7 ± 4.7	0.527
Surgical time (minutes)	147.7 ± 19.7	133.5 ± 14.9	0.046
Incidence of VTE, n (%)	6 (33.3)	1 (5.6)	0.035

DAA: direct anterior approach, BMI: body mass index, VTE: venous thromboembolism. Data represent mean ± SD or number of patients.

decreased in the acetabulum preparation position with a retractor over the anterior wall during acetabular preparation, compared with preincision during THA using DAA [15]. Several studies showed that, because there were leaning curves for THA using the DAA, surgeons who introduced DAA have an increased risk of complications and worse outcomes [16–18]. Considering that VTE cases were concentrated in the first half of the period after DAA introduction and that the surgical time of the first half group was also significantly longer in the present study, VTE was likely to occur due to the longer time of femoral vein occlusion by the retractors. Therefore, the operator should relax retractors when not actively working on acetabular preparation.

To the best of our knowledge, this is the first report to show the possibility of VTE occurrence after THA using DAA, especially in the early period after introducing the DAA. In particular, the present study is a valuable report that shows shortening the preparation time of the acetabulum with retractors can lead to VTE prevention. Therefore, surgeons should become able to prepare the acetabulum in a shorter time using retractors while gaining experience. However, this study had several limitations. First, we did not investigate the degree of hip dysplasia such as "Crowe classification" which may affect the surgical indication of DAA [19]. Second, femoral venous cross-sectional area could not be measured during the operation with ultrasound. Evaluation of blood flow using ultrasound was a useful method; however, it was difficult from the perspective of preventing infection during surgery. Third, the time using a retractor was not measured. Thus, we have to next evaluate the risk of VTE occurrence due to using a retractor by precisely measuring the retractor time and determining the VTE occurrence rate. Fourth, the interobserver and intraobserver agreements of the diagnosis by enhanced CT or lower extremity US were not investigated.

In conclusion, a larger number of VTEs occurred after THA using DAA, especially in the early period than using the DLA. It may be important to shorten the time of using retractors during THA through DAA. In addition, careful monitoring for VTE after surgery and aggressive anticoagulation therapy may be required in the early stage of introducing the DAA until the surgeon becomes familiar with the procedure.

References

[1] J. Hill and T. Treasure, "Reducing the risk of venous thromboembolism in patients admitted to hospital: summary of NICE guidance," *BMJ*, vol. 340, no. 2, p. c95, 2010.

[2] M. A. Mont, J. J. Jacobs, L. N. Boggio et al., "AAOS clinical practice guideline: preventing venous thromboembolic disease in patients undergoing elective hip and knee arthroplasty," *American Academy of Orthopaedic Surgeon*, vol. 19, no. 12, pp. 768–776, 2011.

[3] G. R. Galakatos, "Direct anterior total hip arthroplasty," *Mo Medical*, vol. 115, no. 6, pp. 537–541, 2018.

[4] S. S. Byun, J. H. Kim, Y. J. Kim, Y. S. Chun, C. H. Park, and W.-H. Kim, "Evaluation of deep vein thrombosis with multidetector row CT after orthopedic arthroplasty: a prospective study for comparison with Doppler sonography," *Korean Journal of Radiology*, vol. 9, no. 1, pp. 59–66, 2008.

[5] M. D. Cham, D. F. Yankelevitz, D. Shaham et al., "Deep venous thrombosis: detection by using indirect CT venography," *Radiology*, vol. 216, no. 3, pp. 744–751, 2000.

[6] K. M. Duwe, M. Shiau, N. E. Budorick, J. H. M. Austin, and Y. M. Berkmen, "Evaluation of the lower extremity veins in patients with suspected pulmonary embolism," *American Journal of Roentgenology*, vol. 175, no. 6, pp. 1525–1531, 2000.

[7] M. Bhatt, C. Braun, P. Patel et al., "Diagnosis of deep vein thrombosis of the lower extremity: a systematic review and meta-analysis of test accuracy," *Blood Advances*, vol. 4, no. 7, pp. 1250–1264, 2020.

[8] A. Funayama, Y. Kitsuta, A. Fujie, T. Tando, A. Kanaji, and Y. Toyama, "Transition and present status of the prevention of VTE in total hip arthroplasty with manual hand massage of the lower extremities after operation," *Hip Joint*, vol. 39, pp. 107–111, 2013, in Japanese.

[9] N. Imai, T. Ito, K. Suda, D. Miyasaka, and N. Endo, "Manual calf massage and passive ankle motion reduce the incidence of deep vein thromboembolism after total hip arthroplasty," *Journal of Orthopaedic Science*, vol. 22, no. 4, pp. 726–730, 2017.

[10] K. Murata and E. Yano, *Medical Statistics for Evidence-Based Medicine with SPBS User's Guide*, Nankodo Publisher, Tokyo, Japan, 2002, in Japanese.

[11] J. D. Stamatakis, V. V. Kakkar, S. Sagar, D. Lawrence, D. Nairn, and P. G. Bentley, "Femoral vein thrombosis and total hip replacement," *BMJ*, vol. 2, no. 6081, pp. 223–225, 1977.

[12] M. Binns and R. Pho, "Femoral vein occlusion during hip arthroplasty," *Clinical Orthopaedics and Related Research*, vol. 255, pp. 168–172, 1990.

[13] L. S. Stryker, J. M. Gilliland, S. M. Odum, and J. B. Mason, "Femoral vessel blood flow is preserved throughout direct anterior total hip arthroplasty," *The Journal of Arthroplasty*, vol. 30, no. 6, pp. 998-1001, 2015.

[14] D. Warwick, A. Martin, D. Glew, and G. Bannister, "Measurement of femoral vein blood flow during total hip replacement. Duplex ultrasound imaging with and without the use of a foot pump," *The Journal of Bone and Joint Surgery. British Volume*, vol. 76-B, no. 6, pp. 918–921, 1994.

[15] R. E. Mednick, H. M. Alvi, C. E. Morgan, M. D. Stover, and D. W. Manning, "Femoral vein blood flow during a total hip arthroplasty using a modified Heuter approach," *The Journal of Arthroplasty*, vol. 30, no. 5, pp. 786–789, 2015.

[16] N. Wayne and R. Stoewe, "Primary total hip arthroplasty: a comparison of the lateral Hardinge approach to an anterior mini-invasive approach," *Orthopedic Reviews (Pavia)*, vol. 1, no. 2, p. e27, 2009.

[17] S. T. Woolson, M. A. Pouliot, and J. I. Huddleston, "Primary total hip arthroplasty using an anterior approach and a fracture table," *The Journal of Arthroplasty*, vol. 24, no. 7, pp. 999–1005, 2009.

[18] Y. M. den Hartog, N. M. C. Mathijssen, and S. B. W. Vehmeijer, "The less invasive anterior approach for total HIP arthroplasty: a comparison to other approaches and an evaluation of the learning curve-a systematic review," *HIP International*, vol. 26, no. 2, pp. 105–120, 2016.

[19] J. F. Crowe, V. J. Mani, and C. S. Ranawat, "Total hip replacement in congenital dislocation and dysplasia of the hip," *The Journal of Bone & Joint Surgery*, vol. 61, no. 1, pp. 15–23, 1979.

17

A Geometric Model to Determine Patient-Specific Cup Anteversion Based on Pelvic Motion in Total Hip Arthroplasty

E. Grant Sutter, Samuel S. Wellman, Michael P. Bolognesi, and Thorsten M. Seyler

Department of Orthopaedic Surgery, Duke University Medical Center, Durham, NC, USA

Correspondence should be addressed to E. Grant Sutter; grant.sutter@duke.edu

Academic Editor: Benjamin Blondel

Introduction. Cup position is critical to stability in total hip arthroplasty and is affected by pelvis motion during positions of daily life. The purpose of this study was to explicitly define the relationship between sagittal pelvic motion and resultant cup functional anteversion and create a tool to guide the surgeon to a patient-specific intra-operative anteversion. *Materials and Methods.* 10,560 combinations of inclination, anteversion, and pelvic tilt were generated using a geometric model. Resultant functional anteversion was calculated for each iteration and variables were correlated. An electronic mobile tool was created that compares inputted patient-specific values to population-based averages to determine pelvic positions and dynamics that may lead to instability. *Results.* A third-degree polynomial equation was used to describe the relationship between variables. The freely downloadable mobile tool uses input from pre-operative plain radiographic measurements to provide the surgeon a quantitative correction to intra-operative cup anteversion based on differences in functional anteversion compared to population-based averages. *Conclusion.* This study provides a geometric relationship between planned cup position, pelvic position and motion, and the resultant functional anteversion. This mathematical model was applied to an electronic tool that seeks to determine an individualized intra-operative cup anteversion based on measured patient-specific pelvic dynamics.

1. Introduction

Total hip arthroplasty (THA) is one of the most common and successful surgeries in medicine, and an accelerating number are performed each year [1]. However, instability remains a major concern, with an estimated 1% dislocation rate in primary surgery and up to 25% in revision surgery [2]. It is the most common cause of revision THA surgery, accounting for 17.3-33% of revision THA indications [1, 3, 4]. There are many factors contributing to implant stability, but component positioning is arguably the most important [5, 6]. The classic acetabular cup position "safe zone" is 40±10° inclination and 15±10° anteversion and was presented by Lewinnek et al. in 1978 [7]. It has been used widely as a baseline for appropriate cup position, though subsequent studies have demonstrated that placement of the cup within this zone does not result in reduction of dislocation rate [8–10]. One study found that in a cohort of patients who dislocated, the cup position was within this safe zone in 60% of patients, compared to 79% of patients who did not dislocate [11].

One proposed reason for this discrepancy is the concept of functional anteversion (FA), which is the resultant cup anteversion during dynamic pelvic positions such as standing and sitting [12–15]. The pelvis acts as an intercalary segment between the spine and lower extremities and rotates during dynamic movements to maintain sagittal balance and avoid bony impingement while providing hip joint stability through its relationship to the femur [16]. Because the implanted cup remains static within the acetabulum, pelvic posture changes during functional positions will uniquely alter cup orientation in space and in relation to the femoral component. This may lead to component impingement, instability, and/or accelerated wear. Previous studies have sought to determine the association between change in pelvic orientation and cup position between standing and sitting. Methods used have included plain radiographic and computed tomography (CT) imaging [17, 18], physical modeling [13, 14], and computer modeling [19–21]. The results of these studies have introduced quantitative relationships. However, these relationships are either simplified linear equations valid over small ranges or

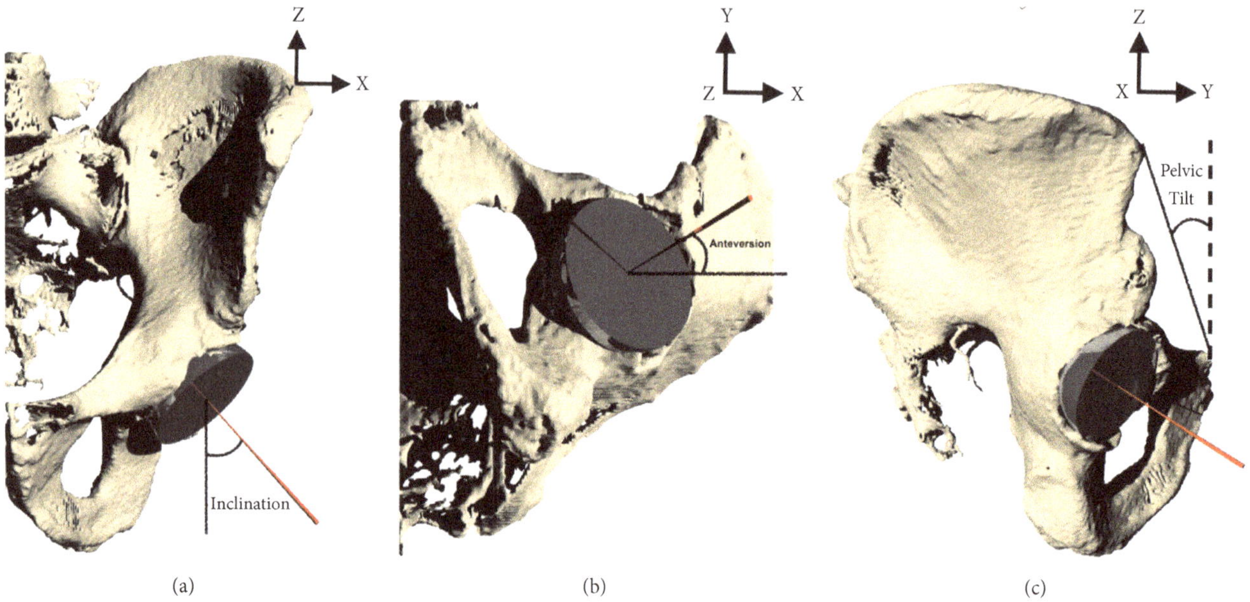

FIGURE 1: Transformations of vector normal to cup flat surface (red line) starting with (a) inclination, then (b) anteversion, and finally (c) pelvic tilt (dotted line is starting orientation and solid line is rotated orientation, with positive tilt being posterior pelvic tilt).

are limited by lack of granularity, making them difficult to interpret and apply clinically. Currently, there is a paucity of data providing a continuous quantitative relationship valid over a large range of cup and pelvic positions. Moreover, some previous studies have used the anterior pelvic plane (APP) [22] as the reference coordinate system rather than the global reference system, which may be more appropriate to assess the dynamic orientation of the pelvis and cup in space.

To the best of our knowledge, there is no study to date that has presented a method to directly calculate FA using an initial cup position and patient-specific sagittal pelvis motion in the global coordinate system. Therefore, the purpose of our study was multifold and included: (1) generate a quantitative relationship between a patient's planned cup position and pelvic motion from standing to sitting and the resultant FA and (2) create an electronic tool that can be used clinically in conjunction with plain radiographic measurements during pre-operative planning to help determine a patient-specific anteversion that can be applied to intra-operative cup placement.

2. Methods

Institutional review board approval was obtained prior to initiation of this study. Following informed consent, 24 subjects without history of inflammatory arthritis, spondyloarthropathies, surgical spinal fusion or neuromuscular disorders underwent lateral standing and sitting radiography of the lumbar spine, pelvis, and proximal femora. Pelvic tilt, sacral slope, and lumbar lordosis were measured as described previously [17, 23]. Increased positive pelvic tilt was defined as increased posterior tilt or pelvic extension i.e. sitting position will result in a higher pelvic tilt compared to standing with normal pelvic motion. Statistical differences were assessed with a paired t-test.

Using numerical computing software (MATLAB, MathWorks, Inc. Natick, MA), a vector-based model was generated in a global coordinate system representing a line normal to the flat plane of an acetabular cup component. Initial cup position was based on neutral pelvic tilt, that is, the initial position of the pelvis was such that the APP was parallel to the coronal plane. The vector was then transformed within this system by adding inclination (rotation in the x-z plane, Figure 1(a)), anteversion (rotation in the x-y plane, Figure 1(b)), and pelvic tilt (rotation in the y-z plane, Figure 1(c)). The vector was then projected onto the axial plane, representing the resultant anteversion. The angle between this vector and the projected vector prior to pelvic tilt was calculated as the change in FA. Iterations of this method were performed at 1° increments from inclination 30-60°, anteversion 15-25°, and pelvic tilt 0-30°, with 10,560 resultant data points. Figure 2 is an example of FA as a function of inclination and change in pelvic tilt when holding planned anteversion constant at 20°. Geometric model accuracy was validated using solid modeling software (Rhinoceros, Robert McNeel and Associates, Seattle, WA). A cup was modeled within a pelvis model and was manually manipulated through random transformations in the same manner as described above and FA was calculated (Figure 3). These values were then compared to the output from the geometric model and results were identical. A polynomial multivariate regression was performed in MATLAB to correlate independent variables planned inclination, planned anteversion, and change in pelvic tilt with the dependent variable being change in FA. Multiple regressions with varying polynomial orders were tested to determine the best fit and minimize error.

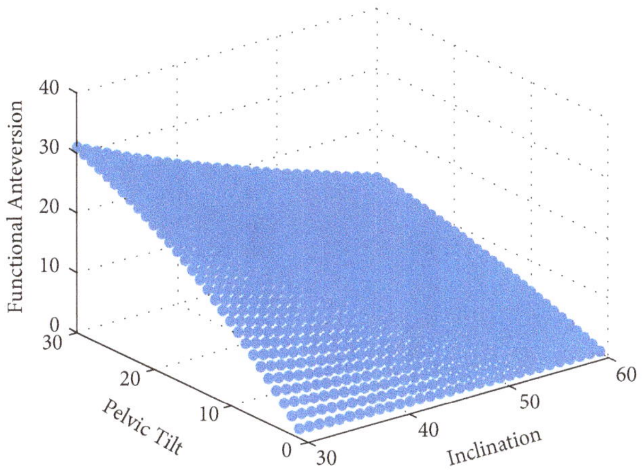

FIGURE 2: Example relationship generated to calculated change in functional anteversion based on inclination, pelvic tilt, and in this graphical example with anteversion held constant at 20°.

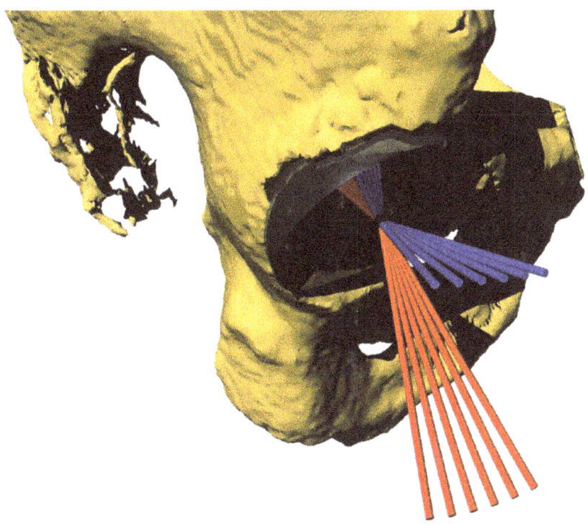

FIGURE 3: Solid modeling of pelvis, cup and vectors generated by changing pelvic tilt (rotation in sagittal plane). Red lines = vectors normal to the flat cup surface. Blue lines = red lines projected onto the axial plane representing functional anteversion.

The mobile application was designed and developed by the authors for iOS (Apple Inc., Cupertino, CA) software using Xcode (Apple Inc.). Data inputs variables for the application are: (a) planned intra-operative cup inclination, (b) planned anteversion, (c) pelvic tilt when standing, and (d) pelvic tilt sitting obtained using radiographic measurements. Using the geometric relationship, the tool calculates the patient's FA when sitting and standing and the change in anteversion from standing to sitting. In addition, population-based pelvic tilt averages are generated using the same equation with inputted inclination and anteversion. Average population values were calculated by combining the data obtained in the current study and prior published data (Table 1) [14, 17, 24–26]. Weighted averages were calculated based on the number of subjects in each study. The average standing pelvic tilt was 0.3°; average sitting pelvic tilt was 25.8°; and average change in pelvic tilt was 25.4°.

Within the tool, patient-specific pelvic tilt when standing, sitting, and the change between standing and sitting are compared to the population-based averages. Eight scenarios of pelvic position and mobility are explored and are addressed with respective clinical recommendations (Table 2). In the case of very limited pelvic mobility, adjustments to cup anteversion may cause unpredictable effects on stability, and additional articulation options (such as dual mobility, constrained liners, or large femoral heads) are recommended. The quantitative adjustment is based on the difference between the concerning patient-specific and population-based FAs, and final output is the suggested new intra-operative cup anteversion target for surgical implantation.

3. Results

Pelvic parameters measured in this study are summarized in Table 3. To determine the geometric relationship, a third-degree polynomial regression was fit to the generated data and found to provide the best fit with $R^2 = 0.999$ and average 0.06° error between modeled and calculated values (Figure 4). The change in FA can be calculated with the following equation:

$$\begin{aligned}
&3.3245 \cdot PT - 0.029675 \cdot PT^2 + 1.4579 \cdot A \\
&\quad - 0.028543 \cdot A \cdot PT - 0.000039528 \cdot A \cdot PT^2 \\
&\quad - 0.065747 \cdot A^2 + 0.000088289 \cdot A^2 \cdot PT \\
&\quad - 0.62941 \cdot I - 0.053399 \cdot I \cdot PT + 0.00042065 \cdot I \\
&\quad \cdot PT^2 - 0.0043096 \cdot I \cdot A + 0.0003293 \cdot I \cdot A \cdot PT \\
&\quad + 0.00019878 \cdot I \cdot A^2 + 0.012728 \cdot I^2 + 0.0001499 \\
&\quad \cdot I^2 \cdot PT - 0.00004212 \cdot I^2 \cdot A + 0.69986 \\
&\quad - 0.000070867 \cdot I^3 + 0.00090945 \cdot A^3 \\
&\quad + 0.000041864 \cdot PT^3
\end{aligned} \tag{1}$$

where PT = difference in pelvic tilt, I = planned inclination, and A = planned anteversion.

The resultant mobile tool is called *SafeTHA* and incorporates the equation, patient-specific and population-based values, and decision algorithm. Output is final suggested intra-operative anteversion with explanation and further details on the patient's FA when sitting, standing, and change from standing to sitting compared to the average population (Figure 5).

4. Discussion

The significance of dynamic pelvic parameters has been established in the literature and is increasingly considered in clinical practice. The current study presents a quantitative relationship describing cup FA from planned cup inclination, anteversion and pelvic tilt when standing, sitting, and change between the two positions. We have applied this relationship

Table 1: Data from the current study and previously studies publishing average and standard deviations of standing and sitting pelvic tilt and either reported or calculated change in pelvic tilt. Overall population-based averages were calculated from the weighted averages of these studies. NR = not recorded.

				Standing Pelvic Tilt (°)				Sitting Pelvic Tilt (°)				Change in Pelvic Tilt (°)	
Study	Year	Number of Subjects	Percentage of Total Patients	Average	Minimum	Maximum	Standard Deviation	Average	Minimum	Maximum	Standard Deviation	Average	Standard Deviation
DiGioa et al. [24]	2006	84	22	-1.2	-27	22.5	8.2	35.9	9	58	12.6	37.1	NR
Phillipot et al. [25]	2009	67	18	4.41	NR	NR	6.68	25.5	NR	NR	9.6	21.1	NR
Lazennec et al. [17]	2011	50	13	2.4	-18	20	7.3	16.9	0	44	9.1	14.5	NR
Kanawade et al. [14]	2014	85	22	-0.4	-26	15	7.4	28.3	48	5	9.1	28.7	8.6
Ranawat et al. [26]	2016	68	18	-3.7	-25	9	8.8	17.7	-7	38	11.6	21.4	12.5
Current Study	2019	24	7	4.2	25.6	-8.3	7.7	23.4	41	5.1	10.6	19.3	9.9

TABLE 2: Clinical scenarios comparing a patient's calculated standing, sitting, and change in functional anteversion to the population-based averages and the respective guidance provided by the mobile application.

Standing Anteversion	Sitting Anteversion	Change in Anteversion	Clinical Outcome	Tool Guidance
Greater than average	Appropriate	Appropriate	Potential for posterior impingement when standing	Decrease intra-operative anteversion
Greater than average	*Less than average*	Appropriate	Unlikely scenario as appropriate pelvic mobility should provide adequate seated anteversion when standing anteversion is increased	This patient has good pelvic mobility and adjustments may cause instability or impingement, maintain anteversion
Appropriate	*Less than average*	Appropriate	Low sitting anteversion may lead to posterior instability when sitting	Increase intra-operative anteversion
Appropriate	*Less than average*	*Less than average*	Low sitting and change in anteversion may lead to posterior instability when sitting	Increase intra-operative anteversion by greater discrepancy
Appropriate	Appropriate	*Less than average*	Low change in anteversion may lead to posterior instability when sitting	Increase intra-operative anteversion
Greater than average	Appropriate	*Less than average*	Decreased pelvic mobility and potential for impingement when standing, but patient can achieve normal sitting anteversion	Decrease intra-operative anteversion (stop if decrease leads to decreased sitting anteversion below average)
Greater than average	*Less than average*	*Less than average*	Patient has very limited pelvic mobility	Cup anteversion adjustments could be detrimental. Consider additional articulation options
Appropriate	Appropriate	Appropriate	Adequate pelvic mobility	No changes required

TABLE 3: Age and spinopelvic measurements of the 24 subjects included in this study. ∗Significant difference between standing and sitting pelvic tilts ($p < 0.001$).

	Average	Minimum	Maximum	Standard Deviation
Age (years)	65.6	48	81	7.1
Standing Pelvic Tilt (°)	4.2	-8.3	25.6	7.7
Sitting Pelvic Tilt (°)	23.4	5.1	41	10.6
Change in Pelvic Tilt (°)∗	19.3	1.6	37.5	9.9
Standing Sacral Slope (°)	41.7	9.8	64.3	14.9
Sitting Sacral Slope (°)	24.3	0.6	53.4	14.7
Change in Sacral Slope (°)	-17.5	-46.3	23.2	15.6
Standing Lumbar Lordosis (°)	45.5	10.6	68.4	17.0
Sitting Lumbar Lordosis (°)	32.3	3.5	67.0	17.0
Change in Lumbar Lordosis (°)	-13.2	-37.4	22.5	14.5

to create a mobile tool for the surgeon during pre-operative planning to help define a new, patient-specific, anteversion that seeks to reduce the risk of instability. This data can be derived from pre-operative standing and sitting plain lateral radiographs and does not require expensive advanced imaging that may also expose the patient to high doses of radiation.

Posterior instability is a risk in the setting of inadequate sitting anteversion and pelvic immobility from standing to sitting. However, this cannot be considered in isolation, and while it is tempting to consistently increase intra-operative anteversion to avoid potential posterior instability when sitting, excessive anteversion can lead to posterior impingement when standing. Our tool seeks to address this interplay and accounts for potential abnormalities throughout the arc of pelvic motion. Similarly, the studies included in the population-based average calculations reported pelvic tilt when standing and sitting, not only magnitude of change between the positions (Table 1). This full description of pelvic orientation is critical to adequately determine at-risk positions and dynamics.

When considering an appropriate population-based standard, there is a normal physiologic range of pelvic mechanics and one could consider a liberal baseline, such as the extremes of ranges measured or based on a subgroup within a standard deviation. In the current study, we chose to use averages for multiple reasons. As these are cross-sectional studies, it is likely that some portion of the population sampled had pathologic pelvic mechanics that are more likely represented at these extremes. It is also difficult to compare standard deviations across studies with varied numbers of subjects and ranges of measurements may vary within the subtleties of radiographic technique. Moreover, there is no guarantee that measurement data will fall into a normal distribution. From

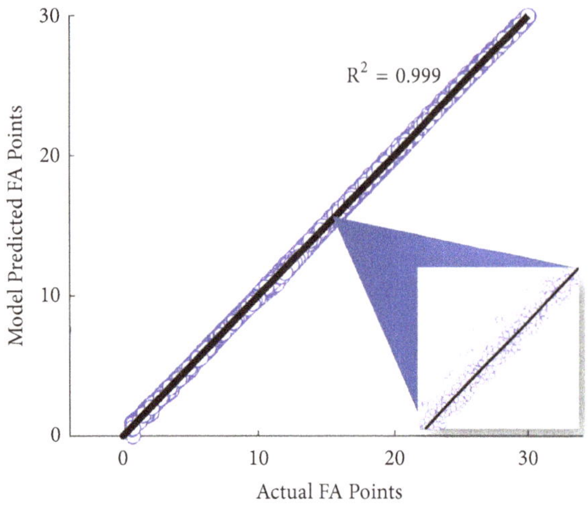

FIGURE 4: Plot of calculated functional anteversion based on the geometric model versus functional anteversion generated by the regression model equation (blue dots). Using 10,560 points, the equation was generated and fits the data (black line) with $R^2 = 0.999$.

a clinical perspective, it is not clear at this time what values (or combination of values) portend a higher risk of instability. However, we believe that aiming for the known mean of the range provides the best opportunity to capture normal pelvic mechanics.

Previous investigations have sought to calculate a FA based on cup and pelvis position using various techniques. Kanawade et al. used a physical phantom model with set pelvic and cup parameters to determine a surrogate measure of anteversion that could be correlated with radiographic measurements [14]. Lazennec et al. used a CT-plane-modifying technique with imaging of post-operative THAs to determine that, with an average change in pelvic tilt of 30°, the average change in FA was 17.3° [18]. This study also presented an equation to determine cup anteversion, however the variables required were post-operative radiographic measurements, limiting the utility of the equation during pre-operative planning. Elkins et al. performed a finite element analysis of various cup and stem positions to determine an ideal "landing zone" of cup position based on cup diameter and stem anteversion [27]. The model is thorough and can be readily clinically applied, but does not account for a patient's unique pelvic mobility, which we believe is critical to provide a patient-specific quantitative anteversion correction.

Other studies have related inclination angle and pelvic tilt to FA. Wan et al. [21] used computer modeling and found that anteversion increased 0.7° for every increase in 1° pelvic tilt. Maratt et al. also estimated that a 1° degree change in pelvic tilt resulted in 0.74° change in FA [19]. We believe that, based on the results of our geometric model, these equations are an over-simplification of this relationship, limited to small ranges of pelvic tilt and do not account for variation in inclination or starting anteversion. Ranawat et al. similarly found a 0.75° increase in FA for every degree of pelvic tilt, but acknowledged that the relationship was accurate for inclination angles limited to 40-45° [26].

Some studies have related FA to larger ranges of discrete values of inclination, starting anteversion and pelvic tilt. However, calculations performed in these studies generated different FA values than those of the current study. For example, Marrat et al. [19] found that 40° inclination, 20° starting anteversion, pelvic and change in pelvic tilt of 15° resulted in FA of 31.1°. In contrast, with the same position, our calculations result in a FA of 34.2°. Malik et al. [20] determined that inclination 35°, anteversion 20°, and 6° of pelvic tilt from standing to sitting resulted in a change in FA of 31.3°, whereas our calculations produce a FA of 27.5°. This discrepancy is due to the difference in the coordinate reference system used to make geometric measurements. Specifically, Maratt et al. and Malik et al. measured angles in the coordinate system defined by the APP [22]. Using the APP is important to define cup placement in relation to the bony anatomy of the pelvis and for successful computer navigation or robotic-assisted surgery to ensure accurate component positioning. However, the APP is defined by the pelvis and does not remain constant in the global coordinate system [28]. We believe that it is more appropriate to use a global reference system to assess the orientation of the pelvis and cup when accounting for dynamic motion and positions in space. Referencing from the APP does account for these dynamic changes and so additional adjustments like those presented in the current study need to be combined with anatomic-based references during intra-operative cup placement [29]. The global reference system is also more applicable when taking into account cup placement with respect to the femoral component and when assessing combined anteversion [30].

Our study is the first to provide a full relationship between pelvic parameters and resultant cup orientation. However, this can be expanded to additional parameters in the dynamic chain, such as lumbar and femoral motion. Esposito et al. showed strong positive correlation between lumbar lordosis and sacral slope in both standing (R^2 = 0.65) and sitting (R^2 = 0.75) positions [23]. Moreover, lumbar and pelvic motion are known to decrease in symptomatic spinal deformity, degenerative spine disease, and lumbar arthrodesis [23, 31–34]. Spinal correction following THA has also shown to reduce anteversion when standing and the change in anteversion to the sitting position [33, 35]. This may account for the increased rate of instability in patients with sagittal deformity and after lumbar fusion [12, 36, 37]. The current study focuses on decreased pelvic mobility, which may be a result of altered spine mechanics, but does not elucidate these effects directly. Future studies should seek to quantitate the consequences of lumbar mobility on instability and to identify which patients may be at risk. In addition, an obligate increase in hip flexion angle when transitioning to the seated position due to loss of lumbar motion has also been demonstrated [23]. High hip flexion is a known high-risk position following THA that can lead to anterior impingement and exacerbate inadequate functional cup anteversion contributing to posterior instability [38, 39].

This study has several limitations. First, it is a modelling study using population-based measurements as standards and has not been validated clinically. However, this study

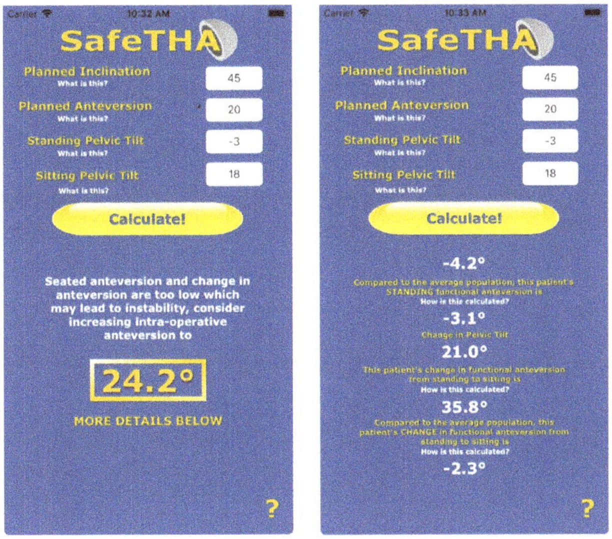

(a) (b)

FIGURE 5: Screenshots of the "*SafeTHA*" app for Apple™ iOS mobile software that provides the user with calculated functional anteversions based on inputted desired planned inclination and anteversion, patient-specific measured standing, sitting, and change in, pelvic tilt using the mathematical relationship presented in this study. The average population-based functional anteversions are also calculated with the same planned cup position and equation. (a) The final output (boxed yellow number) is the resultant recommended new intra-operative anteversion based on these calculations and the presented algorithm. (b) Additional specifics regarding patient's anteversions compared to averages are also presented.

provides a full geometric relationship based on variables that can be known and controlled prior to surgery and, therefore, provides a tool that can help guide pre-operative component position planning. We hope that future work will assess the clinical application of this tool and its effects on instability rate and on specific populations that may be at increased risk for dislocation. Given the relatively low event rate of instability in modern THA, this will require a large multi-center study.

We sought to address FA during positions of daily life based on patient mechanics, not pelvic position in the operating room. The surgeon cannot use this tool in a vacuum and must still understand the pelvic position intra-operatively to accurately place the cup in the desired position. We acknowledge that this tool is a simple guide to help "find the target" but that it needs to be combined with methods to "hit the target" whether via anatomic references [29, 40], computer-aided navigation [41], robotic-guided instrumentation [42], or specialized jigs [43]. Currently this method focuses on FA as it relates to posterior instability or impingement, primarily associated with the posterior approach. However, we believe that this is an appropriate starting point as posterior instability can occur in high-risk positions following both anterior and posterior approaches [44]. Moreover, the posterior approach accounts for most THAs performed throughout the world [45].

This study is the first to present a quantitative relationship and an inexpensive method to provide guidance in cup positioning to minimize instability. We believe that this method will aid the surgeon in cup position planning and may ultimately help define a new safe zone for those patients with abnormal spinopelvic motion. Further work is needed to validate this method clinically and to incorporate intra-operative tools to accurately position the component in the desired orientation. We encourage surgeons to download the free mobile application and incorporate it in their preoperative planning routine.

Acknowledgments

This study was presented at the American Academy of Orthopaedic Surgeons Annual Meeting March 12, 2019 in Las Vegas, NV, USA.

References

[1] K. J. Bozic, S. M. Kurtz, E. Lau, K. Ong, D. T. P. Vail, and D. J. Berry, "The epidemiology of revision total hip arthroplasty in the united states," *The Journal of Bone & Joint Surgery*, vol. 91, no. 1, pp. 128–133, 2009.

[2] P. D. Patel, A. Potts, and M. I. Froimson, "The dislocating hip arthroplasty. prevention and treatment," *The Journal of Arthroplasty*, vol. 22, no. 4, pp. 86–90, 2007.

[3] M. Dobzyniak, T. K. Fehring, and S. Odum, "Early failure in total hip arthroplasty," *Clinical Orthopaedics and Related Research*, no. 447, pp. 76–78, 2006.

[4] C. U. Gwam, J. B. Mistry, N. S. Mohamed et al., "Current epidemiology of revision total hip arthroplasty in the United States: national inpatient sample 2009 to 2013," *The Journal of Arthroplasty*, vol. 32, no. 7, pp. 2088–2092, 2017.

[5] B. M. Jolles, P. Zangger, and P.-F. Leyvraz, "Factors predisposing to dislocation after primary total hip arthroplasty: a multivariate analysis," *The Journal of Arthroplasty*, vol. 17, no. 3, pp. 282–288, 2002.

[6] J. Parvizi, K.-I. Kim, G. Goldberg, G. Mallo, and W. J. Hozack, "Recurrent instability after total hip arthroplasty: Beware of subtle component malpositioning," *Clinical Orthopaedics and Related Research*, no. 447, pp. 60–65, 2006.

[7] G. E. Lewinnek, J. L. Lewis, R. Tarr, C. L. Compere, and J. R. Zimmerman, "Dislocations after total hip-replacement arthroplasties," *The Journal of Bone & Joint Surgery*, vol. 60, no. 2, pp. 217–220, 1978.

[8] M. P. Abdel, P. von Roth, M. T. Jennings, A. D. Hanssen, and M. W. Pagnano, "What safe zone? The vast majority of dislocated THAs are within the Lewinnek safe zone for acetabular component position," *Clinical Orthopaedics and Related Research*, vol. 474, no. 2, pp. 386–391, 2016.

[9] J. R. Danoff, J. T. Bobman, G. Cunn et al., "Redefining the acetabular component safe zone for posterior approach total hip arthroplasty," *The Journal of Arthroplasty*, vol. 31, no. 2, pp. 506–511, 2016.

[10] K. G. Seagrave, A. Troelsen, H. Malchau, H. Husted, and K. Gromov, "Acetabular cup position and risk of dislocation in primary total hip arthroplasty," *Acta Orthopaedica*, vol. 88, no. 1, pp. 10–17, 2016.

[11] R. Biedermann, A. Tonin, M. Krismer, F. Rachbauer, G. Eibl, and B. Stöckl, "Reducing the risk of dislocation after total hip arthroplasty: the effect of orientation of the acetabular component," *The Journal of Bone and Joint Surgery—British Volume*, vol. 87, no. 6, pp. 762–769, 2005.

[12] D. J. Blizzard, C. Z. Sheets, T. M. Seyler et al., "The impact of lumbar spine disease and deformity on total hip arthroplasty outcomes," *Orthopedics*, vol. 40, no. 3, pp. e520–e525, 2017.

[13] T. A. Kalteis, M. Handel, B. Herbst, J. Grifka, and T. Renkawitz, "*In vitro* investigation of the influence of pelvic tilt on acetabular cup alignment," *The Journal of Arthroplasty*, vol. 24, no. 1, pp. 152–157, 2009.

[14] V. Kanawade, L. D. Dorr, and Z. Wan, "Predictability of acetabular component angular change with postural shift from standing to sitting position," *The Journal of Bone and Joint Surgery-American Volume*, vol. 96, no. 12, pp. 978–986, 2014.

[15] J. Lazennec, P. Boyer, M. Gorin, Y. Catonné, and M. A. Rousseau, "Acetabular anteversion with CT in supine, simulated standing, and sitting positions in a THA patient population," *Clinical Orthopaedics and Related Research*, vol. 469, no. 4, pp. 1103–1109, 2011.

[16] J. L. Husson, J. F. Mallet, H. Parent et al., "Applications in spinal imbalance," *Orthopaedics & Traumatology: Surgery & Research*, vol. 96, no. 4, pp. S1–S9, 2010.

[17] J. Lazennec, M. Rousseau, A. Rangel et al., "Pelvis and total hip arthroplasty acetabular component orientations in sitting and standing positions: measurements reproductibility with EOS imaging system versus conventional radiographies," *Orthopaedics & Traumatology: Surgery & Research*, vol. 97, no. 4, pp. 373–380, 2011.

[18] J. Y. Lazennec, N. Charlot, M. Gorin et al., "Hip-spine relationship: a radio-anatomical study for optimization in acetabular cup positioning," *Surgical and Radiologic Anatomy*, vol. 26, no. 2, pp. 136–144, 2004.

[19] J. D. Maratt, C. I. Esposito, A. S. McLawhorn, S. A. Jerabek, D. E. Padgett, and D. J. Mayman, "Pelvic tilt in patients undergoing total hip arthroplasty: when does it matter?" *The Journal of Arthroplasty*, vol. 30, no. 3, pp. 387–391, 2015.

[20] A. Malik, Z. Wan, B. Jaramaz, G. Bowman, and L. D. Dorr, "A validation model for measurement of acetabular component position," *The Journal of Arthroplasty*, vol. 25, no. 5, pp. 812–819, 2010.

[21] Z. Wan, A. Malik, B. Jaramaz, L. Chao, and L. D. Dorr, "Imaging and navigation measurement of acetabular component position in THA," *Clinical Orthopaedics and Related Research*, vol. 467, no. 1, pp. 32–42, 2009.

[22] D. Murray, "The definition and measurement of acetabular orientation," *The Journal of Bone & Joint Surgery (British Volume)*, vol. 75-B, no. 2, pp. 228–232, 1993.

[23] C. I. Esposito, T. T. Miller, H. J. Kim et al., "Does degenerative lumbar spine disease influence femoroacetabular flexion in patients undergoing total hip arthroplasty?" *Clinical Orthopaedics and Related Research*, vol. 474, no. 8, pp. 1788–1797, 2016.

[24] A. M. DiGioia, M. A. Hafez, B. Jaramaz, T. J. Levison, and J. E. Moody, "Functional pelvic orientation measured from lateral standing and sitting radiographs," *Clinical Orthopaedics and Related Research*, no. 453, pp. 272–276, 2006.

[25] R. Philippot, J. Wegrzyn, F. Farizon, and M. Fessy, "Pelvic balance in sagittal and Lewinnek reference planes in the standing, supine and sitting positions," *Orthopaedics & Traumatology: Surgery & Research*, vol. 95, no. 1, pp. 70–76, 2009.

[26] C. S. Ranawat, A. S. Ranawat, J. D. Lipman, P. B. White, and M. Meftah, "Effect of spinal deformity on pelvic orientation from standing to sitting position," *The Journal of Arthroplasty*, vol. 31, no. 6, pp. 1222–1227, 2016.

[27] J. M. Elkins, J. J. Callaghan, and T. D. Brown, "The 2014 frank stinchfield award: the 'landing zone' for wear and stability in total hip arthroplasty is smaller than we thought: a computational analysis," *Clinical Orthopaedics and Related Research*, vol. 473, no. 2, pp. 441–452, 2015.

[28] J. Y. Lazennec, F. Thauront, C. B. Robbins, and A. E. Pour, "Acetabular and femoral anteversions in standing position are outside the proposed safe zone after total hip arthroplasty," *The Journal of Arthroplasty*, vol. 32, no. 11, pp. 3550–3556, 2017.

[29] M. Meftah, A. Yadav, A. C. Wong, A. S. Ranawat, and C. S. Ranawat, "A novel method for accurate and reproducible functional cup positioning in total hip arthroplasty," *The Journal of Arthroplasty*, vol. 28, no. 7, pp. 1200–1205, 2013.

[30] C. Amuwa and L. D. Dorr, "The combined anteversion technique for acetabular component anteversion," *The Journal of Arthroplasty*, vol. 23, no. 7, pp. 1068–1070, 2008.

[31] S. Mendoza-Lattes, Z. Ries, Y. Gao, and S. L. Weinstein, "Natural history of spinopelvic alignment differs from symptomatic deformity of the spine," *The Spine Journal*, vol. 35, no. 16, pp. E792–E798, 2010.

[32] J. Lazennec, A. Brusson, and M. Rousseau, "Lumbar-pelvic-femoral balance on sitting and standing lateral radiographs," *Orthopaedics & Traumatology: Surgery & Research*, vol. 99, no. 1, pp. S87–S103, 2013.

[33] J. Y. Lazennec, I. C. Clark, D. Folinais, I. N. Tahar, and A. E. Pour, "What is the impact of a spinal fusion on acetabular implant orientation in functional standing and sitting positions?" *The Journal of Arthroplasty*, vol. 32, no. 10, pp. 3184–3190, 2017.

[34] M. Stefl, W. Lundergan, N. Heckmann et al., "Hip arthroplasty: avoiding and managing problems spinopelvic mobility and acetabular component position for total hip arthroplasty," *The*

Bone & Joint Journal, vol. 99B, no. 1, pp. 37–45, 2017.

[35] A. J. Buckland, J. Vigdorchik, F. J. Schwab et al., "Acetabular anteversion changes due to spinal deformity correction: bridging the gap between hip and spine surgeons," *Journal of Bone and Joint Surgery - American Volume*, vol. 97, no. 23, pp. 1913–1920, 2014.

[36] E. M. DelSole, J. M. Vigdorchik, R. Schwarzkopf, T. J. Errico, and A. J. Buckland, "Total hip arthroplasty in the spinal deformity population: does degree of sagittal deformity affect rates of safe zone placement, instability, or revision?" *The Journal of Arthroplasty*, vol. 32, no. 6, pp. 1910–1917, 2017.

[37] V. V. G. An, K. Phan, B. S. Sivakumar, R. J. Mobbs, and W. J. Bruce, "Prior lumbar spinal fusion is associated with an increased risk of dislocation and revision in total hip arthroplasty: a meta-analysis," *The Journal of Arthroplasty*, vol. 33, no. 1, pp. 297–300, 2018.

[38] T. F. McCarthy, J. Nevelos, R. K. Elmallah et al., "The effect of pelvic tilt and femoral head size on hip range-of-motion to impingement," *The Journal of Arthroplasty*, vol. 32, no. 11, pp. 3544–3549, 2017.

[39] A. Stephens, S. Munir, S. Shah, and W. L. Walter, "The kinematic relationship between sitting and standing posture and pelvic inclination and its significance to cup positioning in total hip arthroplasty," *International Orthopaedics*, vol. 39, no. 3, pp. 383–388, 2015.

[40] D. Beverland, "The transverse acetabular ligament: optimizing version," *Orthopedics*, vol. 33, article 631, 2010.

[41] D. Davenport and V. Kavarthapu, "Computer navigation of the acetabular component in total hip arthroplasty: a narrative review," *EFORT Open Reviews*, vol. 1, no. 7, pp. 279–285, 2016.

[42] V. Kanawade, L. D. Dorr, S. A. Banks, Z. Zhang, and Z. Wan, "Precision of robotic guided instrumentation for acetabular component positioning," *The Journal of Arthroplasty*, vol. 30, no. 3, pp. 392–397, 2015.

[43] S. B. Murphy and A. O. Thomas, "Smart mechanical navigation: assuring cup positioning," *Seminars in Arthroplasty*, vol. 25, no. 2, pp. 135–139, 2014.

[44] R. Y. G. Woo and B. F. Morrey, "Dislocations after total hip arthroplasty," *The Journal of Bone & Joint Surgery—American Volume*, vol. 64, no. 9, pp. 1295–1306, 1982.

[45] O. Chechik, M. Khashan, R. Lador, M. Salai, and E. Amar, "Surgical approach and prosthesis fixation in hip arthroplasty world wide," *Archives of Orthopaedic and Trauma Surgery*, vol. 133, no. 11, pp. 1595–1600, 2013.

18

Interobserver and Intraobserver Reliabilities of Three-Dimensional Postoperative Evaluation Software in Total Hip Arthroplasty

Kenta Konno, Shigeo Hagiwara, Junichi Nakamura, Yuya Kawarai, Sumihisa Orita, Yawara Eguchi, and Seiji Ohtori

Department of Orthopaedics Surgery, Graduate School of Medicine, Chiba University, 1-8-1 Inohana, Chuo-ku, Chiba 260-8670, Japan

Correspondence should be addressed to Kenta Konno; johnclapton20000@gmail.com

Academic Editor: Benjamin Blondel

Background. In primary and revision total hip arthroplasty, to prevent perioperative complications, the prediction of the optimal implant size is essential. Using three-dimensional computed tomography-based postoperative evaluation software, we explored the accuracy and the precision of measurement of the size, alignment, and position of the prosthetic components after total hip arthroplasty. *Methods.* Using postoperative evaluation software, the postoperative computed tomography data from 20 hips in 20 patients were evaluated. The component size, alignment, and three-dimensional positioning of the cup and stem were assessed. The concordance rates of the component, repeatability (intraobserver reliability), and reproducibility (interobserver reliability) of postoperative evaluation were calculated. The radiographic inclination and radiographic anteversion of the cup, anteversion, varus–valgus angle, and flexion–extension angles of the stem were measured for alignment. The implant positioning was measured along three axes, namely, *X*-axis (transverse), *Y*-axis (sagittal), and *Z*-axis (longitudinal). *Results.* The concordance rates of all parts are above 94%. The intraobserver and interobserver intraclass correlation coefficients of alignment measurement were very good for both cup (0.879–0.964) and stem (0.973–0.996). The intraobserver and interobserver intraclass correlation coefficients of cup positioning were very good (0.961–0.987) for all axes. The intraobserver and interobserver intraclass correlation coefficients of implant positioning were very good for the stem (0.879–0.995) for all axes. *Conclusions.* Computed tomography-based postoperative evaluation software was able to evaluate the size and position of total hip implants with high reproducibility.

1. Introduction

In primary and revision total hip arthroplasty (THA), appropriate implant size and placement are necessary to prevent complications such as dislocation [1, 2], wear of the polyethylene liner, and loosening of the components [3–5]. Lewinnek et al. proposed a "safe zone" of cup alignment, and Widmer et al. proposed an optimal combination of cup alignment and stem anteversion to minimize the risk of impingement [6]. To achieve precise implant placement, the use of a navigation system and a fluoroscopy-guided technique have been reported [7, 8]. Present, the gold standard for the postoperative assessment of component orientation, inclination, anteversion of the acetabular component, and varus–valgus angle of the femoral component is conventional plain radiography [9–11]. Although using these measurement methods, implant alignment accurately can be evaluated, these methods can be less reliable in assessing the components' exact size, position, and alignment in the acetabulum and femur [12, 13] because evaluating three-dimensional (3D) implant alignment using a two-dimensional plain radiograph or intraoperative measurement is challenging [1, 3]. In the case of revision THA without detail implant size and medical record due to long periods of time or moving, predicting the implant size and alignment accurately would be very helpful. It has been reported that a computed tomography- (CT-) based method using low-dose digital stereoradiography, commercialized as the EOS imaging system, has good reliability [14–16].

Recently, a CT-based 3D preoperative planning and postoperative evaluation software, which can measure the alignment and 3D position of the implant, has become available and has shown good reliability for preoperative planning [17, 18]. In total knee arthroplasty, good reliability has been reported regarding the femoral and tibial component positions and alignment [19]. Although the reliability of measurement might be a part of the clinical study, no study has reported the whole reliability of the evaluation software, including component size, alignment, and three-dimensional positioning. The present study aimed to evaluate the accuracy, intraobserver reliability, and interobserver reliability of the CT-based postoperative evaluation software in THA.

2. Materials and Methods

2.1. Study Design. We conducted a retrospective study using CT-based 3D preoperative planning and postoperative analysis software for THA. The study protocol was in compliance with the Helsinki Declaration, approved by the institutional review board, and all patients provided written informed consent before any study-related procedures were conducted.

2.2. Subjects. We selected perioperative CT data from 20 hips in 20 patients who underwent primary THA for osteoarthritis (OA) of the hip and osteonecrosis of the femoral head (ONFH). The planning and operations were all performed by one senior surgeon (N.J.). All patients underwent a unilateral THA between March 2016 and December 2017. Fifteen right and five left hips in eight male and 12 female patients were included in the present study. R3 cementless acetabular cup (Smith and Nephew, Memphis, TN) and Profemur *Z* cementless stem (Microport Orthopedics, Arlington, TN) were implanted in all cases. Exclusion criteria for this study included previous hip surgery including THA, osteotomy, and osteosynthesis, subluxation of Crowe type 2 or greater, and ankylosis. There were 15 hips with OA and five hips with ONFH each in stage 3B and stage 4 of the Japanese Ministry of Health, Labor, and Welfare stage classification [20]. Table 1 provides the mean age at postoperative CT scan, mean height, body weight, and body mass index. The shape of the femoral canal [21] was classified as champagne flute (canal flare index (CFI) > 4.7) in three hips, normal (3.0 ≤ CFI ≤ 4.7) in 14 hips, and stovepipe (CFI < 3.0) in three hips.

2.3. Planning and Analysis. Both preoperative and postoperative CT scans from the bilateral iliac wing to the tibial plateau were performed with a slice thickness of 1 mm using a helical CT scanner (Aquilion ONE; TOSHIBA Medical Systems Corporation, Tokyo, Japan). The CT data were transferred to ZedHip (Lexi Corporation, Tokyo, Japan). This preoperative planning software enables the surgeon to simulate the placement of the prosthetic components into their proper positions in the 3D space of the CT data by using a computer-aided design model [17]. Using this software, the postoperative component size and position can also be compared with the position planned preoperatively. Using skeletal reference points, the coordinates of the acetabular and femoral sides can be determined. Each coordinate was also adapted for postoperative implant positioning and alignment evaluation. The cup positioning and alignment were evaluated using a functional pelvic plane coordinate system (Figure 1), and the stem was evaluated using the coordinate system recommended by the International Society of Biomechanics (Figure 2) [22, 23]. Preoperative and postoperative coordinates were unified by an "image matching" system mounted on postoperative evaluation software. The "Image matching" system can automatically superimpose the preoperative and postoperative CT images (Figure 3). The following parameters, that is, implant alignment and positioning were calculated automatically, whereas the component size was calculated manually using postoperative evaluation software [1].

Table 1: Demographics of all patients for the postoperative analysis.

Characteristic ($n = 20$)	Mean (SD)
Age at CT (years)	64.8 (11.5)
Sex (male), n	8
Weight (kg)	59.2 (12.6)
Height (m)	1.53 (11.5)
Body mass index (kg/m^2)	25.1 (4.2)
Diagnosis	Number (rate)
Osteoarthritis	15 (75%)
Osteonecrosis	5 (25%)
Shape of the femoral canal	Number (rate)
Champagne flute (CFI > 4.7)	3 (15%)
Normal (3.0 ≦ CFI ≦ 4.7)	14 (70%)
Stovepipe (CFI < 3.0)	3 (15%)

CFI, canal flare index.

2.4. Component Size Accuracy. We investigated the concordance rates of each component size (femoral head, cup, and stem) between 3D CT-based postoperative templating and the actual implant used.

2.5. Alignment Measurement. Radiographic inclination (RI) and radiographic anteversion (RA) were evaluated for the acetabular component alignment. RI is the angle between the acetabular axis and the *Z*-axis projected onto the *XZ* plane, and RA is the angle between the acetabular axis and the *Y*-axis projected onto the *XZ* plane (Figure 4). The definition of three-dimensional acetabular coordinate system was as follows:

X-axis: the line passing through the left and right ASIS. Positive direction from left to right of the pelvis.

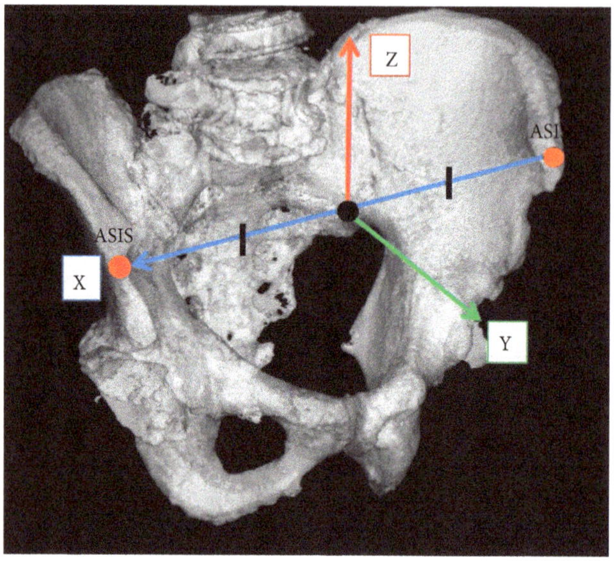

FIGURE 1: Functional pelvic plane coordinate system. The origin (white point) coincident with the middle point of the left and right anterior superior iliac spine (ASIS).

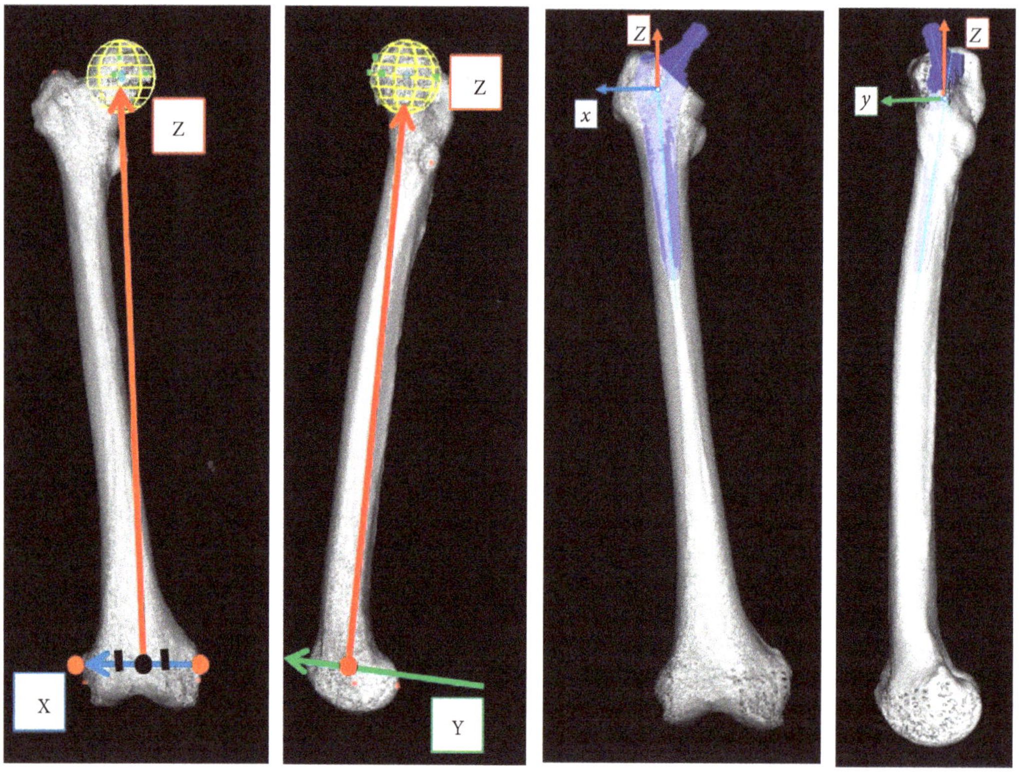

FIGURE 2: The femoral coordinate system recommended by the International Society of Biomechanics (ISB). The origin (black point) coincident with the middle point of the medial femoral epicondyle (ME) and lateral femoral epicondyle (LE).

Y-axis: the line perpendicular to the *X*-axis and the CT coordinate system *Z*-axis and passing through the origin. Positive direction is from the posterior to the anterior of the pelvis.

Z-axis: A straight line perpendicular to the *X* and *Y* axes. Positive direction is from the inferior to the superior aspect of the pelvis.

Anteversion, varus–valgus angle, and flexion–extension angles were evaluated for the femoral component alignment. Anteversion is the angle between the posterior condylar line and the line from the center of the stem head to the stem axis. The varus–valgus angle is the angle between the proximal bone axis and the femoral component on the coronal plane. The flexion–extension angle is the angle between the

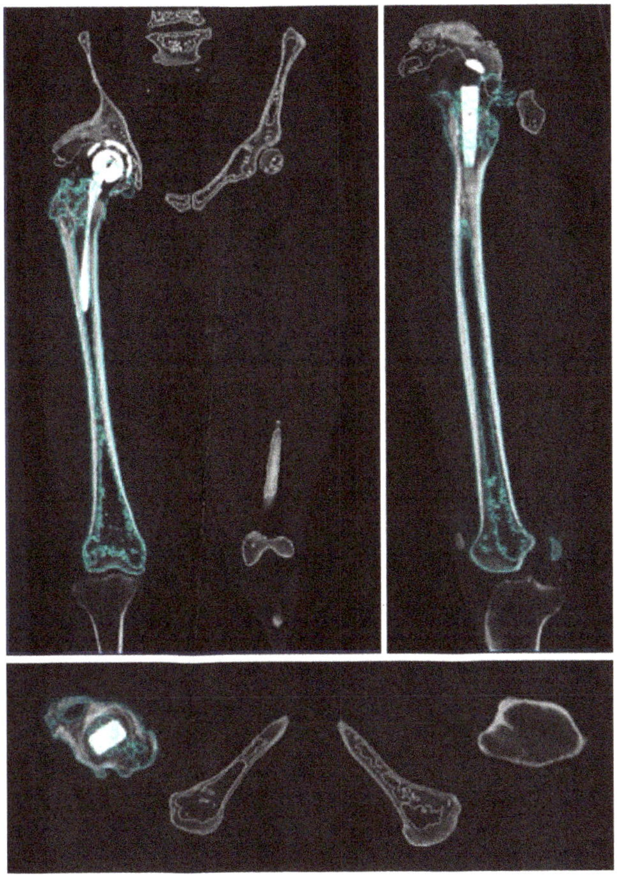

FIGURE 3: Image matching of the preoperative and postoperative CT images. Preoperative CT images (blue line) were fused to the postoperative images (white line) automatically as bone surfaces matched.

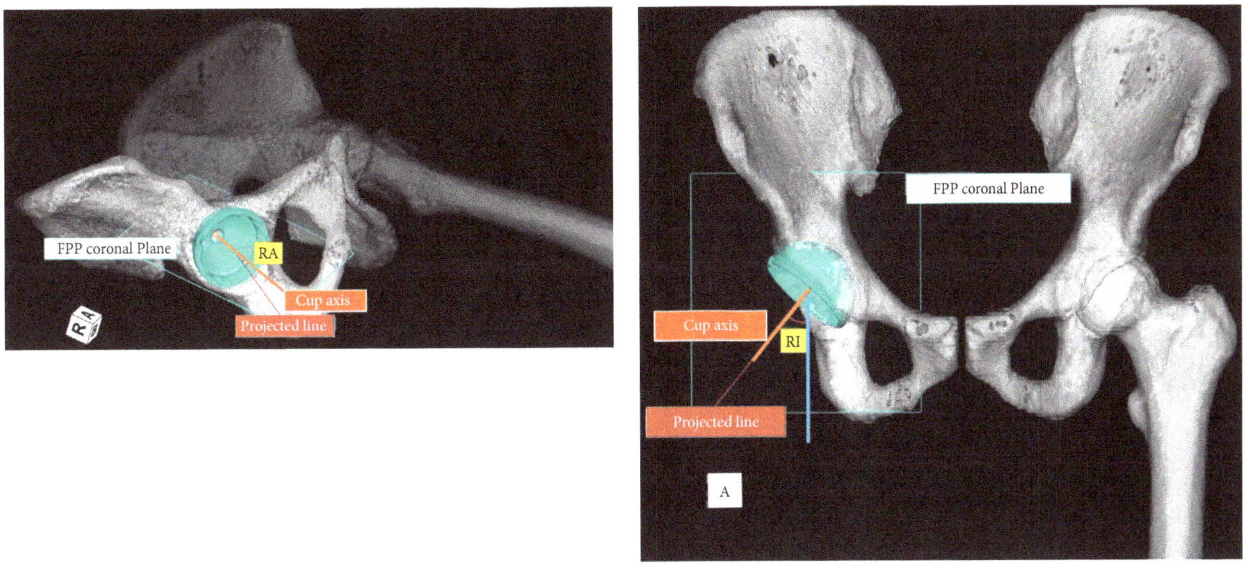

(a) (b)

FIGURE 4: Continued.

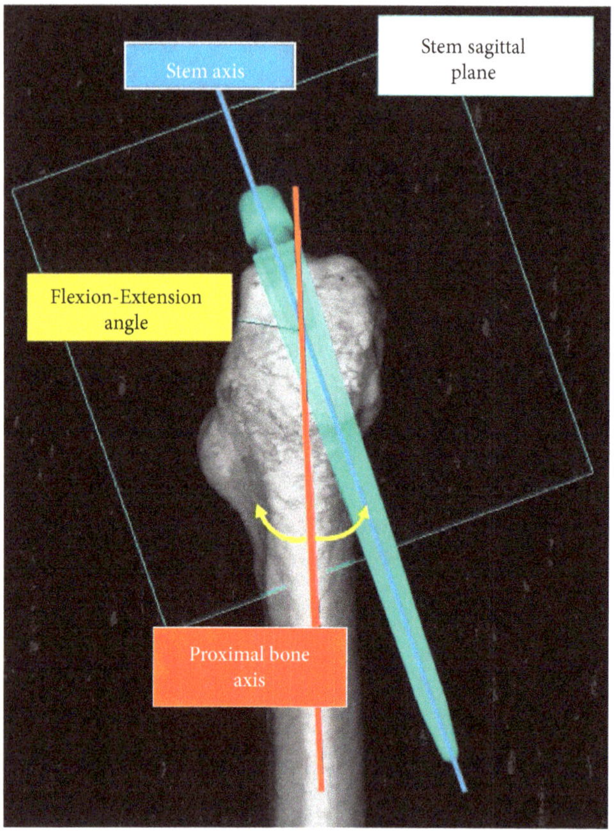

(c)

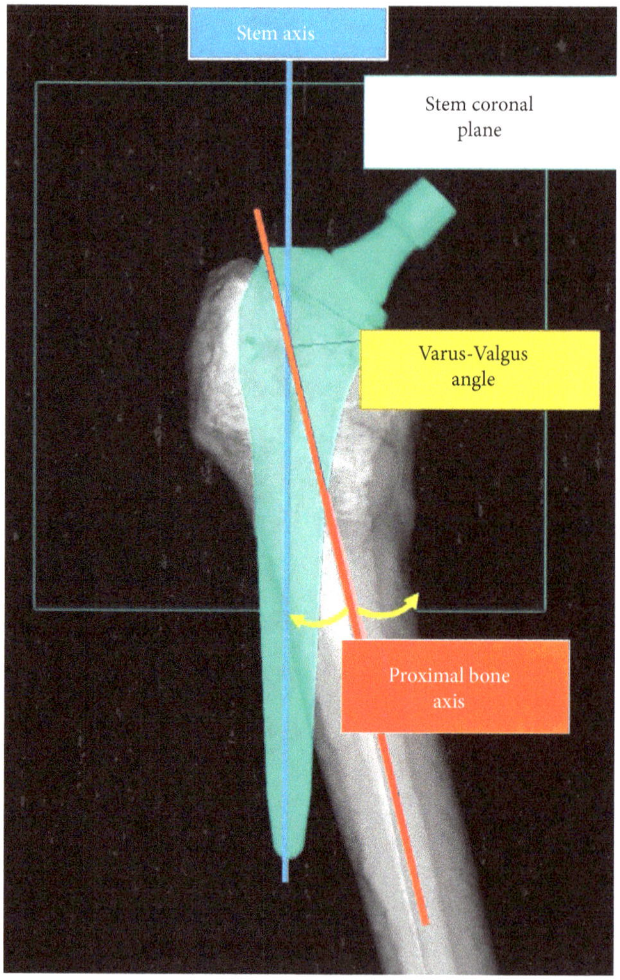

(d)

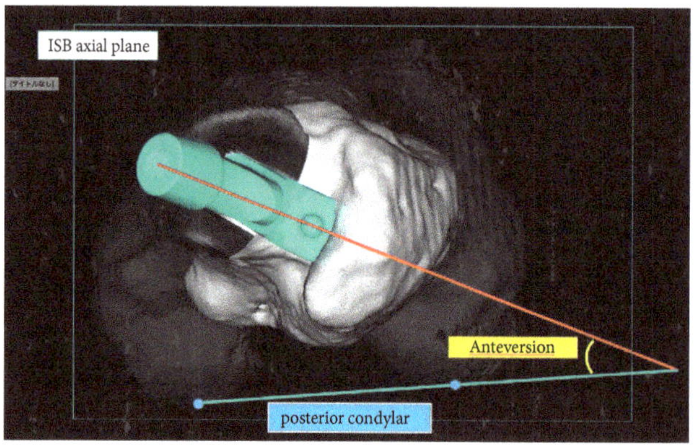

(e)

Figure 4: Alignment of components. The radiographic inclination (RI) (a) and radiographic anteversion (RA) (b) of the cup measured according to the acetabular coordinate system. The alignment of the stem measured according to femoral coordinate systems (c), (d), (e).

proximal bone axis and the femoral component on the sagittal plane (Figure 4). The definition of three-dimensional femoral coordinate systems was as follows.

X-axis: the line perpendicular to the Z-axis and passing through the origin on the plane created by the three points of CFH, ME, and LE. Positive direction is from left to right of the body.

Y-axis: the line perpendicular to the Z and X axes and passing through the origin. Positive direction is from the posterior to the anterior of the body.

Z-axis: the line connecting the center of the femoral head (CFH) and the origin. Positive direction is from distal to proximal femur.

2.6. Implant Positioning. For the three-dimensional positioning of the acetabular and femoral components, the distance between the postoperative implant position and the preoperatively planned position was measured. The software used the preoperative plan as a reference point for the coordinates. Three-dimensional distance axes were defined according to acetabular and femoral component coordinate systems: *X*-axis (transverse), *Y*-axis (sagittal), and *Z*-axis (longitudinal) (Figures 1 and 2).

2.7. Statistics. The statistical analysis was conducted with JMP® 14 (SAS Institute Inc., Cary, NC, USA). To evaluate the component size accuracy, eight observers performed 3D CT-based postoperative templating without knowing the clinical information. The accuracy was measured with concordance rates of postoperative templating and the actual implant size within a range of ±1 size. The repeatability (intraobserver reliability) and reproducibility (interobserver reliability) of the postoperative evaluation software were calculated using intraclass correlation coefficients (ICC). The measurements were performed by three independent observers (*A*, *B*, and *C*), and two successive measurements were performed at 2-week intervals by one observer (*A*) for the 20 patients. The intraobserver and interobserver differences of alignment measurements and implant position for acetabular and femoral components were calculated. An ICC value of 1 indicated perfect reliability, 0.81–1 was very good, 0.61–0.80 was good, 0.41–0.60 was moderate, and <0.40 indicated poor reliability [24].

3. Results

3.1. Component Size Accuracy. Table 2 provides the concordance rates of each part. The exact concordance rates of the head, cup, and stem were 96.6% (309/320), 94.7% (303/320), and 97.8% (313/320), respectively. The concordance rates of postoperative templating within a range of ±1 size was 100% in all components.

3.2. Alignment Measurement. Table 3 provides the intraobserver and interobserver ICC for alignment measurement. The intraobserver and interobserver ICC were 0.964 and 0.969 in RA, respectively, and 0.879 and 0.827 in RI, respectively, for the acetabular component. The intraobserver and interobserver ICC were 0.996 and 0.995, respectively, in anteversion; 0.973 and 0.970, respectively, in varus–valgus angle; and 0.993 and 0.989, respectively, in flexion–extension angle for the femoral component.

3.3. Implant Positioning. Table 4 provides the interobserver and intraobserver ICC for implant positioning. For the acetabular component, the intraobserver and interobserver ICC were, respectively, 0.987 and 0.987 in the *X*-axis

Table 2: Component size accuracy of templating.

	−1 size	0 size	+1 size
Head	2 (0.6%)	309 (96.6)	9 (2.8)
Cup	0 (0%)	303 (94.7%)	17 (5.3%)
Stem	5 (1.6%)	313 (97.8%)	2 (0.6%)

(transverse), 0.988 and 0.987 in the *Y*-axis (sagittal), and 0.961 and 0.958 in the *Z*-axis (longitudinal). For the femoral component, the intraobserver and interobserver ICC were, respectively, 0.879 and 0.841 in the *X*-axis (transverse), 0.993 and 0.956 in the *Y*-axis (sagittal), and 0.995 and 0.965 in the *Z*-axis (longitudinal).

4. Discussion

The present study investigated the component size accuracy and the intraobserver and interobserver reliabilities of CT-based postoperative evaluation software in THA. The results showed that postoperative evaluation software can evaluate postoperative implant size and orientation with perfect to very good reliability.

The use of two-dimensional plain radiography has been the standard for the evaluation of the acetabular component. RI is measured between the long axis of the implant and the tear-drop line. The ratio of the short and long axes of the implant is widely used for assessing the anteversion [11]. Some reports have suggested that the reliability of the acetabular component measurement on plain radiographs using a normal PACS system is high [25–27]. The EOS system is a novel imaging method that uses biplanar low-dose X-rays, which can evaluate implant alignment semiautomatically [15]. Lazennec et al. reported that the reliability of conventional acetabular component measurement on plain radiographs was lower than the performance of the EOS system [12]. However, the measurement of RA is an issue that is yet to be addressed. In the present study, we demonstrated very good reproducibility for RA. Since the pelvic coordinate axis is set after CT imaging and is available as a reference, it is not affected by posture and limb position. We found a slight decrease in the reliability of inclination. With this system, the reference point for the distal implant edge can affect the inclination and positioning on the *Z*-axis. The relatively lower reliability of the inclination and *Z*-axis indicates that the reference point may vary.

Although several reports on the reliability of evaluation methods after THA have concerned acetabular components, there are a few reports on the femoral component [15, 16, 26]. Some studies focused on the stability of the component and the bone reaction of the femur [28, 29]; however, there have been no studies that explore the reliability of the femoral component varus–valgus and flexion–extension angles. The alignment of the femoral component is, however, assumed to be important in preventing impingement and dislocation of the femoral head [30]. Lee et al. reported that the reliability of identifying stem anteversion by plain radiographs is high; intraobserver reliability was 0.944, and interobserver reliability was 0.934

Table 3: Interobserver and intraobserver reliabilities for alignment measurement.

		Average (SD)	Intraobserver reliability (CI)	Interobserver reliability (CI)		
				A1-B	A1-C	B-C
Cup	RA	17.6 (4.3)	0.972 (0.933–0.989)	0.978 (0.943–0.991)	0.970 (0.915–0.989)	0.982 (0.955–0.993)
	RI	36.6 (3.8)	0.955 (0.893–0.982)	0.898 (0.765–0.958)	0.965 (0.913–0.986)	0.892 (0.753–0.956)
Stem	Anteversion	27.6 (13.1)	0.993 (0.984–0.997)	0.999 (0.998–0.999)	0.999 (0.997–1.000)	0.999(0.997–0.999)
	Varus–valgus angle	−1.2 (1.7)	0.956 (0.894–0.982)	0.987 (0.877–0.995)	0.991 (0.977–0.996)	0.995 (0.988–0.998)
	Flexion–extension angle	1.8 (2.3)	0.991 (0.980–0.997)	0.994 (0.985–0.998)	0.995 (0.986–0.998)	0.997 (0.992–0.999)

SD, standard deviation; CI, 95% confidence interval; RA, radiographic anteversion; RI, radiographic inclination.

Table 4: Intraobserver and interobserver reliabilities for implant positioning.

		Average (SD)	Intraobserver reliability (CI)	Interobserver reliability (CI)		
				A1-B	A1-C	B-C
Cup	*x* (transverse)	0.8 (2.8)	0.992 (0.981–0.997)	0.987 (0.965–0.998)	0.989 (0.974–0.996)	0.948 (0.875–0.979)
	y (sagittal)	0.2 (2.5)	0.992 (0.979–0.997)	0.987 (0.968–0.995)	0.982 (0.952–0.993)	0.853 (0.665–0.939)
	z (longitudinal)	−1.2 (2.0)	0.966 (0.917–0.986)	0.947 (0.865–0.979)	0.960 (0.900–0.984)	0.834 (0.626–0.931)
Stem	*x* (transverse)	−0.9 (2.0)	0.976 (0.943–0.991)	0.977 (0.938–0.991)	0.978 (0.946–0.991)	0.987 (0.965–0.995)
	y (sagittal)	1.0 (2.8)	0.993 (0.983–0.997)	0.993 (0.983–0.997)	0.992 (0.981–0.997)	0.995 (0.988–0.998)
	z (longitudinal)	0.2 (5.1)	0.996 (0.990–0.998)	0.996 (0.990–0.998)	0.996 (0.990–0.998)	0.997 (0.992–0.999)

SD, standard deviation; CI, 95% confidence interval.

[26]. Another study that used the EOS system reported an intraobserver reliability of 0.998 and an interobserver reliability of 0.997. The reliability of femoral component anteversion in the present study is equal to or better than other methods. Additionally, with this method, the proximal bone axis and 3D coordinate system of the femur can be placed automatically from the CT image, so it is not affected by the orientation of the lower limbs.

The 3D position of each implant is assumed to affect the biomechanics of the joint [31], the impingement of components, and leg length [32]. Therefore, the 3D position of each implant is also measured and installed via navigation [33]. Nevertheless, there are few reports on its positional evaluation method [34]. Leg length is measured from the transverse line, and femoral offset is measured from the hip center on the X-ray. However, the sagittal positional shift (*Y*-axis, in this study) cannot be evaluated without a 3D approach. This method, therefore, can be useful in evaluating the leg length discrepancy or postoperative biomechanics of the hip joint.

This system allows us to simulate the range of motion and evaluate impingement after surgery. Precise evaluation of the implant position and alignment with residual osteophytes after surgery, identified by postoperative CT, can enable the assessment of the risk of dislocation due to impingement. It can also provide information that is useful for patient guidance. Another potential clinical advantage of this system is the long-term evaluation of implant stability because this method can evaluate implant alignment and position three-dimensionally; it would be possible to detect even slight loosening. In the case of revision THA, knowledge of the diameter of the existing cup can be very important. The knowledge of the correct size of the acetabular cup can decrease intraoperative complications by having the correct implant removal equipment size selected.

Our method has several limitations. First, our evaluation involved only one type of implant, and we do not know what the results of the evaluation with other implants would show. Most acetabular components are spherical; therefore, our results might be generalizable to other acetabular components. Second, the implant size was blinded. Knowing the size, however, might improve reliability because we could calibrate for the implant size making it easier to determine the location of the implant edge. However, we believe that, compared with most studies, the present study has been performed under stricter conditions.

5. Conclusion

The CT-based postoperative evaluation software was able to evaluate the position of the implant with high reproducibility. It can, therefore, be a useful tool for evaluating the accuracy of implant size and placement after primary THA and before revision THA.

Disclosure

The preliminary version of this study was already published as a non-peer reviewed article in the preprint server with DOI: 10.21203/rs.3.rs-42569/v1.

Acknowledgments

This work was supported by JSPS KAKENHI (19K18487), Takeda Science Foundation, the Japan Osteoporosis Foundation, and the Futaba Foundation and Novartis Research Grant.

References

[1] D. D. D'Lima, A. G. Urquhart, K. O. Buehler, R. H. Walker, and C. W. Colwell, "The effect of the orientation of the acetabular and femoral components on the range of motion of the hip at different head-neck ratios," *Journal of Bone and Joint Surgery American Volume*, vol. 82, no. 3, pp. 315–321, 2000.

[2] S. T. Woolson and Z. O. Rahimtoola, "Risk factors for dislocation during the first 3 months after primary total hip replacement," *The Journal of Arthroplasty*, vol. 14, no. 6, pp. 662–668, 1999.

[3] J. G. Kennedy, W. B. Rogers, K. E. Soffe, R. J. Sullivan, D. G. Griffen, and L. J. Sheehan, "Effect of acetabular component orientation on recurrent dislocation, pelvic osteolysis, polyethylene wear, and component migration," *The Journal of Arthroplasty*, vol. 13, no. 5, pp. 530–534, 1998.

[4] B. M. Wroblewski, P. D. Siney, and P. A. Fleming, "Effect of reduced diameter neck stem on incidence of radiographic cup loosening and revisions in charnley low-frictional torque arthroplasty," *The Journal of Arthroplasty*, vol. 24, no. 1, pp. 10–14, 2009.

[5] R. Biedermann, A. Tonin, M. Krismer, F. Rachbauer, G. Eibl, and B. Stöckl, "Reducing the risk of dislocation after total hip arthroplasty," *Journal of Bone & Joint Surgery, British Volume*, vol. 87-B, no. 6, pp. 762–769, 2005.

[6] K.-H. Widmer and B. Zurfluh, "Compliant positioning of total hip components for optimal range of motion," *Journal of Orthopaedic Research*, vol. 22, no. 4, pp. 815–821, 2004.

[7] K. Yamada, H. Endo, T. Tetsunaga, T. Miyake, T. Sanki, and T. Ozaki, "Accuracy of cup positioning with the computed tomography-based two-dimensional to three-dimensional matched navigation system: a prospective, randomized controlled study," *The Journal of Arthroplasty*, vol. 33, no. 1, pp. 136–143, 2018.

[8] J. Nakamura, S. Hagiwara, S. Orita et al., "Direct anterior approach for total hip arthroplasty with a novel mobile traction table -a prospective cohort study," *BMC Musculoskeletal Disorders*, vol. 18, no. 1, p. 49, 2017.

[9] G. E. Lewinnek, J. L. Lewis, R. Tarr, C. L. Compere, and J. R. Zimmerman, "Dislocations after total hip-replacement arthroplasties," *Journal of Bone and Joint Surgery*, vol. 60, no. 2, pp. 217–220, 1978.

[10] R. Y. Woo and B. F. Morrey, "Dislocations after total hip arthroplasty," *Journal of Bone and Joint Surgery*, vol. 64, no. 9, pp. 1295–1306, 1982.

[11] D. Murray, "The definition and measurement of acetabular orientation," *Journal of Bone & Joint Surgery, British Volume*, vol. 75-B, no. 2, pp. 228–232, 1993.

[12] J. Y. Lazennec, M. A. Rousseau, A. Rangel et al., "Pelvis and total hip arthroplasty acetabular component orientations in sitting and standing positions: measurements reproductibility with EOS imaging system versus conventional radiographies," *Orthopaedics & Traumatology: Surgery & Research*, vol. 97, no. 4, pp. 373–380, 2011.

[13] L. D. Dorr, Z. Wan, A. Malik, J. Zhu, M. Dastane, and P. Deshmane, "A comparison of surgeon estimation and computed tomographic measurement of femoral component anteversion in cementless total hip arthroplasty," *Journal of Bone and Joint Surgery*, vol. 91, no. 11, pp. 2598–2604, 2009.

[14] T. Kalteis, M. Handel, T. Herold, L. Perlick, C. Paetzel, and J. Grifka, "Position of the acetabular cup-accuracy of radiographic calculation compared to CT-based measurement," *European Journal of Radiology*, vol. 58, no. 2, pp. 294–300, 2006.

[15] A. L. Demzik, H. M. Alvi, D. E. Delagrammaticas, J. M. Martell, M. D. Beal, and D. W. Manning, "Inter-rater and intra-rater repeatability and reliability of EOS 3-dimensional imaging analysis software," *The Journal of Arthroplasty*, vol. 31, no. 5, pp. 1091–1095, 2016.

[16] B. Guenoun, F. El Hajj, D. Biau, P. Anract, and J.-P. Courpied, "Reliability of a new method for evaluating femoral stem positioning after total hip arthroplasty based on stereoradiographic 3D reconstruction," *The Journal of Arthroplasty*, vol. 30, no. 1, pp. 141–144, 2015.

[17] Y. Wako, J. Nakamura, M. Miura, Y. Kawarai, M. Sugano, and K. Nawata, "Interobserver and intraobserver reliability of three-dimensional preoperative planning software in total hip arthroplasty," *The Journal of Arthroplasty*, vol. 33, no. 2, pp. 601-607, 2018.

[18] M. Miura, S. Hagiwara, J. Nakamura, Y. Wako, Y. Kawarai, and S. Ohtori, "Interobserver and intraobserver reliability of computed tomography-based three-dimensional preoperative planning for primary total knee arthroplasty," *The Journal of Arthroplasty*, vol. 33, no. 5, pp. 1572–1578, 2018.

[19] K. Yoshino, S. Hagiwara, J. Nakamura, T. Tsukeoka, Y. Tsuneizumi, and S. Ohtori, "Intra- and interobserver reliability and agreement in three-dimensional computed tomography measurements of component positions after total knee arthroplasty," *The Knee*, vol. 26, no. 5, pp. 1102–1110, 2019.

[20] N. Sugano, T. Atsumi, K. Ohzono, T. Kubo, T. Hotokebuchi, and K. Takaoka, "The 2001 revised criteria for diagnosis, classification and staging of idiopathic osteonecrosis of the femoral head," *Journal of Orthopaedic Science*, vol. 7, no. 5, pp. 601–605, 2002.

[21] P. C. Noble, J. W. Alexander, L. J. Lindahl, D. T. Yew, W. M. Granberry, and H. S. Tullos, "The anatomic basis of femoral component design," *Clinical Orthopaedics and Related Research*, vol. NA, no. 235, pp. 148–165, 1988.

[22] G. Wu, S. Siegler, P. Allard et al., "ISB recommendation on definitions of joint coordinate system of various joints for the reporting of human joint motion-part I: ankle, hip, and spine," *Journal of Biomechanics*, vol. 35, no. 4, pp. 543–548, 2002.

[23] S. Nishihara, N. Sugano, T. Nishii, K. Ohzono, and H. Yoshikawa, "Measurements of pelvic flexion angle using three-dimensional computed tomography," *Clinical Orthopaedics & Related Research*, vol. 411, pp. 140–151, 2003.

[24] S. D. Walter, M. Eliasziw, and A. Donner, "Sample size and optimal designs for reliability studies," *Statistics in Medicine*, vol. 17, no. 1, pp. 101–110, 1998.

[25] J. Lahy, J. Stevens, D. McKenzie, and R. de Steiger, "The reliability of measuring acetabular component position on radiographs using everyday diagnostic imaging software," *Journal of Orthopaedic Surgery (Hong Kong)*, vol. 25, 2017.

[26] M. Lu, Y.-X. Zhou, H. Du, J. Zhang, and J. Liu, "Reliability and validity of measuring acetabular component orientation by plain anteroposterior radiographs," *Clinical Orthopaedics & Related Research*, vol. 471, no. 9, pp. 2987–2994, 2013.

[27] T. Nomura, M. Naito, Y. Nakamura et al., "An analysis of the best method for evaluating anteversion of the acetabular component after total hip replacement on plain radiographs," *The Bone & Joint Journal*, vol. 96-B, no. 5, pp. 597–603, 2014.

[28] C. Engh, J. Bobyn, and A. Glassman, "Porous-coated hip replacement. The factors governing bone ingrowth, stress shielding, and clinical results," *Journal of Bone & Joint Surgery, British Volume*, vol. 69-B, no. 1, pp. 45–55, 1987.

[29] Y. K. Lee, T. Y. Kim, Y. C. Ha, B. J. Kang, and K. H. Koo, "Radiological measurement of femoral stem version using a modified Budin method," *The Bone & Joint Journal*, vol. 95-B, no. 7, pp. 877–880, 2013.

[30] M. Müller, D. Crucius, C. Perka, and S. Tohtz, "The association between the sagittal femoral stem alignment and the resulting femoral head centre in total hip arthroplasty," *International Orthopaedics*, vol. 35, no. 7, pp. 981–987, 2011.

[31] S. L. Delp, R. L. Wixson, A. V. Komattu, and J. H. Kocmond, "How superior placement of the joint center in hip arthroplasty affects the abductor muscles," *Clinical Orthopaedics and Related Research*, vol. 328, pp. 137–146, 1996.

[32] H. D. Huddleston, "An accurate method for measuring leg length and hip offset in hip arthroplasty," *Orthopedics*, vol. 20, no. 4, pp. 331-332, 1997.

[33] A. S. Wasterlain, J. A. Buza, S. C. Thakkar, R. Schwarzkopf, and J. Vigdorchik, "Navigation and robotics in total hip arthroplasty," *JBJS Reviews*, vol. 5, 2017.

[34] S. T. Woolson, J. M. Hartford, and A. Sawyer, "Results of a method of leg-length equalization for patients undergoing primary total hip replacement," *The Journal of Arthroplasty*, vol. 14, no. 2, pp. 159–164, 1999.

19

Prevalence of Anterior Femoral Neck Osteophyte in a Total Hip Arthroplasty Population: Analysis of Preoperative Surgical Plans

Adam M. Katchky,[1] **Mitchell L. Smith**,[2] **Andrew J. Shimmin**,[2,3] **Stephen J. McMahon**,[3,4] **Jeremy Latham**,[5] **and Jonathan V. Baré**[2,3]

[1] *Department of Orthopedics and Rehabilitation, University of Vermont, Burlington, VT, USA*
[2] *Melbourne Orthopaedic Group, Windsor, VIC, Australia*
[3] *Department of Surgery, Monash University, Melbourne, VIC, Australia*
[4] *Malabar Orthopaedic Clinic, Windsor, VIC, Australia*
[5] *Spire Southampton Hospital, Southampton, UK*

Correspondence should be addressed to Adam M. Katchky; adam.katchky@mail.utoronto.ca

Guest Editor: Yasushi Oshima

Despite strongly positive results of total hip arthroplasty (THA), patients remain at risk for complications including dislocation. Spinopelvic motion and the hip-spine relationship have been recognized as important factors in surgical planning and implant positioning in THA. Periarticular osteophytes are one of the hallmark pathoanatomic features of osteoarthritis and may influence implant positioning and joint stability; residual osteophytes at the anterior femoral neck may cause anterior impingement and posterior instability. No studies have been identified which establish the prevalence of anterior femoral neck osteophyte for incorporation into THA planning. 413 consecutive patients scheduled for THA underwent preoperative planning taking into account spinopelvic motion to establish optimal component position. Each surgical plan was reviewed retrospectively by four independent raters who were blinded to other imaging and intraoperative findings. Anterior femoral neck osteophytes were rated as being absent, minor, or extensive for each case. A single outlying rater was excluded. Inter-rater reliability was calculated manually. The patient group comprised 197 male and 216 female hips, with a mean age of 63 years (range 32–91). The presence of anterior femoral neck osteophytes was identified in a mean of 82% of cases (range 78–86%). A significant number of patients were found to have large or extensive osteophytes present in this location (mean 27%; range 23–31%). Inter-rater reliability was 70%. A large majority of our THA patients were found to have anterior femoral neck osteophytes. These must be considered during preoperative planning with respect to the spinopelvic relationship. Failure to identify and address osteophytes intraoperatively may increase the risk of impingement in flexion and/or internal rotation, leading to decreased range of motion, joint instability, and possibly dislocation. Planned future directions include incorporation of an impingement and instability model into preoperative planning for THA.

1. Introduction

Total hip arthroplasty (THA) is a common surgical procedure to treat osteoarthritis (OA) and other hip conditions, with over 91,000 cases reported in the UK in 2017 [1]. Despite significant advances in surgical technique and implant design, patients remain at risk of joint instability and dislocation following THA. Estimates for the rate of dislocation following primary THA have ranged from 0.3 to 10% [2–6]. Numerous patient, surgical, and implant factors may augment the risk of dislocation [2, 3, 6]. Impingement is defined as the abnormal contact between the femoral and acetabular sides during physiologic hip range of motion. Among the multiple causes of dislocation following THA, impingement may be a significant contributing factor [7]. THA impingement may result from contact of the implant, bony, or soft tissue structures. In addition to dislocation, THA impingement may lead to restricted range of motion, subluxation, edge loading, accelerated wear, and increased pain [7]. Impingement may occur at any location around the acetabulum, most commonly at the anterior or posterior walls. Anterior impingement following THA is often caused by residual anterior osteophyte on the femoral or acetabular side. Anterior impingement tends to cause increased edge loading and asymmetric wear at the posterior aspect of the acetabulum, as well as posterior subluxation or dislocation.

Implant positioning is critically important to ensure THA stability [2, 7]. The landmark paper by Lewinnek [8] established the gold standard "safe zone" for acetabular component positioning as 40° ± 10° abduction (inclination) and 15° ± 10° anteversion. However, even the Lewinnek cohort included patients within the safe zone who suffered THA dislocation, and other papers have further questioned the presence and location of a true "safe zone" to prevent dislocation [9]. One explanation for this may lie in the spinopelvic relationship. The pelvis is known to tilt forward and backward (flex/extend) with activities of daily living, including climbing stairs, lying, sitting, or rising from a seated position [10]. Further, considerable variation has been demonstrated between individuals including the pattern, direction, and degree of pelvic motion [10]. Differences in spinopelvic motion may significantly impact the instantaneous functional position of a THA acetabular component [11, 12]. For example, anterior rotation (flexion) of the pelvis will lead to an effectively more flat and retroverted cup position, increasing the risk of anterior impingement and posterior instability.

In view of this evolving understanding of the impact of the spinopelvic relationship on THA, numerous techniques and technologies have been developed which accommodate for pelvic motion in the placement of THA implants. One such technology is the Optimized Positioning System (OPS™, Corin Group, Gloucestershire, UK). This system utilizes preoperative lateral pelvic radiographs in multiple functional positions, as well as a low-dose CT scan, to assess patient-specific anatomy and spinopelvic motion and guide THA positioning to maximize range of motion and minimize impingement [13]. A surgical plan is developed for each patient, including 2D imaging and 3D reconstructions of patient anatomy, and planned implant positions.

In spite of the importance of bony anatomy and implant positioning to the stability of THA, no studies have been identified which assess the presence and size of anterior femoral neck osteophytes in patients undergoing THA. The identification of osteophytes in this area may be particularly important in patients with certain patterns of spinopelvic motion, specifically those who display increased pelvic flexion when sitting. This study aimed to use presurgical templating documents to establish the prevalence of anterior femoral neck osteophytes for incorporation into THA planning.

2. Materials and Methods

Surgical plans were retrospectively reviewed for all patients who underwent primary THA using the OPS™ system at a single hospital in Australia between November, 2015, and December, 2016. All patients had previously undergone standardized preoperative assessment including routine radiographs of the pelvis and operative hip, lateral pelvic radiographs in 3 stances (standing, seated, and contralateral leg step-up), and low-dose computerized tomography (CT) scan of the operative hip. Preoperative surgical plans were generated using the OPS™ system, taking into account spinopelvic motion in order to establish the optimal component positions to minimize impingement and maximize range of motion and stability. Each surgical plan includes an AP pelvic radiograph, two CT cuts (coronal plane, central implant axis; axial plane, level of planned femoral neck cut), and three 3D reconstruction images of the proximal femur (coronal, sagittal, and axial views) with the planned femoral implant in situ. An example of the surgical plan generated is shown in Figure 1.

Each planning document was reviewed by four independent assessors (one orthopaedic registrar, one fellow in lower extremity reconstruction, and two fellowship trained arthroplasty surgeons). Assessors were permitted to inspect all images contained within the plan, in the order of their choosing. Assessors were blinded to patient identity, any other imaging which may have been conducted, and any intraoperative findings. Each assessor examined each case to assess the presence and size of osteophytes at the anterior aspect of the femoral neck. In each case, osteophyte was judged to be absent (no bone extending beyond anterior cortex), minor (osteophyte encompassing ≤50% of anterior neck and extending ≤ 5 mm), or extensive (encompassing >50% of anterior neck and/or extending >5 mm). Examples of cases with no, minor, and extensive anterior neck osteophytes are displayed in Figure 2. Scores from each of the four assessors were compiled for each patient case. Descriptive statistics and inter-rater reliability were calculated manually in Apple Numbers [version 5.3 (5989)]. A single assessor was found to be significantly divergent from the other three. Analyses were repeated with all four assessors included and again with the single outlying assessor excluded.

3. Results and Discussion

3.1. Patient Demographics. A total of 413 cases were identified with surgical planning documents available. No patient cases were excluded. The group comprised 197 (48%) male hips and 216 (52%) female hips. Mean age of patients at the time of surgery was 63 years (SD = 10, range 32–91 years). 227 cases (55%) were planned for right THA, compared to 186 cases (45%) on the left hip. Descriptive data on the patient cohort is summarized in Table 1.

3.2. Anterior Femoral Neck Osteophyte. A summary of ratings for all 4 assessors is included in Table 2. All four assessors identified the presence of anterior femoral neck osteophytes in the majority of cases (range 69–86%). After exclusion of Rater #2 as an outlier, a mean of 82% (78-86%) of cases were found to have osteophytes in this location. A significant proportion of patients (mean 27%, range 23–31%) were found to have large or extensive osteophytes there.

3.3. Inter-Rater Reliability (IRR). Inter-rater reliability was calculated manually in Apple Numbers [version 5.3 (5989)].

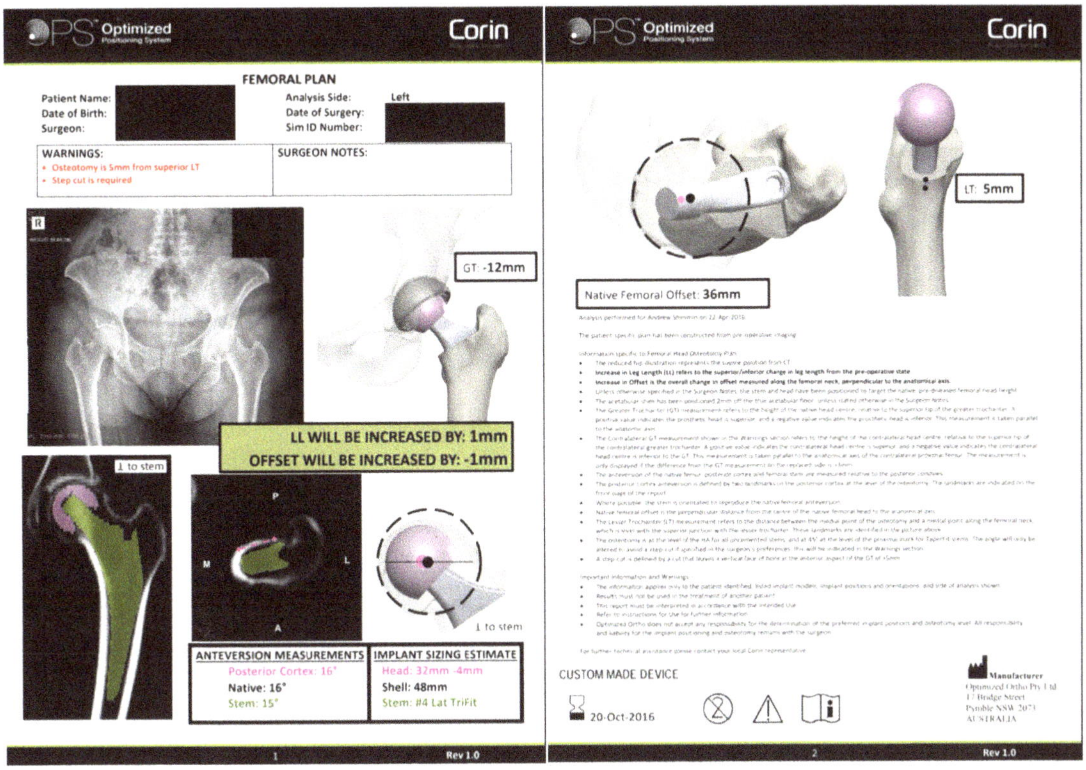

FIGURE 1: Case example of a presurgical plan developed using the OPS™ system, analyzed to assess the presence and size of anterior femoral neck osteophytes.

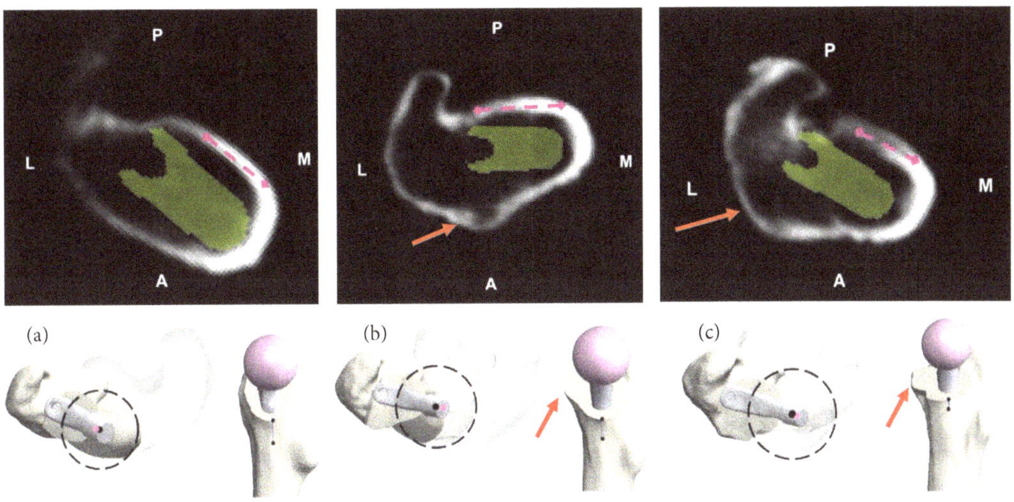

FIGURE 2: Case examples showing axial CT scan slices in the plane of the planned femoral neck osteotomy, with corresponding 3D reconstructions in the axial and sagittal planes (red arrows indicate anterior femoral neck osteophyte): (a) no anterior femoral neck osteophyte; (b) minor osteophyte; (c) extensive osteophyte.

Table 1: Descriptive statistics of patient cohort.

Patient Parameter	N = 413
Age (years) [mean, range]	63 (32-91)
Gender [n, %]	
Male	216 (52%)
Female	197 (48%)
Laterality [n, %]	
Right	227 (55%)
Left	186 (45%)

With all 4 assessors included, inter-rater reliability was calculated to be 68%. After exclusion of a single divergent assessor, IRR exceeded 70%.

4. Discussion

This study identified the presence of anterior femoral neck osteophyte in the large majority of this Australian cohort of THA patients. This finding was unanimous among all raters who assessed the preoperative plans. This finding is not surprising, given the experience of the authors and the inclusion of periarticular osteophyte formation as one of the hallmark radiographic features of osteoarthritis. If not addressed at the time of surgery, the presence of osteophytes at the anterior aspect of the femoral neck may significantly increase the risk of anterior bony impingement and subsequent posterior instability.

The ability to visualize osteophytes and assess the risk of impingement intraoperatively maybe depends on the choice of surgical approach. In particular, osteophytes at the anterior femoral neck may be more difficult to visualize during cases done via the posterior approach to the hip, when compared to the direct anterior, anterolateral, or direct lateral approaches. In its 2015 annual report, the UK National Joint Registry reported the use of the posterior approach in 62% of all primary total hip arthroplasty cases [14]. Given the commonality of both the posterior approach and anterior femoral neck osteophytes, a significant risk of unaddressed osteophytes remains. Numerous factors may be considered in the selection of a surgical approach, and surgeons may be hesitant to alter their approach in order to facilitate access to anterior osteophytes. Surgeons who utilize the posterior approach may elect to focus specific attention on assessing for and resecting anterior osteophytes during femoral preparation.

The impact of unaddressed anterior neck osteophytes likely also depends on a given patient's pattern of pelvic motion. It has been estimated that 52% of patients experience increased anterior pelvic tilt when sitting compared to standing [15]. These patients would be at particularly high risk of posterior instability in flexion and internal rotation due to the presence of anterior femoral neck osteophytes. A further analysis of this study cohort reveals a similar pattern, in that approximately half of the patients in each group exhibit anterior pelvic tilt with sitting (no osteophyte: 46%; minor: 58%; extensive: 50%) [unpublished data].

One limitation of this study is the utilization of an Australian cohort. This population may not be reflective of other global populations. There were no patient exclusions during analysis of a consecutive series, however, so this cohort is likely to represent the true local population. In addition, the images included in the surgical plans were generated for the purpose of implant positions and sizing and were not optimized for assessment of osteophytes. The relatively low resolution may limit the accuracy of this assessment and may have contributed to the moderate inter-rater reliability. The outlying rater was the most junior member of the research team. Differences in training may have contributed to variability among assessors.

5. Conclusions

A large majority of total hip arthroplasty patients may be expected to exhibit osteophyte formation at the anterior aspect of the femoral neck. Approximately 27% were found to exhibit large or extensive osteophytes in this area. These pathoanatomic variations must be incorporated into surgical planning and addressed intraoperatively in order to mitigate the risk of postoperative impingement and instability. Patients who experience anterior pelvic tilt with sitting will be at particularly high risk. During procedures performed via the posterior approach, focused effort and attention may be required to visualize and resect anterior femoral neck osteophytes. Planned future directions include incorporation of an impingement and instability model into preoperative surgical planning for THA.

Disclosure

No industry partners were involved in study funding, nor in the preparation or publishing of the manuscript. No specific funding was attributed to this study. Two authors (Adam M. Katchky and Mitchell L. Smith) were paid stipends as clinical fellow and registrar, respectively, by the Melbourne Orthopaedic Group, which included research time to complete this study.

Conflicts of Interest

Adam M. Katchky declares that there are no conflicts of interest regarding the publication of this paper. Mitchell L. Smith declares that there are no conflicts of interest regarding the publication of this paper. Andrew J. Shimmin works for Matortho (royalties; paid consultant), Corin (royalties; paid consultant), Smith & Nephew (paid consultant), and Knee360 (unpaid consultant; shareholder). Stephen McMahon works for Smith & Nephew (unpaid consultant), Corin (shareholder; paid consultant; royalties), Knee360 (unpaid consultant; shareholder), and Stryker (consultant). Jeremy Latham works for Zimmer (paid speaker) and Lima LTO (royalties). Jonathan V. Baré works for Corin (shareholder; royalties; consultant; paid presentations; institutional support), Knee360 (shareholder; consultant), and Matortho (institutional support).

TABLE 2: Summary of ratings for presence of anterior femoral neck osteophyte, by assessor. Analysis was repeated with Rater #2 excluded due to divergence from the others.

Assessor	Absent [n, % of cases]	Minor [n, % of cases]	Extensive [n, % of cases]	Any osteophyte (minor + extensive) [n, % of cases]
#1	56 (14%)	230 (56%)	127 (31%)	357 (86%)
#2	**128 (31%)**	**224 (54%)**	**61 (15%)**	**285 (69%)**
#3	75 (18%)	243 (59%)	95 (23%)	338 (82%)
#4	89 (22%)	210 (51%)	113 (27%)	323 (78%)

References

[1] NJR Editorial Board, "National Joint Registry for England, Wales, Northern Ireland and Isle of Man, 15th Annual Report," National Joint Registry, 2018, http://www.njrreports.org.uk/Portals/0/PDFdownloads/NJR%2015th%20Annual%20Report%202018.pdf.

[2] Y. Kim, Y. Choi, and J. Kim, "Influence of patient-, design-, and surgery-related factors on rate of dislocation after primary cement less total hip arthroplasty," *The Journal of Arthroplasty*, vol. 24, no. 8, pp. 1258–1263, 2009.

[3] K. J. Bozic, K. Ong, E. Lau et al., "Risk of complication and revision total hip arthroplasty among medicare patients with different bearing surfaces," *Clinical Orthopaedics and Related Research*, vol. 468, no. 9, pp. 2357–2362, 2010.

[4] J. Parvizi, E. Picinic, and P. F. Sharkey, "Revision total hip arthroplasty for instability: surgical techniques and principles," *The Journal of Bone and Joint Surgery*, vol. 90, no. 5, pp. 1134–1142, 2008.

[5] D. J. Berry, M. Von Knoch, C. D. Schleck, and W. S. Harmsen, "The cumulative long-term risk of dislocation after primary charnley total hip arthroplasty," *The Journal of Bone and Joint Surgery*, vol. 86A, no. 1, pp. 9–14, 2004.

[6] D. J. Berry, M. von Knoch, C. D. Schleck, and W. S. Harmsen, "Effect of femoral head diameter and operative approach on risk of dislocation after primary total hip arthroplasty," *The Journal of Bone and Joint Surgery*, vol. 87, no. 11, pp. 2456–2463, 2005.

[7] A. Malik, A. Maheshwari, and L. D. Dorr, "Impingement with total hip replacement," *The Journal of Bone & Joint Surgery*, vol. 89, no. 8, pp. 1832–1842, 2007.

[8] G. E. Lewinnek, J. L. Lewis, R. Tarr, C. L. Compere, and J. R. Zimmerman, "Dislocations after total hip-replacement arthroplasties," *The Journal of Bone & Joint Surgery*, vol. 60, no. 2, pp. 217–220, 1978.

[9] M. P. Abdel, P. von Roth, M. T. Jennings, A. D. Hanssen, and M. W. Pagnano, "What safe zone? The vast majority of dislocated THAs are within the Lewinnek safe zone for acetabular component position," *Clinical Orthopaedics and Related Research*, vol. 474, no. 2, pp. 386–391, 2016.

[10] A. M. DiGioia, M. A. Hafez, B. Jaramaz, T. J. Levison, and J. E. Moody, "Functional pelvic orientation measured from lateral standing and sitting radiographs," *Clinical Orthopaedics and Related Research*, no. 453, pp. 272–276, 2006.

[11] A. Stephens, S. Munir, S. Shah, and W. L. Walter, "The kinematic relationship between sitting and standing posture and pelvic inclination and its significance to cup positioning in total hip arthroplasty," *International Orthopaedics*, vol. 39, no. 3, pp. 383–388, 2015.

[12] S. Parratte, M. W. Pagnano, K. Coleman-Wood, K. R. Kaufman, and D. J. Berry, "The 2008 frank stinchfield award: variation in postoperative pelvic tilt may confound the accuracy of hip navigation systems," *Clinical Orthopaedics and Related Research*, vol. 467, no. 1, pp. 43–49, 2009.

[13] Corin Group, "OPS™ Optimized Positioning System: product overview and surgical technique," Corin USA, 2018, https://www.coringroup.com/assets/product-resources/optimized-positioning-system-ops/Resources-Product-Information-OPS-Surgical-Technique-USA.PDF.

[14] J. Palan and A. Manktelow, "Surgical approaches for primary total hip replacement," *Journal of Orthopaedics and Traumatology*, vol. 32, no. 1, pp. 1–12, 2018.

[15] J. Pierrepont, L. Walter, B. Miles et al., "Pelvic tilt in the standing, supine and seated positions," *The Bone and Joint Journal*, vol. 98-B, supplementary 9, 2018.

20

Intraoperative Patella Dimension Measurement in Asian Female Patients and its Relevance in Patellar Resurfacing in TKA

Shaifuzain Ab Rahman,[1] **Amran Ahmed Shokri**,[1] **Muhammad Rajaie Ahmad**,[1] **Ahmad Filza Ismail**,[2] **and Nur Syahida Termizi**[1]

[1]*Department of Orthopedic, Hospital Universiti Sains Malaysia, 16150 Kubang Kerian, Kelantan, Malaysia*
[2]*Department of Community Medicine, Hospital Universiti Sains Malaysia, 16150 Kubang Kerian, Kelantan, Malaysia*

Correspondence should be addressed to Shaifuzain Ab Rahman; shaifuzain@usm.my

Academic Editor: Benjamin Blondel

Background. Implants used for total knee arthroplasty (TKA) in Asian patients are mostly produced based on anthropometry of the Western population, thus causing problem with patella sizing, especially in Asian females where the patellae are regarded to be smaller. This study is to define intraoperative patella dimensions in our female populations and compare them with current prosthetic systems available at our institution. *Methods.* This is a cross-sectional study involving 156 TKA female patients with normal patellae. The patella height, width, thickness, medial and lateral articular facets' width and thickness, and the dome position were measured. The smallest implant size from 3 manufacturers was compared to the data obtained. Analysis using descriptive statistics was used to get the mean and median of anatomical patella dimensions, whereas the independent *T* test and one-way ANOVA test were used to compare the Malaysian female's patella dimensions with various implant sizes. *Results.* The articular surface of the patella was found to have an oval shape with a width-height ratio of 1.31. The mean (SD) patella thickness, width, and height were 20.7 (1.85) mm, 40.7 (3.79) mm, and 31.3 (2.81) mm, respectively. Only 17.9% fit for smallest implant size from all 3 manufacturers. The oval-shape implant was suitable in 53.8% patients based on their width-height ratio. The dome position is 2.2 mm medial to centre. *Conclusion.* These female patients have thinner and smaller patella, which are generally unable to accommodate patellar components based on the Caucasian database. Therefore, orthopaedic implant manufacturers should consider optimizing the thicknesses as well as widths of their patellar prostheses.

1. Introduction

The patella is the largest sesamoid bone, which shields over the anterior surface of femoral condyles [1]. Its posterior surface can be divided into superior articulating surface and inferior nonarticulating surface. A vertical ridge further subdivides the superior part into medial and lateral facets. Wiberg has classified patella into 3 types, which is based on the width dimensions of the medial (MAF) and lateral articular facets (LAF) [2].

The patella is a part of the patella-femoral joint, which is essential to provide knee stability through its role in the extensor mechanism, whereby it improves mechanical property of extensor muscles. This is conducted via transmitting the extensor force across the knee at a greater distance from the centre of rotation. The magnification of moment arm reduces quadriceps force to extend the knee by 15% to 30% [3, 4].

Patella replacement in total knee arthroplasty (TKA) is not a universal procedure for all arthroplasty surgeons; thus, ample knowledge on its science is required. This includes knowledge of the patella anatomy and understanding the pathological changes that affect it [5]. Anthropometric measurements of the patella and patella ligament are crucial in the diagnoses and surgical corrections of knee-related injuries [4, 6].

A success in functionality of TKA with patella replacement highly depends on appropriate size and thickness of the chosen patella implant [6]. Poor design characteristics of the implants and technical errors were related to early patellar failures in a tricompartment TKA [7].

Various patella components are currently available in the market, which allow the prostheses to be onset or inset by using symmetrical or asymmetrical domes [7]. Most systems highlight on replacing the articular surface, correct positioning of the dome, and restoring the patella thickness. However, they do not focus on maximizing the anatomic bony coverage of the patella [7].

Implant components used for TKA in Asian patients are mostly produced based on anthropometry of the Western population. There would be differences in terms of conformity of implants to the patient's anatomy and clinical results after TKA due to anatomic features and life styles dissimilarities between Western and Asian populations. For that reason, surgeons in Asia are particularly concerned in related surgical techniques and implant designs that are being used in TKA for better quality clinical results as well as patient satisfaction [8, 9].

This study was conducted to define intraoperative anatomy of patella dimensions in female patients undergoing TKA and compare them with the commonly used prosthetic component systems. The goal is to get practical anatomic patella data in our female population. It is also to help in the development and improvement of patella component design and implantation for TKA in this population.

2. Materials and Methods

This was a cross-sectional study carried out at our centre for a period of 12 months from July 2016 to Jan 2018. Ethical approval from the institutional review board (IRB) was obtained before the study was conducted. All female patients who underwent TKA at our institution during this period of study were recruited with exclusion. We excluded patients with severe patella deformity from previous trauma, severe osteoarthritis of patellofemoral joint, or congenital deformity that normal anatomy could not be determined.

Initial detailed and thorough explanation regarding the TKA procedure was carried out by an arthroplasty surgeon during preoperative consultation at the orthopaedic clinic of our institution. Verbal and written consents from participants were obtained prior to the TKA.

Intraoperative anatomic measurement of patella was carried out by one of the two arthroplasty surgeons by using a surgical vernier caliper which is sensitive up to 0.1 mm.

The patella dimensions were measured after the marginal osteophytes were properly removed. The dimensions were inclusive of the patella height, which was from the edge of the superior articular surface to the margin of the inferior articular surface; the patella width, which was from the border of the medial articular surface to the border of lateral articular surface; and the patella thickness, which was the maximum thickness measured at the centre of the dome [7]. Finally, the widths of medial articular facet (MAF) and lateral articular facet (LAF) as well as their thickness were also measured (Figure 1 and 2). The average time taken for the measurement was less than 5 minutes, which was added to the normal time taken for TKA procedure. All measurements were recorded in the data collection sheet (Study Proforma).

The anthropometric data obtained intraoperatively were compared with the smallest patella component size from 3 commonly used manufacturers at our centre.

Data were analyzed using software IBM SPSS version 22 including descriptive statistics and compared the means using the independent T test and one-way ANOVA. Confidence interval was set at 95%, and p value <0.05 was considered statistically significant.

3. Results

There were 128 female patients undergoing 186 TKAs during the period of this study. However, following our inclusion and exclusion criteria, we ended up collecting data from 156 patellae of 102 patients who underwent TKA. The patients were between 45 to 79 years old with a mean age of 62.5 years old (SD 7.41). Out of 156 patients, 144 (92.3%) are Malays, 9 (5.8%) are Chinese, and 3 patients (1.9%) are from Indian ancestry.

The patella thickness ranges from 18 to 26 mm with mean 20.74 (1.85) mm. Patella height ranges from 22 to 38 mm with mean 31.33 (2.81) mm. Patella width ranges from 31 to 51 mm with mean 40.76 (3.79) mm. MAF width ranges from 13 to 27 mm with mean 19.38 (2.70) mm. LAF width ranges from 15 to 28 mm with mean 21.30 (2.27) mm. MAF thickness ranges from 11 to 20 mm with mean 15.90 (2.24) mm. LAF thickness ranges from 12 to 22 mm with mean 16.93 (2.16) mm. Width-height ratio ranges from 0.97 to 1.68 with mean 1.31 (0.13). These results are summarized in Table 1.

Out of 156 patients, 82 (52.6%) were measured from right knees, while 54 (47.4%) were from left knees. Based on Wiberg Classification [3], 94 (60.3%) patellae were type 1 patella, 53 (34.0%) were type 2, and 9 (5.7%) were type 3 patella. The mean dome position is 2.2 mm (3.4 mm) medial to the centre of the patella. This is consistent with the overall finding of Wiberg type 1 in this population.

The mean patella dimensions including patella height, patella width, patella thickness, MAF width, and LAF width between right side and left side was not statistically significant different ($p > 0.05$) (Table 2). The mean patella thickness and patella width between Wiberg types were also not statistically different (p value >0.05) (Table 3).

Based on the measurement of patella dimensions, further analysis comparing patients' patella with the smallest patella components from the 3 commonly used manufacturers were carried out. The smallest patella size (diameter) for implants A and C is 30 mm. The smallest size for implant B is 32 mm. Out of 156 patellae, 66 (42.4%) patellae fit for the smallest implant size from manufacturers A and C, while only 28 patellae fit for the smallest implant size from manufacturer B. Thus, there were 90 (57.6%) patellae that did not fit all smallest implants (A and C) used at our centre.

Based on their width-height ratio, there were 84 patellae (53.8%), which were suitable for oval-shape implants, while

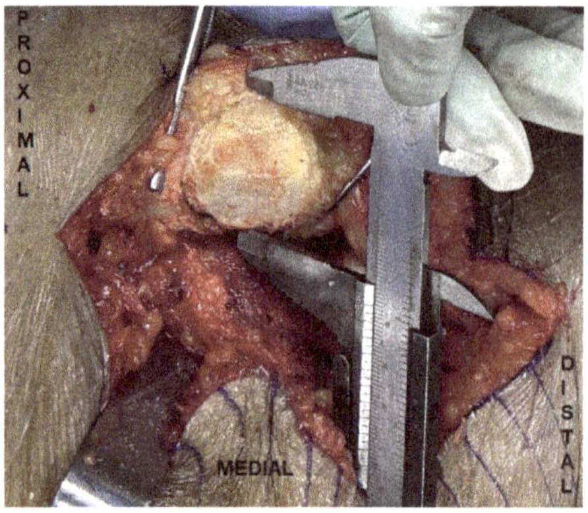

Figure 1: Measurement of left patella's width using a vernier caliper.

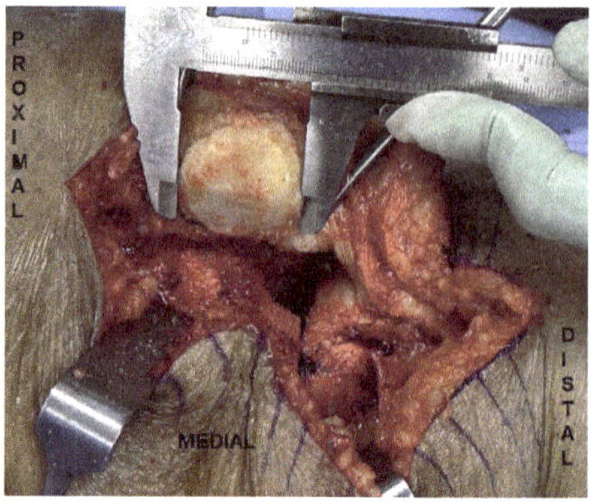

Figure 2: Measurement of left patella's height using a vernier caliper.

another 72 (46.2%) were suitable for round-shape implants. The mean width-height ratio between group of patients suitable for oval-shape implants and round-shape implants was statistically significant different with p value <0.001.

The mean patella height between the group of patients suitable for oval-shape implants and round-shape implants was statistically significantly different (p value <0.001). The mean patella height of patients suitable for round-shape implants was higher compared to the mean patella height of patients suitable for oval-shape implants, with 2.50 mean difference between these two groups (Table 4).

Table 1: Age and dimensions of patellae ($n = 156$).

Variables	Mean (SD)
Age (years)	65.50 (7.41)
Patella thickness (mm)	20.74 (1.85)
Patella height (mm)	31.33 (2.81)
Patella width (mm)	40.76 (3.79)
MAF width (mm)	19.38 (2.70)
LAF width (mm)	21.30 (2.27)
MAF thickness (mm)	15.90 (2.24)
LAF thickness (mm)	16.93 (2.16)
Width-height ratio	1.31 (0.13)

MAF = medial articular facets; LAF = lateral articular facets.

4. Discussion

A success in functionality of knee arthroplasty is highly dependent on appropriate size and thickness of the chosen patella implant [6]. This includes avoiding overstuffing or oversizing of the patella. This study aimed to document the anthropometric measurement of patella dimensions among our female patients receiving TKA and compare them with the available current patella implants size.

We only include female patients in this study since majority (>89%) of TKA patients at our centre are females. In addition, following previous studies, female is expected to have smaller patella dimensions [6, 7, 10–12]. Therefore, it is appropriate to assess if this female population will have issue fitting the smallest available patella component from the 3 commonly used TKA systems.

In the present study, the mean patella thickness, patella width, and patella height were 20.7 mm, 40.7 mm, and 31.3 mm, respectively. In an American study [7], the mean patella thickness was 21.8 mm, the mean patella width was 42.7 mm, and the mean patella height was 35.0 mm in their female samples. Another study among the South African females with European ancestry showed the mean patella thickness, patella width, and patella height were 22.8 mm, 42.7 mm, and 41.0 mm, respectively [11]. Based on the above data, it is concluded that our female population have thinner and smaller patellae than the Westerners.

In this study, Wiberg type I patellae, in which the MAF and LAF widths are concave and equal, were the most prevalent with 60.3% of the patients as compared to 34% of Wiberg type II patellae. This is different from the study by Wiberg himself in 1941 that reported type II patellae were the most prevalent [2]. This finding was supported by Fucentese et al. which also showed Wiberg type II as the majority in his series [13].

The average dome of the articular surface of the patella in this study is located at 2.2 mm medial of centre, which is consistent with Wiberg type I patellae. Aglietti et al. [14] showed that, in their series, the mean dome position was 4.0 mm medially. While in the Hofmann et al. [15] series, the mean dome was 5.4 mm medially. These patellae are consistent with Wiberg type II or III. Baldwin and House series has the closest mean dome position (at 3.7 mm) to this study's findings [7]. However, the series still showed predominantly Wiberg II patella in their study. Based on the above findings, previous studies had agreed on the benefits of medialization of the patella during the patellar resurfacing [15, 16]. However, in our series, medialization of the patella is not usually necessary since most of our patellae are Wiberg I.

In patellofemoral arthritis, the chondral wear is the most prominent in the lateral patellar facet, which points out that the lateral patellar facet receives higher load than the central or medial aspect of the patella [13]. Since majority of our patients had almost equal MAF and LAF widths, the higher load exerted on lateral facet may lead to a higher risk of developing patellofemoral arthritis in our population. Another supportive evidence is that the highest compressive

Table 2: Comparison of patella dimensions between the right and left side ($n = 156$).

Variables (mm)	Right side, mean (SD)	Left side, mean (SD)	Mean difference (95% CI)	t statistics (df)	p value
Patella height	31.41 (2.88)	31.24 (2.77)	0.17 (−1.11, 1.45)	0.27 (76)	0.790
Patella width	40.67 (3.62)	40.85 (4.02)	−0.18 (−1.90, 1.54)	−0.21 (76)	0.835
Patella thickness	20.82 (2.06)	20.65 (1.61)	0.17 (−0.67, 1.01)	0.40 (76)	0.691
MF width	19.22 (2.66)	19.55 (2.77)	−0.33 (−1.56, 0.89)	−0.54 (76)	0.588
LF width	21.30 (2.35)	21.30 (2.20)	0.01 (−1.02, 1.04)	0.02 (76)	0.988

MF = medial facet; LF = lateral facet.

Table 3: Comparison of patella thickness and width with Wiberg type ($n = 156$).

Variable (mm)	Wiberg type 1, mean (SD) ($n = 90$)	Wiberg type 2, mean (SD) ($n = 53$)	Wiberg type 3, mean (SD) ($n = 9$)	F-statistics (df)	p value*
Patella thickness	20.71 (1.67)	20.81 (2.29)	20.60 (1.14)	0.04 (2)	0.965
Patella width	41.03 (3.81)	40.02 (3.85)	42.00 (3.32)	0.88 (2)	0.418

*One-way Anova. Since p value is not significant, the post hoc test is not performed.

load is found primarily beneath the lateral facet, which are related to the higher subchondral bone densities [17]. It has been described that the patellar trabecular bone architecture over the lateral facet is nonhomogenous stacking up of sheets resulting from improved remodelling process because of the constant pressure in situ [18].

This current study shows moderate to good correlation between patella width and patella thickness, which is consistent with the results of Iranpour et al. [10] and Olateju et al. [11]. This finding explains that, in general, smaller patellae will not only have problem fitting the implant but also face problem to maintain minimum bone thickness upon resection. Patella width has been proposed to be a dependable factor for predicting the normal size of patella thickness, which helps the surgeons to decide on the thickness of the patella prosthesis during TKA [10].

This study also shows that 90 patients (57.6%) do not fit the smallest available patella component (size 30 mm) used at out institution. Although we did not have patella component smaller than size 30 mm during the period of this study, we further analyzed the number of patients that would fit smaller component sizes. For a size 28 mm, 101 (64.7%) of our patellae fit the patella component. Furthermore, the theoretical analysis shows that a component size of 26 mm fits 149 (95.5%) patellae of this series.

Our findings is different from an American study [19] that showed only one-third of their female patients were unable to accommodate their smallest patella implant without overhang. The study also showed that the native patellae which measured about 17 to 21 mm thick may have problem fitting prosthesis between 26 mm and 33 mm in diameter. Thus, in order to avoid over-resection of remaining bone stock and at the same time restore the original patella thickness, the authors suggested prostheses in the diameter range of about 26 to 33 mm need to be available in thicknesses of approximately 5 to 7 mm [19].

Other authors have reported that the patella articular surface is oval, with the width being larger than the height [2–4, 6–8, 10]. The ratio of width to height in this series was 1.31, similar to findings by Aglietti [14], which was also 1.31 and ratio of 1.34 by Zaffagnini et al. [1]. The point that the mean articular surface of patella is 25% wider than its height could be a significant consideration in patella prosthesis design. An American study by Baldwin and House [7] showed that there is potential to improve maximum patellar coverage by 9.1% if the surgeon uses an oval patella implant, with 11.5% improvement of coverage in men and 7.7% in women, which will improve the load transfer through the implant.

Our study relies on an intraoperative direct measurement for the patellae dimension as compared to some studies where measurements were taken from cadavers or from radiographs. Although a radiographic study allows the availability of large sample size, it is usually related to male samples following trauma or sport injury. Furthermore, there is also limitation in accuracy of the measurements due to magnification in radiograph as well as thickness of the patella cartilage that cannot be measured on radiograph. However, for cadaveric study, the limited number of cadavers is the negative point.

There were several limitations present in this study. First, regarding the number of patients involved in this study, we require a larger sample size with multicentre involvement to get better results. Second, a surgical caliper was used to measure the patella dimensions. Even though caliper measurements are commonly used in anthropometric studies, a question raised regarding the accuracy of smooth caliper measurements [20]. Thus, a digital vernier caliper would be a better option. Third, although we consider the effect of pre-arthritic thickness of the patellae involved in this study by eliminating all the deformed and misshapen patellae, the local effect and the extent of patella surface thinning due to arthritis at the time of operation are unknown.

TABLE 4: Comparison of width-height ratio and patella height between the group of patients suitable for oval-shape implants and round-shape implants ($n = 156$).

Variable	Oval, mean (SD) ($n = 84$)	Round, mean (SD) ($n = 72$)	Mean difference (95% CI)	t statistics (df)	p value*
Width-height ratio	1.40 (0.09)	1.20 (0.06)	0.20 (0.16, 0.23)	11.18 (76)	<0.001
Patella height (mm)	30.18 (2.51)	32.68 (2.56)	−2.50 (−3.64, −1.36)	−4.35 (76)	<0.001

*Independent T-test.

5. Conclusion

As a conclusion, the implant manufacturers will have to consider ideal size of patella component for Asian patients, especially for the female. This is to provide optimum patella coverage during the patella resurfacing in a tri-compartmental TKA in order to achieve optimum biomechanical integrity of the patellofemoral joint after TKA. The Malaysian female knees have thinner native patella and generally accommodate smaller patellar components than the Caucasian female counterparts.

Acknowledgments

This project was supported by the research university grant of Universiti Sains Malaysia (Grant no. 1001/PPSP/8012312).

References

[1] S. Zaffagnini, D. Dejour, A. Grassi et al., "Patellofemoral anatomy and biomechanics: current concepts," *Joints*, vol. 1, no. 2, pp. 15–20, 2013.

[2] G. Wiberg, "Roentgenographic and anatomic studies on the femoropatellar joint: with special reference to chondromalacia patellae," *Acta Orthopaedica Scandinavica*, vol. 12, no. 1-4, pp. 319–410, 1941.

[3] J. P. Goldblatt and J. C. Richmond, "Anatomy and biomechanics of the knee," *Operative Techniques in Sports Medicine*, vol. 11, no. 3, pp. 172–186, 2003.

[4] B. C. Bengs and R. D. Scott, "The effect of patellar thickness on intraoperative knee flexion and patellar tracking in total knee arthroplasty," *The Journal of Arthroplasty*, vol. 21, no. 5, pp. 650–655, 2006.

[5] T. K. Kim, B. J. Chung, Y. G. Kang, C. B. Chang, and S. C. Seong, "Clinical implications of anthropometric patellar dimensions for TKA in Asians," *Clinical Orthopaedics and Related Research*, vol. 467, no. 4, pp. 1007–1014, 2009.

[6] J. H. Yoo, S. R. Yi, and J. H. Kim, "The geometry of patella and patellar tendon measured on knee MRI," *Surgical and Radiologic Anatomy*, vol. 29, no. 8, pp. 623–628, 2007.

[7] J. L. Baldwin and C. K. House, "Anatomic dimensions of the patella measured during total knee arthroplasty," *The Journal of Arthroplasty*, vol. 20, no. 2, pp. 250–257, 2005.

[8] T. Schmalzried, "Orthopedic surgeon's guide to total knee systems," *Orthopedics Today*, vol. 22, no. 41, 2002.

[9] D.-K. Kim, M.-C. Seo, S.-J. Song, and K.-I. Kim, "Are Korean patients different from other ethnic groups in total knee arthroplasty?" *Knee Surgery & Related Research*, vol. 27, no. 4, pp. 199–206, 2015.

[10] F. Iranpour, A. M. Merican, A. A. Amis, and J. P. Cobb, "The width:thickness ratio of the patella: an aid in knee arthroplasty," *Clinical Orthopaedics and Related Research*, vol. 466, no. 5, pp. 1198–1203, 2008.

[11] O. I. Olateju, I. Philander, and M. A. Bidmos, "Morphometric analysis of the patella and patellar ligament of South Africans of European ancestry," *South African Journal of Science*, vol. 109, no. 9/10, pp. 1-6, 2013.

[12] R. Muhamed, V. V. Saralaya, B. V. Murlimanju, and G. K. Chettiar, "In vivo magnetic resonance imaging morphometry of the patella bone in South Indian population," *Anatomy & Cell Biology*, vol. 50, no. 2, pp. 99–103, 2017.

[13] S. F. Fucentese, A. von Roll, P. P. Koch, D. R. Epari, B. Fuchs, and P. B. Schottle, "The patella morphology in trochlear dysplasia—a comparative MRI study," *The Knee*, vol. 13, no. 2, pp. 145–150, 2006.

[14] P. Aglietti, J. N. Insall, P. S. Walker, and P. Trent, "A new patella prosthesis," *Clinical Orthopaedics and Related Research*, vol. 107, pp. 175–187, 1975.

[15] A. A. Hofmann, T. K. Tkach, C. J. Evanich, M. P. Camargo, and Y. Zhang, "Patellar component medialization in total knee arthroplasty," *The Journal of Arthroplasty*, vol. 12, no. 2, pp. 155–160, 1997.

[16] J. C. Bayley, R. D. Scott, F. C. Ewald, and G. B. Holmes, "Failure of the metal-backed patellar component after total knee replacement," *The Journal of Bone & Joint Surgery*, vol. 70, no. 5, pp. 668–674, 1988.

[17] F. Eckstein, M. Muller-Gerbl, and R. Putz, "Distribution of subchondral bone density and cartilage thickness in the human patella," *Journal of Anatomy*, vol. 180, pp. 425–433, 1992.

[18] P. R. Townsend, R. E. Miegel, R. M. Rose, P. Raux, and E. L. Radin, "Structure and function of the human patella: the role of cancellous bone," *Journal of Biomedical Materials Research*, vol. 10, no. 4, pp. 605–611, 1976.

[19] H. D. Clarke and M. J. Spangehl, "Gender optimized patellar component designs are needed to better match female patellar anatomy," *The Knee*, vol. 21, no. 6, pp. 1250–1253, 2014.

[20] M. A. Rauh, M. Bayers-Thering, C. M. Buyea, M. Phillips, and K. A. Krackow, "Reliability and validity of a new caliper for measuring patellar thickness," *The Journal of Arthroplasty*, vol. 17, no. 1, pp. 105–107, 2002.

21

Clinical and Radiological Outcomes of Total Knee Arthroplasty Performed with Midvastus and Medial Parapatellar Approaches in Obese Patients

Olcay Guler, [1] **Gürkan Gümüşsuyu**, [2] **Hakan Sofu**, [1] **and Hüseyin Bahadır Gökçen** [2]

[1] *Department of Orthopedics and Traumatology, Medical Faculty, Altınbaş University, Istanbul, Turkey*
[2] *Department of Orthopedics and Traumatology, Medical Faculty, Istinye University, Istanbul, Turkey*

Correspondence should be addressed to Olcay Guler; olcayguler77@gmail.com

Academic Editor: Francesco Liuzza

Background. The use of total knee arthroplasty (TKA) for primary osteoarthritis of the knee has remarkably increased recently. We aimed to compare the clinical and radiological outcomes of TKA in obese patients (>30 kg/m^2) operated with midvastus (MV) or medial parapatellar (MPP) approaches. *Methods.* This retrospective study was performed using data derived from 80 patients (70 women; 10 men) with an average age of 66.17 ± 5.42 (range: 54 to 77). Patients were allocated into 2 groups as for the type of approach conducted during TKA: group I ($n = 41$) underwent TKA by MV approach, while the MMP technique was used in group II ($n = 39$). *Results.* Demographic, clinical, and radiological parameters included age, side of involvement, sex, BMI, diameters of thigh and calf, length of incision, duration of operation, amount of bleeding and transfusion, duration of hospitalization and follow-up, complications, and range of motion, as well as Knee Society Score (KSS) and Knee Society Function Score (KSFS). Patients with a higher BMI (≥35 kg/m^2) experienced more profound bleeding and needed more transfusion of erythrocyte suspension. The range of motion was more favorable in groups with BMI <35 kg/m^2. The functional outcomes as reflected in KSS and KSFS were much better in patients with BMI <35 kg/m^2. *Conclusions.* Our data indicated that obesity can adversely influence the clinical and radiological outcomes after TKA performed by both MV and MPP approaches. A careful analysis of patient characteristics and selection of appropriate operative procedures is critical. Further randomized, controlled trials on larger series must be designed to elucidate the relationship between obesity and therapeutic outcomes after TKA with different approaches.

1. Introduction

Total knee arthroplasty (TKA) is considered the best treatment method for end-stage osteoarthritis [1]. It is performed to correct deformity, relieve pain, and restore joint function in arthritic knees [2]. The medial parapatellar (MPP) approach is accepted as a simple and standard approach for TKA, which provides adequate exposure of the joint [2, 3]. Nevertheless, this method brings about risks such as the split of the quadriceps tendon, reduction of the patellar blood supply, and diminution of extensor strength. These drawbacks may lead to complications such as patellar fracture and patellofemoral instability [2, 3]. On the other hand, the midvastus (MV) approach was developed as an option to MPP, and it allows the preservation of the quadriceps tendon intact. The MV offers advantages such as better quadriceps control, earlier functional outcomes, less pain, and better patellar tracking. On the other hand, MV may be associated with problems like neurovascular injury and insufficient exposure. There is still controversy on the preference of MPP and MV routes for TKA [2–4].

Obesity is a frequent condition that increases the need for TKA. There is debate on the risks, benefits, and complications of TKA in obese patients. An accurate understanding of the medical and surgical complications associated with TKA in the obese patients will enhance research efforts and improve outcomes [5].

The purpose of the present study was to compare the clinical and radiological outcomes of TKA with MV and MPP approaches in obese patients.

2. Patients and Methods

2.1. Study Design. This retrospective study was performed in the orthopedics and traumatology department of our tertiary care center. The approval of the local institutional review board was obtained before the study. Data was gathered from the medical files of a total of 80 patients (70 women; 10 men) who underwent TKA for primary osteoarthritis of the knee using MV or MPP approaches. The average age of our series was 66.17 ± 5.42 (range: 54 to 77). Patients had undergone surgery between January 2014 and January 2019. Patients were allocated into 2 groups as for the type of approach conducted during TKA: group I ($n = 41$) underwent TKA by MV approach while the MMP technique was used in group II ($n = 39$).

Patients aged 18 to 80 years with a body mass index (BMI) >30 kg/m^2 were included. Patients with BMI <35 were termed group Ia and group IIa, whereas patients with BMI ≥35 were named as group Ib and group IIb. Exclusion criteria were collagen vascular diseases, history of high tibial osteotomy, flexion angle <80°, valgus and varus deformity >30°, previous history of infection of knee joint, neurological deficit such as diabetic neuropathy, previous history of fracture or surgery of the femur and tibia, and osteoarthritis of the ipsilateral or contralateral hip joint.

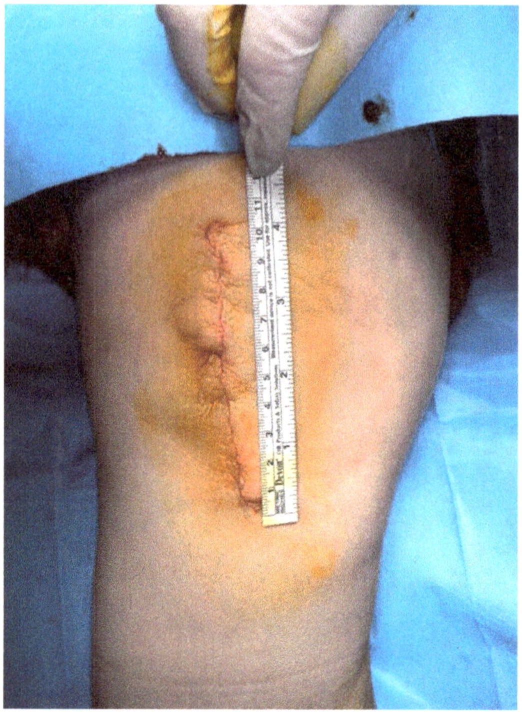

FIGURE 1: The measurement of incision length at extension of the knee.

2.2. Surgical Procedure. Spinal or epidural anesthesia was routinely used in all patients. An anterior cruciate ligament preserving total knee replacement prosthesis (*Genesis 2, Smith & Nephew, Memphis, TN, USA*) was utilized. Tourniquet was not used in any of our patients.

In group I, a skin incision passing through 1/3 medial of the patella, which starts from 1 to 2 cm proximal of the patellar upper pole, extends toward 2 cm distal to knee joint line, and ends at the medial border of tibial tuberosity, was performed (Figure 1).

The exposure to the patellar retinaculum was provided longitudinally; starting 1 cm medial to the patella, the capsular incision was extended from 2 cm proximal to the upper pole of the patella. The incision passed 2–4 cm inside the vastus medialis oblique (VMO) muscle bundles. Patella was dislocated laterally without eversion. In group I, specially designed small instruments were used to carry out distal femoral incisions for allowing 6° of valgus in the coronal plane and providing 90° exposure to the anterior-posterior distal femur in the sagittal plane. The femoral rotation was adjusted using posterior condylar and epicondylar axes. Tibial incisions were performed 90° on the coronal plane and 7° on the posterior tibial slope on the sagittal plane. An extramedullary guide was used on the tibia and an intramedullary guide was used on the femur. Lateral release and patellar resurfacing were not performed in any patients. No thumb test was performed to assess patellar alignment.

In group II, a straight incision that passes through the midpatellar line was performed while the knee was maintained at flexion. After the patellar retinaculum was incised longitudinally through the medial patella, a capsular incision was extended proximally to the union of rectus femoris and VMO muscles and 2 cm below tibial tuberosity distally. Patella was dislocated laterally without eversion and the knee joint was maintained at flexion. Using specially designed instruments, femoral incisions were performed with an intramedullary guide with a 90° angle in the sagittal plane on the anterior and posterior distal femur. The femoral rotation was arranged using posterior condylar and epicondylar axes. After exposure to the tibia, tibial incisions were carried out using an extramedullary guide. Lateral release and patellar resurfacing were not performed in any patients. Patella tracking was evaluated using a no thumb test.

All patients received tranexamic acid at a dose of 1 g via the intravenous route (*Transamine®, Mefar Pharmaceuticals, Istanbul, Turkey*) before and after the operation. Moreover, periarticular tranexamic acid injections were performed perioperatively. All patients had low molecular weight heparin (*Clexane®, Sanofi, Istanbul, Turkey*) for 21 days for prophylaxis against deep venous thrombosis.

2.3. Postoperative Care and Follow-Up. The drain was removed on the 1st day postoperatively and the patient was mobilized with crutch Canadian canes. In addition to the initiation of passive joint motion with a continuous passive motion (CPM) device, isometric quadriceps and active knee flexion and extension exercises were started on the first postoperative day.

For the relief of postoperative pain, narcotic analgesics were administered with patient-controlled analgesia (PCA) on the first postoperative day. On the following, intravenous and oral analgesics were administered. Prophylactic antibiotics were given for 24 hours. Patients were controlled on 15 days, 6 weeks, 3 months, 6 months, 12 months, and annually every year after the procedure. Evaluation of the axis using low extremity roentgenography and calculation of mechanical femorotibial angle were carried out before surgery and on the 3rd month postoperatively.

All radiological measurements were performed on Picture Archiving and Communication System (PACS). These steps were carried out by 2 experienced surgeons who were not involved in the surgical team and who were blinded to patient data. These surgeons conducted measurements twice with 1-month intervals.

Superficial infections were treated with oral antibiotics. In patients with a patellar tendon injury, knee pads were used for 4 weeks since patients could perform active straight leg raise.

2.4. Outcome Measures. The main outcome measures were age, side of involvement, sex, BMI, diameters of thigh and calf, length of incision, duration of operation, amount of bleeding and transfusion, duration of hospitalization and follow-up, complications, time of straight leg raise (days), pre- and postoperative mechanical femorotibial angle measurements in terms of coronal and sagittal femoral and tibial slopes, range of motion, Knee Society Score (KSS), and Knee Society Function Score (KSFS) [6, 7].

The parameters of the radiographic evaluation system were coronal femur alpha (medial distal femoral angle: MDFA), coronal tibia (beta), sagittal femur (lambda), and sagittal tibia (gamma) (Figure 2) [8, 9].

The range of motion was assessed in terms of flexion and extension and the clinical and functional outcomes after TKA as for KSS and KSFS were evaluated preoperatively, on 2 weeks, 6 weeks, 3 months, 6 months, 12 months, and on the final visit.

The diameters of the thigh and calf were measured in the midthigh and midcalf, respectively. The duration of surgery was described as the interval between the onset of incision and the placement of the final suture (Figure 3). The amount of intraoperative bleeding (mL) was calculated using the blood collected in suction (the volume of irrigation fluid was excluded), the weight of gauze, and blood collected in the drain. The length of the incision was measured at extension.

2.5. Statistical Analysis. Our data were analyzed with Statistical Package for Social Sciences version 21.0 for Windows software (*SPSS Inc., Chicago, Illinois, USA*). Descriptive data were presented as counts and percentages. Quantitative data were expressed as mean, standard deviation, median, minimum, and maximum. The normal distribution of variables was tested using the Kolmogorov–Smirnov test. For continuous variables, the student's t-test was employed as a parametric test, whereas Mann–Whitney U and Kruskal–Wallis tests were used as nonparametric tests. The Pearson chi-square test was utilized for the evaluation of categorical variables. A p value less than 0.05 was considered statistically significant.

3. Results

A comparative overview of demographic variables under investigation is presented in Table 1. Our population consisted of 80 patients (70 women; 10 men) with an average age of 66.17 ± 5.42 (range: 54 to 77). Groups I and II were further classified into 2 groups as for BMI. Patients with BMI <35 were termed group Ia and group IIa, whereas patients with BMI ≥35 were named as group Ib and group IIb.

The clinical and perioperative variables in 2 groups are demonstrated in Table 2. Radiographic parameters before and after TKA and the range of motion and functional scores before and after surgery are shown in Tables 3 and 4, respectively.

These 4 groups revealed similar results in terms of age ($p = 0.171$), sex distribution ($p = 0.293$), side of involvement ($p = 0.674$), duration of follow-up ($p = 0.634$), preoperative mechanical femorotibial angle ($p = 0.383$), preoperative flexion ($p = 0.779$), extension on postoperative 2nd week ($p = 0.166$), and diameters of thigh ($p = 0.573$) and calf ($p = 0.639$) (Tables 1–4).

Remarkably, the amount of bleeding was more profound ($p < 0.001$), BMI was higher ($p < 0.001$), postoperative mechanical femorotibial angle results were increased ($p = 0.001$), and the preoperative extension range was more extensive ($p = 0.029$) in groups Ib and IIb. The length of the incision was longer in group Ib ($p = 0.001$). The amount of erythrocyte suspension transfusion was higher in groups Ib and IIb ($p < 0.001$) (Table 2).

Flexion on the 2nd week, 6th week, and 3rd month postoperatively was higher in group IIa ($p < 0.001$, for all). Flexion on the 3rd month postoperatively was higher in group IIa ($p < 0.001$) (Table 4).

Extension on the 3rd month postoperatively was higher in group IIb ($p = 0.012$). Flexion on the 6th and 12th months postoperatively was higher in groups Ia and IIa ($p = 0.001$) (Table 4).

Extension on 6th and 12th months postoperatively was higher in groups Ib and IIb ($p = 0.012$ and $p = 0.028$, respectively). Flexion on the final control visit was remarkably lower in groups Ib and IIb ($p = 0.001$). On the other hand, the extension on the final control visit was higher in groups Ib and IIb ($p = 0.048$) (Table 4).

Radiographic parameters such as coronal femoral alpha, coronal tibia beta, sagittal femoral lambda, and sagittal tibial gamma displayed remarkable differences in both measurements performed by 2 independent observers.

The KSS and KSFS preoperatively, on 6 weeks, 3 months, 6 months, 12 months, and on the final visit postoperatively were remarkably higher in groups Ia and IIa (Table 4).

In group I, a skin blister was detected in 1 patient and a superficial infection treated successfully with oral antibiotics was diagnosed in 1 patient. In group II, skin blisters were observed in 2 patients and superficial infection was identified in 1 patient.

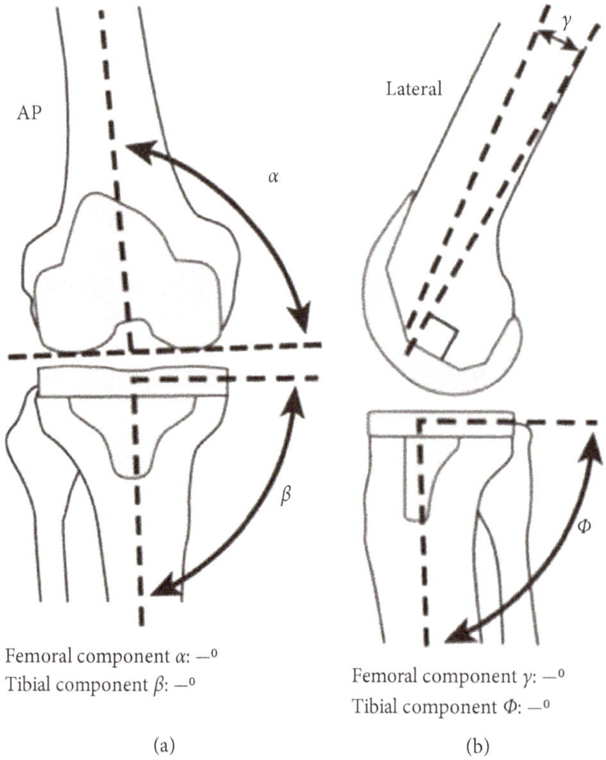

FIGURE 2: Roentgenographic evaluation parameters after total knee arthroplasty (TKA) (Ewald FC).

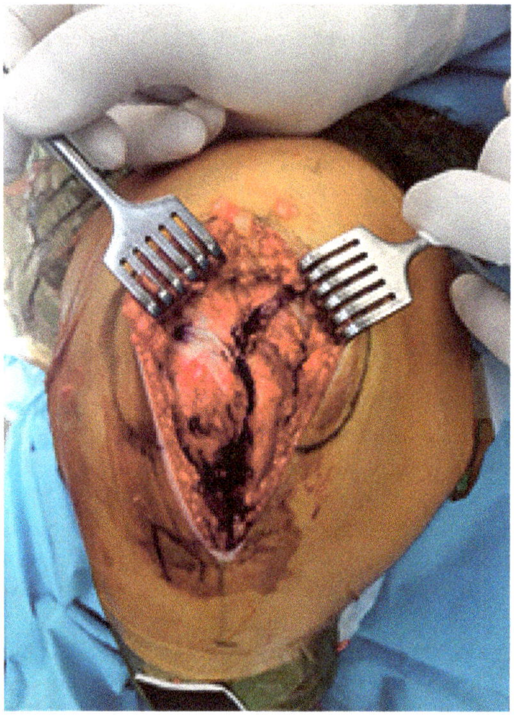

FIGURE 3: Preoperative image demonstrating midvastus approach.

4. Discussion

TKA provides satisfactory and reproducible results, and the MPP approach has been used as the standard technique before minimally invasive approaches were devised. Despite the fact that MP is a successful method, the recovery period can be prolonged and a rehabilitation period of up to 1 year can be necessary before prompt functional recovery. The midvastus method is one of the minimally invasive techniques and it may allow faster functional recovery, shorter duration of hospitalization, and more favorable ROM. However, the debate on the advantages and disadvantages of minimally invasive techniques is not resolved [10].

Our findings yielded that bleeding and the need for transfusion of erythrocyte suspension were more frequent in obese patients who underwent TKA. The functional outcomes as reflected in KSS and KSFS were more favorable in nonobese patients. Similarly, nonobese patients displayed better outcomes in terms of the range of motion and radiography compared to that of obese patients.

Efforts have been spent to determine the optimal surgical modality with satisfactory safety and effectivity in TKA [11]. The prevalence of obesity was found to be increased in patients undergoing primary, revision, and infected TKA. The obesity epidemic seems to be linked with the increased likelihood of revision and infection after surgery. Since the rates of obesity may further increase, it can be estimated that the burden of revision and infection related to obesity may be more obvious [12].

Li et al. suggested that MV offers a better range of motion and more effective pain control than MPP in the immediate postoperative period after TKA [2]. Postoperative knee function is the most important criterion for the assessment of the effectiveness of the procedure. The MV approach can

TABLE 1: A comparative overview of demographic variables under investigation.

Variable	Group				p value
	Ia	Ib	IIa	IIb	
Age (years)	63.67 ± 5.95	68.53 ± 5.18	66.57 ± 5.07	66.00 ± 5.69	0.171
Sex (F/M)	22/2	14/3	26/2	8/3	0.293
Body mass index (kg/m^2)	32.79 ± 1.47	36.65 ± 1.00	33.18 ± 1.61	36.91 ± 0.83	**<0.001**
Side of involvement (R/L)	15/9	13/4	17/11	8/3	0.674

TABLE 2: A comparative overview of clinical and perioperative variables under investigation.

Variable	Group				p value
	Ia	Ib	IIa	IIb	
Bleeding (mL)	31.35 ± 12.62	54.80 ± 17.04	28.73 ± 9.44	66.23 ± 20.95	**<0.001**
Follow-up (months)	38.58 ± 10.96	35.12 ± 14.20	36.21 ± 13.52	39.09 ± 11.38	0.634
Diameter of thigh (cm)	52.92 ± 3.59	62.41 ± 4.46	52.64 ± 5.89	63.82 ± 4.28	0.573
Diameter of calf (cm)	34.83 ± 4.00	44.59 ± 3.68	37.04 ± 5.37	43.82 ± 3.63	0.639
ES transfusion (units)	1.25 ± 0.61	2.06 ± 0.56	1.25 ± 0.70	2.36 ± 0.51	**<0.001**

TABLE 3: Radiographic parameters before and after TKA.

Preoperative MFTA (°)		190.63 ± 3.63	190.29 ± 2.73	190.50 ± 3.25	193.27 ± 4.82	0.383
Postoperative MFTA (°)		180.54 ± 1.38	181.47 ± 1.62	180.54 ± 1.17	182.45 ± 1.57	**0.001**
Coronal femur (alpha)*	I	122.50 ± 5.32	120.59 ± 3.48	124.46 ± 4.97	117.73 ± 5.18	**0.002**
Coronal tibia (beta)*	I	89.42 ± 1.18	88.88 ± 1.17	89.64 ± 1.16	88.45 ± 0.93	**0.008**
Sagittal femur (lambda)*	I	0.79 ± 1.02	1.59 ± 1.23	1.11 ± 1.42	2.55 ± 1.37	**0.002**
Sagittal tibia (gamma)*	I	84.88 ± 0.68	84.65 ± 0.79	85.21 ± 0.88	84.36 ± 1.63	**0.018**
Coronal femur (alpha)*	II	64.58 ± 3.27	62.06 ± 2.54	72.86 ± 6.00	67.27 ± 4.67	**<0.001**
Coronal tibia (beta)*	II	88.71 ± 1.33	89.29 ± 1.16	89.39 ± 1.29	89.82 ± 0.60	**0.045**
Sagittal femur (lambda)*	II	1.54 ± 1.06	0.88 ± 1.22	1.21 ± 1.26	2.36 ± 0.92	**0.021**
Sagittal tibia (gamma)	II	85.21 ± 0.98	85.06 ± 1.03	84.75 ± 0.97	84.91 ± 0.70	0.302
Coronal femur (alpha)$	I	95.25 ± 0.85	94.88 ± 0.86	95.07 ± 0.72	95.00 ± 0.78	0.378
Coronal tibia (beta)$	I	95.08 ± 0.83	94.94 ± 0.80	89.54 ± 0.96	89.09 ± 1.22	**<0.001**
Sagittal femur (lambda)$	I	1.42 ± 1.28	1.41 ± 0.94	1.75 ± 1.04	1.18 ± 1.25	**<0.001**
Sagittal tibia (gamma)$	I	89.54 ± 1.41	89.29 ± 1.05	85.46 ± 0.79	85.55 ± 0.79	**<0.001**
Coronal femur (alpha)$	II	85.04 ± 0.95	84.76 ± 1.15	95.07 ± 0.72	95.27 ± 1.10	**<0.001**
Coronal tibia (beta)$	II	88.78 ± 1.27	89.12 ± 1.07	89.54 ± 1.00	89.55 ± 1.21	**<0.001**
Sagittal femur (lambda)$	II	1.38 ± 0.77	1.24 ± 1.03	1.64 ± 1.13	1.55 ± 0.93	**<0.001**
Sagittal tibia (gamma)$	II	85.25 ± 0.94	85.00 ± 1.12	84.93 ± 1.02	85.27 ± 0.90	0.516

TABLE 4: Range of motion and functional scores before and after surgery.

Preoperative flexion	94.38 ± 6.81	96.47 ± 6.56	96.61 ± 6.81	93.18 ± 7.17	0.779
Preoperative extension	5.00 ± 3.90	8.24 ± 2.46	5.71 ± 4.24	8.18 ± 4.62	**0.029**
Flexion (postoperative 2 weeks)	82.92 ± 5.88	80.00 ± 5.86	91.43 ± 8.70	83.18 ± 6.03	**<0.001**
Extension (postoperative 2 weeks)	3.33 ± 3.18	5.00 ± 3.54	3.21 ± 3.39	5.45 ± 4.16	0.166
Flexion (postoperative 6 weeks)	105.21 ± 7.44	100.00 ± 5.86	113.39 ± 7.82	104.55 ± 10.60	**<0.001**
Extension (postoperative 6 weeks)	0.63 ± 1.69	1.47 ± 2.35	0.36 ± 1.89	2.73 ± 3.44	**0.037**
Flexion (postoperative 3 months)	118.75 ± 5.16	117.06 ± 3.98	123.21 ± 4.76	116.82 ± 5.13	**<0.001**
Extension (postoperative 3 months)	0.42 ± 1.41	1.18 ± 2.19	0.18 ± 1.66	2.73 ± 3.44	**0.012**
Flexion (postoperative 6 months)	120.53 ± 5.02	118.97 ± 3.60	123.26 ± 4.50	117.42 ± 5.10	**0.001**
Extension (postoperative 6 months)	0.40 ± 0.92	1.10 ± 2.05	0.16 ± 1.40	2.40 ± 2.70	**0.011**
Flexion (postoperative 12 months)	122.92 ± 5.30	120.88 ± 3.18	124.64 ± 4.45	118.18 ± 5.14	**0.001**
Extension (postoperative 12 months)	0.40 ± 1.37	1.14 ± 2.10	0.34 ± 1.67	2.73 ± 3.12	**0.048**
Preoperative KSS	40.88 ± 6.95	38.88 ± 5.48	42.75 ± 6.94	35.55 ± 3.42	**0.014**
Preoperative KSFS	37.92 ± 5.70	37.06 ± 5.32	39.64 ± 5.08	32.73 ± 5.18	**0.010**
KSS (postoperative 6 weeks)	83.00 ± 3.50	80.00 ± 2.12	83.61 ± 3.76	78.55 ± 4.89	**<0.001**
KSFS (postoperative 6 weeks)	81.67 ± 4.34	78.82 ± 3.76	82.50 ± 3.72	76.82 ± 4.62	**0.001**
KSS (postoperative 3 months)	86.33 ± 2.87	83.35 ± 1.77	87.86 ± 2.80	83.36 ± 2.58	**<0.001**

Table 4: Continued.

KSFS (postoperative 3 months)	86.88 ± 3.85	83.24 ± 3.03	86.79 ± 4.13	82.27 ± 5.18	**0.002**
KSS (postoperative 6 months)	87.29 ± 2.48	84.41 ± 1.80	88.32 ± 2.37	84.64 ± 3.26	**<0.001**
KSFS (postoperative 6 months)	87.29 ± 3.60	85.29 ± 2.78	87.32 ± 4.19	82.73 ± 5.64	**0.015**
KSS (postoperative 12 months)	87.46 ± 2.38	84.82 ± 1.42	88.71 ± 2.36	85.73 ± 2.00	**<0.001**
KSFS (postoperative 12 months)	86.42 ± 2.66	85.53 ± 2.34	87.62 ± 4.01	81.73 ± 4.28	**0.002**
KSS (final control)	87.63 ± 2.34	84.88 ± 1.45	88.86 ± 2.42	85.73 ± 2.00	**<0.001**
KSFS (final control)	87.75 ± 2.91	85.59 ± 2.42	87.68 ± 4.19	82.73 ± 5.64	**0.003**

yield more favorable outcomes in the early recovery period compared to the MPP method. On the other hand, restoration of appropriate patella tracking is crucial for postoperative recovery. The midvastus approach can provide more acceptable patella tracking due to the preservation of patellar tendons which keep the patella in its original position. No remarkable differences were noted between the 2 approaches in terms of alignments of the knee, tibial and femoral components, posterior slope, and bone-patellar angle [2].

Bourke et al. proposed that trials should have an adequate sample size, preoperative baseline assessment of pain and function, physical measurements of the knee, intraoperative data including operative time and blood loss, follow-up for at least 6 to 12 months, and length of hospitalization [13].

It must be remembered that the duration of hospitalization after TKA can be affected by many factors including the overall healthcare system, demographic features, social and environmental factors, and perioperative management [6]. We suggest that loss of weight may lead to improved functional outcomes as reflected in KSS and KSFS. The KSS, which is an outcome measure related to the range of motion, was reported as the primary concern by the patients [11]. Our data imply that the musculoskeletal system and joint procedures such as TKA are directly affected by weight gain and an increase in BMI.

Xu et al. reported that the MV approach was more effective in an improvement of VAS and ROM in short term. However, it was associated with prolonged operative time. These aspects must be remembered during tailoring the treatment strategy for primary osteoarthritis of the knee [11].

Obesity is supposed to make surgery more challenging in TKA, and it has been termed a potential contraindication to the subvastus approach [14, 15]. We compared the MV and MPP approaches and our preliminary data is insufficient to address obesity as a contraindication for these 2 methods. Notably, we detected that the amount of erythrocyte suspension transfusion was higher in patients with BMI of ≥35. These findings are important since it reminds that risks of obesity will be further amplified by risks associated with increased likelihood for transfusion.

The single-use instruments offer advantages like the reduction of costs, timely turnover of operating rooms, and decreased rate of infection. No difference has been observed between single-use and conventional instruments as for clinical outcomes and radiographic parameters. These data imply that SUI can be an alternative to conventional instruments; however, further trials are warranted to compare the clinical outcomes [16].

To the best of our knowledge, this is the first study focusing on the comparison of 2 surgical methods in obese patients scheduled for TKA. The main limitations of the present study include retrospective design, heterogeneity of gender distribution, relatively small sample size, and data restricted to the experience of a single center. The main strengths of this trial were simultaneous evaluation of clinical, radiological, and perioperative parameters. In other words, both physical and functional measures were included in the evaluation of therapeutic outcomes. These points should be considered during the interpretation of our results.

5. Conclusion

Obesity is a growing health problem, and it may directly affect the surgical outcomes in TKA. This procedure can be carried out using MV and MPP approaches. We noted that obesity could influence the clinical and radiological outcomes after TKA performed by using MV and MPP approaches. A careful analysis of patient characteristics and selection of operative procedure is critical, and BMI is an important parameter to be considered during the establishment of the treatment plan. Further multicentric, randomized, controlled trials on larger series must be designed to verify our findings and to understand the association between obesity and therapeutic outcomes after TKA.

Abbreviations

F: Female
M: Male
R: Right
L: Left
ES: Erythrocyte suspension
MFTA: Mechanical femorotibial angle
I: Initial measurement
II: Second measurement
*: First independent researcher
§: Second independent researcher
KSS: Knee Society Score
KSFS: Knee Society Function Score.

Authors' Contributions

OG was the principal investigator of the study. GG and HS participated in the design of the study and performed the statistical analysis. OG and HBG wrote the study protocol. All authors read and approved the final manuscript.

References

[1] Y. Wu, Y. Zeng, X. Bao et al., "Comparison of mini-subvastus approach versus medial parapatellar approach in primary total knee arthroplasty," *International Journal of Surgery*, vol. 57, pp. 15–21, 2018.

[2] T. Li, Q. Zhuang, K. Xiao, L. Zhou, and X. Weng, "Comparison of the clinical and radiological outcomes following midvastus and medial parapatellar approaches for total knee arthroplasty: a meta-analysis," *Chinese Medical Journal*, vol. 127, pp. 2982–2990, 2014.

[3] J. R. Berstock, J. R. Murray, M. R. Whitehouse, A. W. Blom, and A. D. Beswick, "Medial subvastus versus the medial parapatellar approach for total knee replacement," *EFORT Open Reviews*, vol. 3, no. 3, pp. 78–84, 2018.

[4] I. Alcelik, M. Sukeik, R. Pollock, A. Misra, A. Naguib, and F. S. Haddad, "Comparing the mid-vastus and medial parapatellar approaches in total knee arthroplasty: a meta-analysis of short term outcomes," *The Knee*, vol. 19, no. 4, pp. 229–236, 2012.

[5] J. R. Martin, J. M. Jennings, and D. A. Dennis, "Morbid obesity and total knee arthroplasty," *Journal of the American Academy of Orthopaedic Surgeons*, vol. 25, no. 3, pp. 188–194, 2017.

[6] Y. Kuroda, T. Matsumoto, K. Takayama, K. Ishida, R. Kuroda, and M. Kurosaka, "Subjective evaluation before and after total knee arthroplasty using the 2011 Knee Society Score," *The Knee*, vol. 23, pp. 964–967, 2016.

[7] A. K. Steinhoff and W. D. Bugbee, "Knee Injury and osteoarthritis outcome score has higher responsiveness and lower ceiling effect than knee society function score after total knee arthroplasty," *Knee Surg Sports Traumatol Arthrosc*, vol. 24, pp. 2627-2633, 2016.

[8] F. C. Ewald, "The knee society total knee arthroplasty roentgenographic evaluation and scoring system," *Clinical Orthopaedics and Related Research*, vol. 248, pp. 9–12, 1989.

[9] R. M. Meneghini, M. A. Mont, D. B. Backstein, R. B. Bourne, D. A. Dennis, and G. R. Scuderi, "Development of a modern knee society radiographic evaluation system and methodology for total knee arthroplasty," *Journal of Arthroplasty*, vol. 30, pp. 2311–2314, 2015.

[10] Z. Liu and H. Yang, "Comparison of the minimally invasive and standard medial parapatellar approaches for total knee arthroplasty: systematic review and meta-analysis," *Journal of International Medical Research*, vol. 39, pp. 1607–1617, 2011.

[11] S. Z. Xu, X. J. Lin, X. Tong, and X. W. Wang, "Minimally invasive midvastus versus standard parapatellar approach in total knee arthroplasty: a meta-analysis of randomized controlled trials," *PLoS One*, vol. 9, Article ID e95311, 2014.

[12] J. George, A. K. Klika, S. M. Navale, J. M. Newman, W. K. Barsoum, and C. A. Higuera, "Obesity epidemic: is its impact on total joint arthroplasty underestimated? an analysis of national trends," *Clinical Orthopaedics and Related Research*, vol. 475, pp. 1798–1806, 2017.

[13] M. G. Bourke, P. J. Buttrum, P. L. Fitzpatrick, P. A. Dalton, G. A. Jull, and T. G. Russell, "Systematic review of medial parapatellar and subvastus approaches in total knee arthroplasty," *Journal of Arthroplasty*, vol. 25, pp. 728–734, 2010.

[14] Y. In, J. M. Kim, N. Y. Choi, and S. J. Kim, Large thigh girth is a relative contraindication for the subvastus approach in primary total knee arthroplasty," *Journal of Arthroplasty*, vol. 22, no. 4, pp. 569–573, 2007.

[15] N. Shah, G. Nilesh, and N. Patel, "Mini-subvastus approach for total knee arthroplasty inobese patients," *Indian Journal of Orthopaedics*, vol. 44, pp. 292–299, 2010.

[16] M. Romeo, G. Rovere, L. Stramazzo et al., "Single use instruments for total knee arthroplasty," *Medicinski Glasnik (Zenica)*, vol. 18, no. 1, pp. 247–251, 2021.

22

Cementless Metaphyseal Sleeve Fixation in Revision Knee Arthroplasty: Our Experience with an Arabic Population at the Midterm

Abdulrahman D. Algarni

Department of Orthopedic Surgery, King Saud University, Riyadh, Saudi Arabia

Correspondence should be addressed to Abdulrahman D. Algarni; abdulrahmanga@gmail.com

Academic Editor: Panagiotis Korovessis

Objective. Metaphyseal sleeve (MS) fixation in revision knee arthroplasty (RKA) among Western populations has been reported with very encouraging outcomes. The aim of this study was to report our experience with the use of MS in RKA among an Arabic population. Clinical and radiographic outcomes and implant survivorship were reported at a minimum follow-up of 2 years and a mean follow-up of 4.1 years. *Methods.* A retrospective analysis was conducted on prospectively collected data of patients who underwent RKA with a MS in combination with a cementless stem (femoral or tibial). Range of motion (ROM) and Knee Society Score (KSS) were obtained pre- and postoperatively. Complications, occurrence of stem-tip pain, and implant survival were documented. Knee radiographs were obtained to evaluate the alignment and osseointegration or loosening of the MS. *Results.* A total of 52 sleeves (27 tibial and 25 femoral) implanted in 27 RKAs (27 patients) were included. The mean follow-up period was 4.1 ± 1.8 (2–7.5) years. Postoperatively, the ROM improved from 89.3 ± 9.2 to 106.3 ± 11.4 ($p = 0.19$) and the KSS also significantly improved, from 102.9 ± 35.6 to 130.2 ± 33.7 ($p < 0.001$). One patient (3.7%) developed heterotopic ossification, and another one (3.7 %) had a stem-tip pain on the tibial side; both were managed conservatively. One patient (3.7 %) sustained a fracture and required reoperation. None of the sleeves showed progressive radiolucent lines, and none required revision. The aseptic survivorship and overall survivorship at a mean of 4.1 years were 100% and 96.3%, respectively. *Conclusion.* MS provided successful midterm outcomes that were maintained in obese patients with different levels of constraint. Our series supports their use as a viable option in RKA.

1. Introduction

The extent of bone loss encountered in revision knee arthroplasty (RKA) is often underestimated on preoperative radiographs and may also increase considerably during the explantation of implants [1]. Bone loss is commonly classified according to the Anderson Orthopaedic Research Institute (AORI) system. AORI type 1 is an epiphyseal defect with an intact metaphysis, type 2 describes a damaged metaphysis involving 1 (2A) or both (2B) femoral condyles or tibial plateaus, and type 3 describes a deficient metaphysis that compromises the major segment of the condyles or plateaus [2].

Depending on the AORI type of bone loss, various methods have been proposed for reconstruction. These usually involve the use of stems, cementless or cemented, combined with several reconstructive options ranging from simple cancellous bone grafting and cement, metal augments and blocks, to total segment replacement of the distal femur and/or proximal tibia. The current literature does not support the superiority of either type of stem; both have obtained comparable outcomes in long-term follow-up studies [3]. While cemented stems offer immediate fixation, they are difficult to remove and have been associated with loosening and metaphyseal bone resorption due to stress shielding [4]. Likewise, cementless stems have an offset option but have been linked with diaphyseal cortical reaction and stem-tip pain [5]. Greene et al. have shown very promising results with the hybrid type of stem fixation, wherein the stem is press-fit in the diaphysis and cemented in the metaphysis [6].

The long-term survival rate in RKA is generally lower than that in primary total knee arthroplasty (TKA); hence, the need for improved fixation still exists [7]. Contemporary RKA systems, both cementless and cemented, increasingly focus on the metaphysis for defect augmentation and implant fixation [8]. Based on the successful experience of cementless metaphyseal fixation in total hip arthroplasty, cementless metaphyseal sleeves (MS) (DePuy Synthes, Warsaw, IN, USA) were introduced in the 1970s along with hinged RKA implants [9]. These are conical, stepped, and coated with titanium beads to encourage osseointegration.

Early to midterm studies of MS in RKA among Western populations have been reported with very encouraging outcomes [10–13]. We found one study among Chinese patients; the authors also reported excellent outcomes at the short-term follow-up [14]. To the best of our knowledge, similar outcomes among patients of Arabic ethnicity have not been reported. Therefore, the aim of this study was to report our experience with the use of MS in RKA among the Arabic population. Clinical and radiographic outcomes and implant survivorship were reported at a minimum follow-up of 2 years and a mean follow-up of 4.1 years.

2. Materials and Methods

Following the Institutional Review Board approval, we conducted a retrospective analysis of prospectively collected data of patients who underwent RKA with a MS (femoral or tibial) under the author's care between June 2012 and May 2018. The preoperative health status of the included patients was evaluated using the American Society of Anaesthesiologists (ASA) score. Details of patient demographics and clinical parameters are shown in Table 1. Patients were included until their latest follow-up date. Range of motion (ROM) and Knee Society Score (KSS) were obtained preoperatively and at the time of the postoperative follow-ups [15]. Complications (intra- or postoperative) and a survey of stem-tip pain were also documented. Implant survival, with failure defined as reoperation with the end point being aseptic loosening and reoperation for any reason, was recorded. Knee radiographs (anteroposterior (AP) in the weight-bearing position as well as lateral and skyline views) and hip-to-ankle (HTA) radiographs were obtained to evaluate the alignment and the presence of progressive radiolucent lines (RLs) at the bone-sleeve interface (level of osseointegration). Radiographic assessment was performed twice within an interval of 6 weeks by an independent observer. Loosening was defined as the presence of continuous two-millimetre RLs around the porous-coated part of the MS [16]. On the tibial side, the osseointegration was assessed in four metaphyseal zones (anterior, posterior, medial, and lateral). On the femoral side, the partially coated sleeve is coated only in the distal part, which is largely obscured in the AP view; therefore, osseointegration was only assessed in two zones (anterior and posterior) on the lateral view. RLs around the noncoated part of the MS or the stem were not considered signs of prosthesis loosening.

Table 1: The patients' demographic and clinical parameters.

Parameter	Value
Age (years)	65.4 ± 10.2 (51–98)
Sex	
Male	5 (18.5%)
Female	22 (81.5%)
Side	
R	16 (59.2%)
L	11 (40.8%)
Height (cm)	155 ± 8.8 (142–173)
Weight (kg)	90.2 ± 20.1 (65–119)
BMI (kg/m^2)	37.6 ± 8.1 (26.7–50.2)
ASA score	
ASA 1	1 (3.7%)
ASA 2	7 (25.9%)
ASA 3	16 (59.3%)
ASA 4	3 (11.1%)
Follow-up (years)	4.1 ± 1.8 (2–7.5)
Time to index revision (years)	9.3 ± 5.6 (0.5–18)

Quantitative variables: mean ± standard deviation; categorical variables: frequency (percentages) with the range in parentheses. TKA = total knee arthroplasty, BMI = body mass index, and ASA = American Society of Anaesthesiologists.

2.1. Surgical Technique. All patients received a revision prosthesis from DePuy Synthes. All RKAs included partially coated MS combined with the shortest cementless stem (length: 75 mm) on both the femoral and tibial sides. We aimed whenever possible not to exceed 14 mm stem-diameter on the tibial side to theoretically ease extraction of the stem and tibial tray through the sleeve if required later. In the case of a periprosthetic femoral fracture, a distal femoral replacement and a cemented stem, without femoral sleeve, were implanted. The DePuy Synthes RKA system offers different levels of constraint: the total condylar III-rotating platform (TC3-RP), which is a varus-valgus constrained implant, the Sivash-range of motion (S-ROM) Noiles, which is a rotating hinge, and the limb preservation system-distal femoral replacement (LPS-DFR), which is reserved for periprosthetic fractures. All the aforementioned femoral options with their respective rotating-platform inserts are compatible with the same mobile-bearing revision tibial tray and with the MS system. The choice of implant and level of constraint were determined by the amount of bone loss and ligamentous involvement. Details of the revision procedures and the components implanted are summarised in Table 2.

Adequate exposure was achieved through the medial parapatellar approach and release of the medial and lateral gutters. Quadriceps snip and/or tibial tubercle osteotomy were performed if further exposure was required. Following removal of the polyethylene (PE) insert, the components were explanted (femoral first) using a small oscillating saw and malleable osteotomes at the implant-cement interface to minimise additional bone loss. The cement was completely removed in all revisions, and thorough debridement with removal of the infected membrane was also performed in second-stage revisions. The AORI type of intraoperative bone loss is summarised in Table 3. The tibial and femoral

Table 2: The details of the RKA and the components implanted.

Parameter	N (%)
RKA	27 (100%)
Indications	
Aseptic loosening	14 (51.9%)
PE wear	4 (14.8%)
Infection (second-stage)	3 (11.1%)
Instability	2 (7.4%)
Malalignment	2 (7.4%)
Femoral periprosthetic fracture/nonunion	2 (7.4%)
Metaphyseal sleeves	
All	52 (100%)
Femoral	25 (48.1%)
Tibial	27 (51.9%)
Sleeve size (median)	
Femoral	34 mm (31–46)
Tibial[b]	29 mm (29–61)
75 mm cementless stem[c]	
All	52 (100%)
Diameter (median)	12 mm (10–16)
Component size (median)	
Femoral[d]	2 (1.5–3)
Tibial	1.5 (1.5–3)
PE insert	12.5 mm (10–22.5)
Type of constraint	
TC3-RP	24 (88.9%)
S-ROM Noiles rotating hinge	1 (3.7%)
LPS-DFR	2 (7.4%)

[a]Femoral sleeve sizes are 20 mm, 31 mm, 34 mm, 40 mm, and 46 mm. [b]Tibial sleeve sizes are 29 mm, 37 mm, 45 mm, 53 mm, and 61 mm. [c]Two cemented stems implanted with the 2 cases of LPS-DFR. [d]Femoral component used in 2 cases of LPS-DFR, and 1 case of S-ROM was the smallest size (xx-small). RKA = revision knee arthroplasty, PE = polyethylene, TC3-RB = total condylar III-rotating platform, S-ROM = Sivash-range of motion, and LPS-DFR = limb preservation system-distal femoral replacement.

Table 3: The intraoperative bone loss as classified by AORI.

AORI	Femur N (%)	Tibia N (%)
Type 1	1 (3.7%)	0 (0%)
Type 2A	6 (22.3%)	10 (37%)
Type 2B	17 (62.8%)	13 (48.2%)
Type 3	3 (11.2%)	4 (14.8%)

AORI = Anderson Orthopaedic Research Institute.

medullary canals were then reamed until cortical diaphyseal contact was achieved. The tibial metaphysis was then prepared using a broach in consecutive sizes to accept the sleeve, using the trial stem to ensure that the broach was centred within the canal. We sometimes undersized the diameter of the trial stem by one to ease the broaching. The sleeve was correctly sized when it had a tight fit with rotational stability. On the femoral side, we aimed to ream and broach the canal as posterior as possible to build up the posterior femoral condylar offset (PFCO) and address the large flexion gap. The rotationally stable femoral sleeve needed to restore the joint line was selected. Femoral condylar augments (distal and posterior) were used as appropriate to address epiphyseal bone loss. Soft tissue release was performed as appropriate to adequately balance the knee, and a trial reduction was carried out. The definitive prosthesis was then assembled on the back table, taking care to match the same rotational orientation of the trial component. Cement was applied to the undersurface of the tibial tray and the femoral component (FC), taking care to avoid the porous-coated part of the MS.

2.2. Statistical Analysis. Data were analysed using SPSS statistical software version 22 (IBM Corp., Armonk, NY, USA). Pre- and postoperative ROM and KSS score values were compared using the dependent-sample Student's t-test. The intraobserver reliability (IOR) of radiographic evaluations was assessed using Cohen's kappa analysis. The correlation between the AORI type and the outcome variables was assessed with the chi-square analysis or Fisher's exact test, as appropriate. Implant survival was assessed using the Kaplan–Meier analysis. A p value of <0.05 was considered statistically significant.

3. Results

We identified a total of 52 sleeves (27 tibial and 25 femoral) in combination with 52 cementless stems implanted in 27 RKAs (27 patients). The mean follow-up period was 4.1 ± 1.8 (2–7.5) years. One patient died (of an unrelated cause), and another was lost to follow-up at 5 and 3 years after the index revision, respectively. Both these patients were included until their latest follow-up. The index revision was first time revision in 25 (92.6%) knees and second time revision in 2 (7.4%) knees.

At the most recent follow-up, the preoperative ROM improved from 89.3 ± 9.2 to 106.3 ± 11.4 ($p = 0.19$). The KSS also significantly improved, from 102.9 ± 35.6 to 130.2 ± 33.7 ($p < 0.001$). There was no significant correlation between the AORI type and the functional outcome, the level of osseointegration, or implant survival ($p = 0.51$, $p = 0.23$, and $p = 0.3$, respectively). There were no intraoperative complications. One patient (3.7 %) (man; 70 years; body mass index (BMI), 31.3 kg/m^2, ASA 3) postoperatively developed heterotopic ossification (HO) at the anterior surface of the distal femur (Figure 1). At his latest 3-year follow-up, he maintained reasonable ROM (5–90), and the HO did not interfere with his function; thus, excision was not required. One patient (3.7 %) (woman; 72 years; BMI, 42.4 kg/m^2, ASA 3) had a stem-tip pain on the tibial side for 5 months postoperatively; however, it completely resolved spontaneously thereafter.

The IOR of radiographic assessment showed substantial agreement (0.79). Postoperative HTA radiographs revealed optimal (±3 of neutral) mechanical alignment (−1.7 ± 2.9) compared to preoperative values (−8.9 ± 4.1) as measured using the hip-knee-ankle angle. One (3.7%) tibial sleeve had RLs <1 mm in 2 zones but did not progress. None of the sleeves showed progressive RLs in the porous-coated part, and none required revision.

One patient (3.7%) (woman; 76 years; BMI, 38.9 kg/m^2, ASA 2) underwent reoperation 2 years after her index revision. She fell and sustained an avulsion fracture of the tibial

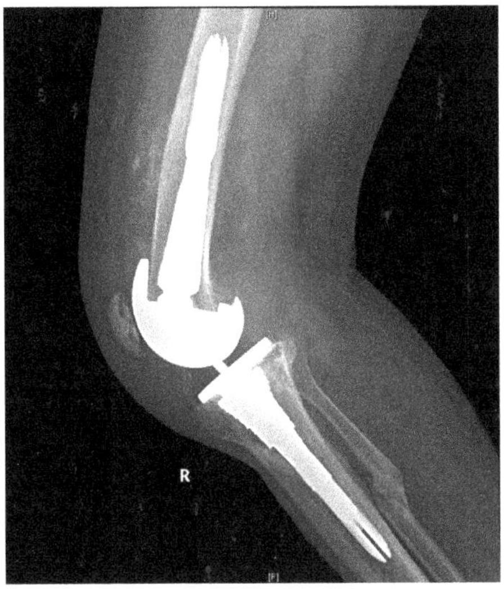

FIGURE 1: Lateral radiograph of the right knee showing the heterotopic ossification.

tuberosity with a subluxated prosthesis in association with an ankle fracture of the contralateral side. She was successfully treated; the tuberosity fracture was reduced and fixed with screws and suture anchors, the prosthetic knee was reduced, and the liner was exchanged. Radiographs after the fall and at the most recent 2-year follow-up are shown in Figure 2. Implant survivorship was therefore 96.3% at 4.1 years, with the end point being reoperation for any reason, and 100% survival at 4.1 years, with the end point being reoperation for aseptic loosening of the MS.

4. Discussion

The main findings of the present study were the excellent rate of functional outcomes, osseointegration, and survival rate. The aseptic survivorship and overall survivorship at a mean of 4.1 years were 100% and 96.3%, respectively.

Bone loss management and secured implant fixation are the two main challenges encountered in RKA [17]. The concept of zonal fixation has been recently proposed to assist in securing the fixation of revision implants [18]. It defined three potential zones for fixation: zone 1 (epiphysis), zone 2 (metaphysis), and zone 3 (diaphysis), and recommended implant fixation in at least 2 of these 3 relevant zones. The MS combined with the stem has enabled implant fixation in two zones (2 and 3), even if the epiphysis is severely compromised. MS enabled direct fixation of the implant and bone loss management in a single step. The osseointegration potential of the sleeve is enhanced by metaphyseal bone loading, which reduces stress shielding, and by the mobile-bearing interface, which reduces the shear forces through the sleeve [19,20]. Porous-metal cones, such as the trabecular metal system, tantalum (Zimmer Biomet, Warsaw, IN, USA), can also address metaphyseal bone loss [21]. As opposed to sleeves, the cones will also need diaphyseal fixation, usually with a cemented stem that also allows fixation of the stem to the cone until the cone is osseointegrated. Therefore, an additional interface exists between the cone and prosthesis. It remains to be seen if this could have a significant impact on long-term fixation. Cones have the advantage of being a more flexible tool to address bone loss, independent of the type of the revision system implanted in contrast to the MS, which are implant-specific, as they are a fixed part of the prosthesis [22]. Midterm studies regarding the use of cones in RKA have shown very encouraging results in terms of functional outcomes, osseointegration, and the aseptic loosening rate that were comparable to those achieved with MS [23,24]. Further long-term studies are needed to determine the superiority of either method.

There is a paucity of studies comparing the MS with a standard diaphyseal stem-based RKA prosthesis. In a recent study by Lai et al., the authors reported comparable clinical and radiographic outcomes of the MS and the constrained condylar knee (CCK) prosthesis (Zimmer Biomet, Warsaw, IN, USA) at a mean of 2-year follow-up [25]. Studies have shown successful outcomes of MS in RKA with significant improvement in functional scores and excellent rate of osseointegration [26–28]. Implant survival rates of 94% to 100% have been reported at the midterm follow-up, with the endpoint being aseptic loosening [29,30]. Bloch et al. recently reported a large series of 227 patients (319 RKA) using the MS (319 tibial and 146 femoral) with a mean follow-up of 7.6 years [30]. The study demonstrated excellent implant survivorships of 99.1% at 3 years, 98.7% at 5 years, and 97.8% at 10 years. None of the MS had progressive RLs, and none were revised for aseptic loosening in this study. Similarly, another recent study by Kim et al. which included 92 patients (93 RKA) with a mean follow-up of 6.3 years also demonstrated satisfactory results. The authors reported average improvements of the Western Ontario and McMaster Universities Osteoarthritis Index (WOMAC) from 55 preoperatively to 9 postoperatively and the Subjective Satisfaction Score (SSS) from 2 preoperatively to 8 postoperatively (both $p < 0.05$) [29]. All patients in their series demonstrated optimal osseointegration at the final follow-up. Our study also demonstrated similar improvement in KSS, osseointegration, and implant survival at a mean follow-up of 4.1 years. In the present study, the cohort consisted predominantly of female patients (81.5%) who were obese (BMI = 37.68.1 kg/m^2; Grade 2: moderate obesity) with the ASA 2-3 score. It seems that obesity did not negatively impact our outcomes; we had successful outcomes among our patients with no case of aseptic loosening at the midterm similar to that published among Caucasians. Comparing our outcomes to those in other patients of Arabic origin was limited by the lack of studies in this context. To the best of our knowledge, ours is the first report on the use of MS in RKA of Arabic patients. The female predominance in our cohort has been observed in other series and was attributed to postmenopausal osteoporosis [31,32]. We believe that this is a reflection of the higher percentage of primary TKA in our female patients as compared to their male counterparts.

Another advantage of the MS we experienced was the ease of intraoperative reconstruction of the PFCO, although postoperative measurement of the PFCO was not analysed in

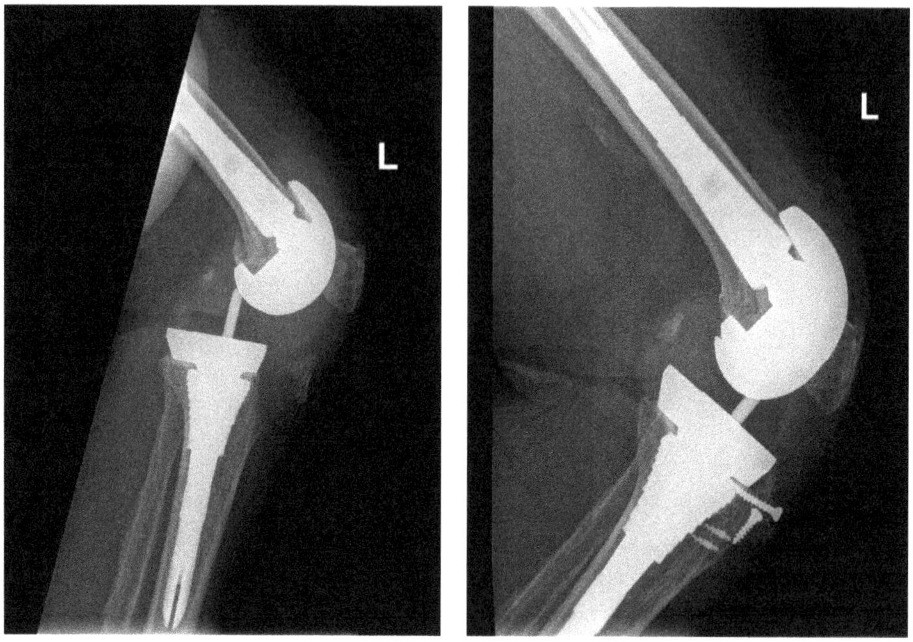

(a) (b)

Figure 2: (a) Lateral radiograph of the left knee showing the posttraumatic tibial tuberosity avulsion fracture and the subluxated prosthesis. (b) Lateral radiograph of the same knee at the most recent 2-year follow-up showing a healed fracture.

this study. The most frequent FC used in our series was size 2, followed by size 1.5 (both are the smallest sizes) because of the documented smaller bone geometry in the knees of people of Arabic ethnicity in contrast to that in Caucasians [33]. Keeping the femoral canal reaming and broaching as posterior as possible and using the largest stable femoral sleeve to restore the distal joint line combined to the shortest stem to stay distal to the femoral bowing allowed us to address a large flexion gap without reverting to larger FC, which is not always possible in patients with small bone geometry, as in our study. It may also cause component overhang with the risk of soft tissue irritation. Wirries et al. reported that they could restore the distal joint line at a mean of 0.36 mm lower to the anatomic level using the MS [34]. We are not aware of any study comparing the amount of PFCO obtained using the MS in contrast to an offset stem. However, it should be remembered that the offset stem sometimes will have only press-fit more proximally, leading to anterior shift of the FC, resulting in a larger flexion gap. Consequently, a higher PFCO is required in contrast to the MS that fits in the metaphysis and distal diaphysis. Using this technique together with the thick tibial tray options (15 and 25 mm) provided by this system and meticulous soft tissue balancing obviates the need for thick PE inserts in most patients in our series (median PE insert was 12.5 mm).

Although MS has advantages, there are some concerns that need to be addressed. As the removal of the osseointegrated sleeve is challenging, a fully porous-coated sleeve should be reserved for selected cases. In addition, using a tibial stem not more than 14 mm in diameter is recommended to theoretically allow explantation of the stem through the osseointegrated MS in case of further revision. In our series, we exclusively used partially coated MS and avoided tibial stems greater than 14 mm when possible. Fortunately, we were not required to remove any osseointegrated MS to date. Intraoperative fracture during metaphyseal broaching is also a potential complication [8]. This complication was not observed in our study. Another concern is stem-tip pain. The rate of stem-tip pain in the current study (3.7%) was comparable to the findings of Graichen et al. (3.2%) and Martin-Hernandez et al. (2.2%) [35,36]. Interestingly, the stem-tip pain in our patient spontaneously resolved within six months after the procedure. It is unknown whether MS osseointegration contributes to pain subsidence. Although it may be possible to use the stemless sleeve construct, it has remained our practice to add the shortest stem to the MS in all cases to achieve 2 zones fixation. The initial stability offered by the stem until the MS is fully osseointegrated and the benign course of the stem-tip pain in our series are also in support of the stem use. Therefore, we recommend the use of the shortest (length: 75 mm) cementless stem with any implanted MS. Nadorf et al. advocated the use of a short tibial stem to reduce micromotors of the tray and sleeve and to reduce proximal stress shielding, which occurs with no stem or long stem use, respectively [19]. Although Thorsell et al. described good midterm results of stemless sleeve fixation, they also had an increased risk for malpositioning of the implant [32]. Scior et al. recently reported successful outcomes of a larger series of stemless sleeve constructs [37]. The authors limited its use to cases in which zone 1 and 2 fixation was sufficient (AORI type 1 and type 2A) together with navigation use in cases with femoral or tibial deformity to prevent malpositioning.

The limitations of the present study are its retrospective design, the lack of a comparative group, and the relatively small number of the cohort. The variety of revision indications and using different levels of constraint also constitute limitations. However, the data were prospectively collected, and the procedures were performed by a single surgeon using the same standardised protocol over the study period. Long-term follow-up is still awaited before definitive conclusions are made.

5. Conclusion

MS provided excellent outcomes in terms of function, osseointegration, and implant survivorship at the midterm. These successful outcomes were maintained in obese patients with different levels of constraint. Our series supports the use of MS as a viable option in RKA.

Acknowledgments

The author would like to extend his appreciation to the Deanship of Scientific Research at King Saud University under research group no. RG-1441-359.

References

[1] M. C. Nadaud, T. K. Fehring, and K. Fehring, "Underestimation of osteolysis in posterior stabilized total knee arthroplasty," *The Journal of Arthroplasty*, vol. 19, no. 1, pp. 110–115, 2004.

[2] G. A. Engh and D. J. Ammeen, "Classification and preoperative radiographic evaluation: Knee," *Orthopedic Clinics of North America*, vol. 29, no. 2, pp. 205–217, 1998.

[3] C. Wang, T. Pfitzner, P. von Roth, H. O. Mayr, M. Sostheim, and R. Hube, "Fixation of stem in revision of total knee arthroplasty: cemented versus cementless-a meta-analysis," *Knee Surgery, Sports Traumatology, Arthroscopy*, vol. 24, no. 10, pp. 3200–3211, 2016.

[4] P. F. Lachiewicz and E. S. Soileau, "A 30-mm cemented stem extension provides adequate fixation of the tibial component in revision knee arthroplasty," *Clinical Orthopaedics and Related Research*, vol. 473, no. 1, pp. 185–189, 2015.

[5] T. P. Gross and F. Liu, "Total knee arthroplasty with fully porous-coated stems for the treatment of large bone defects," *The Journal of Arthroplasty*, vol. 28, no. 4, pp. 598–603, 2013.

[6] J. W. Greene, S. M. Reynolds, J. D. Stimac, A. L. Malkani, and M. A. Massini, "Midterm results of hybrid cement technique in revision total knee arthroplasty," *The Journal of Arthroplasty*, vol. 28, no. 4, pp. 570–574, 2013.

[7] K. L. Ong, E. Lau, J. Suggs, S. M. Kurtz, and M. T. Manley, "Risk of subsequent revision after primary and revision total joint arthroplasty," *Clinical Orthopaedics and Related Research*, vol. 468, no. 11, pp. 3070–3076, 2010.

[8] B. P. Chalmers, N. M. Desy, M. W. Pagnano, R. T. Trousdale, and M. J. Taunton, "Survivorship of metaphyseal sleeves in revision total knee arthroplasty," *The Journal of Arthroplasty*, vol. 32, no. 5, pp. 1565–1570, 2017.

[9] S. Agarwal, D. S. Neogi, and R. Morgan-Jones, "Metaphyseal sleeves in revision total knee arthroplasty: minimum seven-year follow-up study," *The Knee*, vol. 25, no. 6, pp. 1299–1307, 2018.

[10] G. E. Alexander, T. L. Bernasek, R. L. Crank, and G. J. Haidukewych, "Cementless metaphyseal sleeves used for large tibial defects in revision total knee arthroplasty," *The Journal of Arthroplasty*, vol. 28, no. 4, pp. 604–607, 2013.

[11] S. L. Barnett, R. R. Mayer, J. S. Gondusky, L. Choi, J. J. Patel, and R. S. Gorab, "Use of stepped porous titanium metaphyseal sleeves for tibial defects in revision total knee arthroplasty: short term results," *The Journal of Arthroplasty*, vol. 29, no. 6, pp. 1219–1224, 2014.

[12] R. Huang, G. Barrazueta, A. Ong et al., "Revision total knee arthroplasty using metaphyseal sleeves at short-term follow-up," *Orthopedics*, vol. 37, no. 9, pp. e804–9, 2014.

[13] K. E. Bugler, R. Maheshwari, I. Ahmed, I. J. Brenkel, and P. J. Walmsley, "Metaphyseal sleeves for revision total knee arthroplasty: good short-term outcomes," *The Journal of Arthroplasty*, vol. 30, no. 11, pp. 1990–1994, 2015.

[14] L. Guo, Y. Du, M. Zhang et al., "Short-term effectiveness of revision total knee arthroplasty with porous-coated metaphyseal Sleeve and MBT implant," *Zhongguo Xiu Fu Chong Jian Wai Ke Za Zhi*, vol. 33, no. 3, pp. 302–306, 2019, in Chinese.

[15] G. Insall, M. Dorr, M. Scott, and F. Norman, "Rationale of the Knee Society clinical rating system," *Clinical Orthopaedics and Related Research*, vol. 248, pp. 13-14, 1989.

[16] R. Agarwal, S. I. S. Azam, H. Morgan-Jones, and F. S. Haddad, "Zonal fixation in revision total knee arthroplasty," *The Bone & Joint Journal*, vol. 97-B, no. 2, pp. 147–149, 2013.

[17] G. Panegrossi, M. Ceretti, M. Papalia, F. Casella, F. Favetti, and F. Falez, "Bone loss management in total knee revision surgery," *International Orthopaedics*, vol. 38, no. 2, pp. 419–427, 2014.

[18] W. Morgan-Jones, A. Oussedik, S. Graichen, and J. Haddad, "A zonal fixation classification in revision total knee arthroplasty: a methodology to aid reconstruction, fixation and implant survival," *Journal of Knee Surgery*, vol. 97-B, no. 1, pp. 45–49, 2015.

[19] R. M. Nadorf, D. G. Kinkel, A. D. Gantz, E. Jakubowitz, and J. P. Kretzer, "Tibial revision knee arthroplasty with metaphyseal sleeves: the effect of stems on implant fixation and bone flexibility," *The Journal of Bone and Joint Surgery-American Volume*, vol. 12, no. 1, Article ID e0177285, 2017.

[20] R. P. Goldstein, A. J. Gordon, O. A. Swope, and S. C. Branson, "Rotating platform revision total knee arthroplasty," *The Journal of Knee Surgery*, vol. 25, no. 1, pp. 45–50, 2012.

[21] A. F. Meneghini, D. G. Lewallen, and A. D. Hanssen, "Porous tantalum metaphyseal cones for severe tibial bone loss in revision knee arthroplasty," *The Journal of Bone and Joint Surgery-American Volume*, vol. 90, no. 3, pp. 78–84, 2008.

[22] G. D. Roach, M. P. Clair, D. G. Behery, A. D. Thakkar, R. Iorio, and A. J. Deshmukh, "Aseptic loosening of porous metaphyseal sleeves and tantalum cones in revision total knee arthroplasty: a systematic review," *The Journal of Knee Surgery*, no. 15, Online ahead of print, 2020.

[23] A. F. Kamath, D. G. Lewallen, and A. D. Hanssen, "Porous tantalum metaphyseal cones for severe tibial bone loss in revision knee arthroplasty: a five to nine-year follow-up," *Journal of Bone and Joint Surgery: American Volume*, vol. 97, pp. 216–223, 2015.

[24] D. F. Potter III, W. P. Abdel, D. G. Lewallen, and A. D. Hanssen, "Midterm results of porous tantalum femoral cones in revision total knee arthroplasty," *The Knee*, vol. 98, pp. 1286–1291, 2016.

[25] T. S. Lai, J. R. Chen, D. L. Liow et al., "Is constraint implant with metaphyseal sleeve a viable option for revision TKR with preoperative coronal plane instability and bone defect?" *The*

Journal of Arthroplasty, vol. 28, no. 2, Article ID 2309499020926313, 2020.

[26] C. J. Dalury and A. F. Barrett, "The use of metaphyseal sleeves in revision total knee arthroplasty," *The Knee*, vol. 23, no. 3, pp. 545–548, 2016.

[27] T. S. Watters, J. R. Martin, D. L. Levy, C. C. Yang, R. H. Kim, and D. A. Dennis, "Porous-coated metaphyseal sleeves for severe femoral and tibial bone loss in revision TKA," *The Journal of Arthroplasty*, vol. 32, no. 11, pp. 3468–3473, 2017.

[28] B. V. Fedorka, O. A. Chen, J. Pagnotto, J. R. A. Crossett, and P. J. Klatt, "Revision total knee arthroplasty with porous-coated metaphyseal sleeves provides radiographic ingrowth and stable fixation," *The Journal of Arthroplasty*, vol. 26, no. 5, pp. 1500–1505, 2018.

[29] G. Klim, V. Amerstorfer, G. Bernhardt et al., "Excellent mid-term osseointegration and implant survival using metaphyseal sleeves in revision total knee arthroplasty," *Knee Surg Sports Traumatol Arthrosc*, vol. 5, no. 4, 2020.

[30] M. Bloch, M. Hedström, M. C. Palan, R. J. Phillips, and P. J. James, "Metaphyseal sleeves in revision total knee arthroplasty provide reliable fixation and excellent medium to long-term implant survivorship," *Acta Orthopaedica*, vol. 35, no. 1, pp. 495–499, 2020.

[31] M. A. Stefani, S. M. Mattiuzzo, and E. S. B. Prestini, "Revision total knee arthroplasty with metaphyseal sleeves without stem: short-term results," *The Journal of Arthroplasty*, vol. 5, pp. 207–211, 2017.

[32] N. Thorsell, H. J. Hedstrom, G. v. Wick, H. Weiss, and M. Skutek, "Good clinical and radiographic outcome of cementless metal metaphyseal sleeves in total knee arthroplasty," *The Journal of Arthroplasty*, vol. 89, no. 1, pp. 84–88, 2018.

[33] H. Hafez, W. Sheikhedrees, and M. Saweeres, "Anthropometry of arabian arthritic knees: comparison to other ethnic groups and implant dimensions," *The Journal of Arthroplasty*, vol. 31, no. 5, pp. 1109–1116, 2016.

[34] C. Wirries, L. J. Winnecken, M. P. Lewinski et al., "Osteointegrative sleeves for metaphyseal defect augmentation in revision total knee arthroplasty: clinical and radiological 5-year follow-up," *The Journal of Arthroplasty*, vol. 34, no. 9, pp. 2022–2029, 2019.

[35] W. Graichen, D. Scior, and H. Strauch, "Direct, cementless, metaphyseal fixation in knee revision arthroplasty with sleeves-short-term results," *The Journal of Arthroplasty*, vol. 30, no. 12, pp. 2256–2259, 2015.

[36] C. Martin-Hernandez, L. J. Floria-Arnal, M. P. Muniesa-Herrero et al., "Mid-term results for metaphyseal sleeves in revision knee surgery," *Knee Surgery, Sports Traumatology, Arthroscopy*, vol. 25, no. 12, pp. 3779–3785, 2017.

[37] W. Scior, D. Chanda, and H. Graichen, "Are stems redundant in times of metaphyseal sleeve fixation?" *The Journal of Arthroplasty*, vol. 34, no. 10, pp. 2444–2448, 2019.

23

Optimizing Acetabular Component Bone Ingrowth: The Wedge-Fit Bone Preparation Method

Dani M. Gaillard-Campbell and Thomas P. Gross

Midlands Orthopaedics & Neurosurgery, 1910 Blanding Street, Columbia, SC 29201, USA

Correspondence should be addressed to Dani M. Gaillard-Campbell; dani.gaillard@midorthoneuro.com

Academic Editor: Benjamin Blondel

We investigate the efficacy of a modified acetabular bone-preparation technique in reducing the incidence of two clinical problems identified in hip resurfacing arthroplasty. The first issue is failure due to lack of bone ingrowth into the acetabular component. The second is a newly recognized phenomenon of early cup shift. We hypothesize that these issues might be resolved by using a "wedge-fit method", in which the component wedges into the peripheral acetabular bone rather than bottoming out and potentially toggling on the apex of the cup. Prior to November 2011, all acetabula were reamed 1 mm under and prepared with a press-fit of the porous coated acetabular component. After November 2011, we adjusted reaming by bone density. In "soft bone" (T-score <-1.0), we underreamed acetabula by 1 mm less than the outer diameter of the cup, as was previously done in all cases. For T-scores greater than -1.0, we reamed line-to-line. Additionally, we began performing an "apex relief" starting June 2012 in all cases by removing 2 mm of apex bone with a small reamer after using the largest reamer. Failure of acetabular ingrowth occurred in 0.5% of cases before the wedge-fit method and <0.1% after. Rate of cup shift was reduced from 1.1% to 0.4%. The rate of unexplained pain between 2 and 4 years postoperatively also declined significantly from 2.6% to 1.3%. Our evidence suggests that wedge-fit acetabular preparation improves initial implant stability, leading to fewer cases of early cup shift, unexplained pain, and acetabular ingrowth failure.

1. Background

Hip resurfacing arthroplasty (HRA) is a less common, alternative method to total hip arthroplasty (THA) for reconstructing the arthritic hip. Its popularity has waxed and waned since its introduction in the 1950s [1, 2]. In the late 1990s, McMinn and Amstutz were instrumental in the introduction of metal-on-metal (MoM) hip resurfacing [2–4]. MoM HRA grew in popularity until 2007 [5–7]; then, it lost popularity for a variety of reasons, including the identification of adverse wear-related failure (AWRF). Some HRA failure modes are unique, but many are the same as for THA. An issue for both uncemented THA and HRA is failure of bone ingrowth into the acetabular component. Its incidence is not well known, and it is difficult to diagnose unless the implant migrates.

Our initial experience with resurfacing was promising, with a 92% 10-year implant survivorship reported in young patients; this compared favorably with registry reports [8, 9]. We therefore chose to redouble our efforts with HRA rather than follow much of the orthopedic community, in which many professionals abandoned MoM bearings after the recall of two faulty systems [10]. Our strategy was to identify modes of failure and implement steady improvements to implant design and surgical techniques. We have now improved 10-year implant survivorship to 96.5% in patients below 50 [11]. In an endeavor to further improve results, we chose to modify acetabular preparation in 2012 with hopes of more stable initial fixation. We anticipated that this would lower the rate of acetabular bone ingrowth, which had prevalence of 0.5% in our database. We hypothesized that creating a "wedge fit" while preparing and implanting the acetabular component might reduce the rate of ingrowth failure. Early asymptomatic cup shift and unexplained pain seem to be related problems that have not previously been addressed in the literature. These problems are related to the quality of the initial implant press-fit [12].

Uncemented acetabular components that fail to achieve bone ingrowth rarely develop complete radiolucent lines [13].

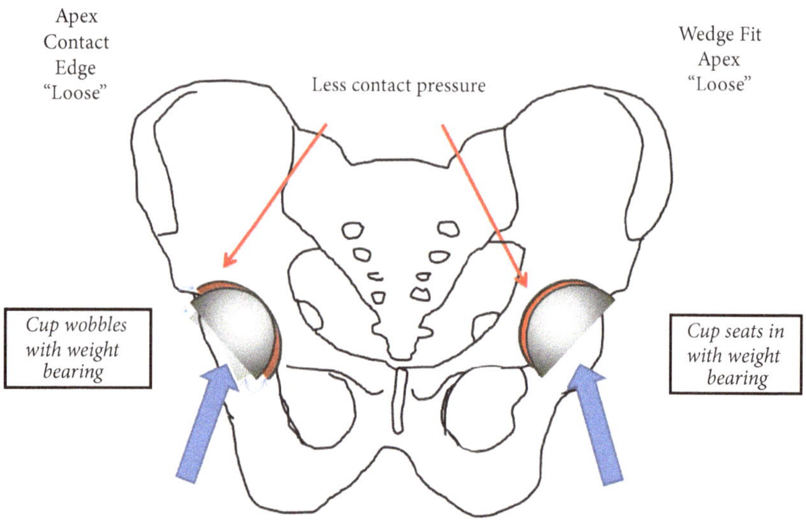

FIGURE 1: Cup fixation variation for two acetabular preparation methods.

Thus, they can be difficult to diagnose unless they shift in position. We have not found bone scans or other tests to be helpful in diagnosing bone ingrowth failure in nonshifted cups. The definitive method to diagnose a loose cup is to test it intraoperatively, but this is not appropriate in most cases. In our experience, there are two basic presentations for failure of acetabular ingrowth. The first is a dramatic spin out of the cup, usually within a few months. In the second, a patient develops persistent pain within the first 2 years postoperatively, and the acetabular component shows a cup shift over a series of standard pelvic x-rays. In our experience, most failures of cup ingrowth become evident by 2 years postoperatively. Therefore, we diagnose symptomatic patients with failure of ingrowth when the cup moves significantly between 6 weeks and 2 years. On the other hand, some patients present excellent initial outcome, but, sometimes after 2 years, they develop persistent pain and cup migration. We consider these late loosening. We suspect that some cases of unexplained pain in THA and HRA may be due to these loose or fibrous ingrown cups [14–16], which we have discovered in some rare cases during surgical exploration for the patient's pain.

We hypothesize that adjusting acetabular preparation by bone density and adding an apex relief will improve acetabular bone ingrowth, unexplained pain, and cup stability. We refer to this collective surgical technique as the "wedge-fit method". We postulate that a wedge fit into peripheral acetabular bone prevents the component from bottoming out and toggling on the apex of the cup, thus providing more stability and better fixation. Herein, we report our clinical outcomes with this new strategy for acetabular bone preparation.

2. Materials and Methods

Between September 2006 and November 2011, we performed 1496 HRAs (Group 1) with the Biomet Magnum™ uncemented acetabular component using a 1 mm under ream press-fit technique in all cases. Between June 2012 and June 2016, we performed 1565 HRAs (Group 2) using the new wedge-fit technique. All patients in both groups received the Biomet Magnum acetabular component. A minimum follow-up of 2 years was available in our prospective database, with a mean follow-up rate of 94%. We compared the two preparation techniques for three endpoints: revision for failure of acetabular ingrowth, residual unexplained pain, and early component shift.

These Biomet implants are relatively stiff with 3-6 mm thick cast cobalt-chrome components with a thin layer of titanium alloy porous plasma spray for bone ingrowth fixation. For the Biomet Magnum system, the porous plasma spray coating is similar to that seen on all other Biomet titanium plasma coated implants. However, THA cups come in a wide variety of thicknesses and coatings [17]. Therefore, it is not clear how well our technique will work in THA implants; further studies are required.

A minimally invasive posterior approach with a 4-5-inch incision was used in most cases. In Group 1, all acetabula were serially reamed up to a size 1 mm smaller than the actual outer diameter (OD) of the component. In Group 2, we reamed bone based on the bone density as determined by DEXA scan. If the bone was hard (femoral neck T-score ≥ -1.0), the acetabulum was reamed line-to-line with the OD of the component. If the bone was soft (T-score < -1.0), the last reamer was 1 mm less than the OD of the implanted cup. In addition, 2 mm of acetabular apex bone was removed in all cases regardless of bone density by finishing with a clean reamer 5 mm smaller than the largest size. A clean reamer was used so that the amount of bone removed from the apex could be easily seen. We performed an apex relief so that the impacted component would "wedge fit" into the peripheral bone and have less chance of bottoming out on the apex (Figure 1). A metal trial component that was approximately line-to-line with the final component was placed into the reamed socket to judge if reaming depth was adequate to allow correct positioning of the component with respect to

TABLE 1: Demographics.

Variable	Group 1 (Before protocol)	Group 2 (Wedge fit)	P value
Date Range	9/2006-11/2011	6/2012-6/2016	- -
# of Cases	1496	1565	- -
# Deceased*	7 (0.5%)	3 (0.2%)	0.1802
Demographics		- -	
#, % Female	383 (25.5%)	415 (26.5%)	0.5619
Mean Follow-Up (Years)	4.7 ± 2.3	2.4 ± 1.3	<0.0001*
Age (Years)	52.4 ± 8.3	54.2 ± 8.6	<0.0001*
BMI	27.6 ± 4.5	27.8 ± 4.8	0.2349
T-Score	0.0 ± 1.3	0.0 ± 1.2	1.000
Femoral Component Size (mm)	49.9 ± 3.5	49.9 ± 3.6	1.000
Diagnoses		- -	
Osteoarthritis	1138 (76.1%)	1276 (81.5%)	0.0002*
Dysplasia	198 (13.2%)	184 (11.8%)	0.2150
Osteonecrosis	76 (5.1%)	70 (4.5%)	0.4295
RA	6 (0.4%)	3 (0.2%)	0.2846
Post-Trauma	33 (2.2%)	17 (1.1%)	0.0147*
LCP/SCFE	31 (2.1%)	26 (1.7%)	0.4009
Other	14 (0.9%)	15 (1.0%)	0.9522

TABLE 2: Failures and complications.

Failure Type	Group 1	Group 2	P value
# Cases	1496	1565	- -
(1) Revisions			
(a) Failure of Acetabular Ingrowth (<2 years)	7 (0.5%)	1 (<0.1%)	0.0271*
(b) Adverse Wear	3 (0.2%)	0 (0.0%)	0.0735
(c) Late Acetabular Loosening (>2 years)	2 (0.1%)	0 (0.0%)	0.1443
(d) Acetabular Component Shift	1 (<0.1%)	1 (<0.1%)	0.9681
(2) Unrevised Cup shift	16 (1.1%)	7 (0.4%)	0.0424*
(3a) Unexplained pain (>2 years, latest F/U)	31 (2.2%)	21 (2.6%)	0.1031
(3b) Unexplained pain (2-4 years, peak pain)	39 (2.6%)	20 (1.3%)	0.0061*

inclination, anteversion, and cup overhang. No attempt was made to judge the quality of fit with the trial component. All patients in both groups received the Biomet Magnum acetabular component.

Table 1 compares demographic data. Group 2 was slightly older, on average, with more cases of osteoarthritis and fewer cases of trauma. Because these groups are consecutive, the follow-up is not equal; however, all cases had a minimum of 2-year follow-up. Therefore, we only include failures of acetabular ingrowth diagnosed prior to 2-year follow-up for our comparison to eliminate time bias in the analysis. Since it can be difficult to diagnose failure of acetabular component ingrowth, we analyzed whether there was a difference in the rate of unexplained pain in the two groups. We defined this as cases where the pain component of the Harris hip score (HHS) [18] was less than or equal to 30 (moderate to disabling pain). We compared pain scores at the latest follow-up for both groups, but because Group 1 has a greater length of follow-up, we also compared the minimum pain score (peak amount of pain) for each patient between 2 and 4 years postoperatively.

This retrospective analysis is exempt from IRB review based on 45 CFR 46, "Collection or Study of Existing Data", considering the HIPPA Privacy Rule (45 CFR 160 and 164a); this has been confirmed by the IRB at Providence Hospital in Columbia, SC.

3. Results

Group 1 comprised 1496 consecutive HRAs in 1276 patients performed between September 2006 and November 2011. After the wedge-fit method was fully implemented, the primary surgeon performed 1565 consecutive uncemented Biomet HRAs in 1365 patients prior to June 2016. The minimum follow-up period for both groups was 2 years, with an average of 4.7 years for Group 1 and 2.4 years for Group 2.

Failures due to lack of bone ingrowth into the acetabular component (Table 2) were significantly reduced after employing

Table 3: Clinical outcomes.

Variable	Group 1	Group 2	P value
Preoperative			
HHS Score	58.6 ± 13.2	57.3 ± 18.7	<0.0001*
Postoperative			
Cases with 2-year FU (#, %)	1407 (94.1%)	1121 (71.6%)	<0.0001*
Cases with any FU	1485 (99.3%)	1496 (95.6%)	<0.0001*
HHS Score	98.1 ± 6.0	97.7 ± 6.2	0.1716
Harris Pain Score	42.8 ± 4.2	42.7 ± 4.1	0.6182
UCLA Score	7.6 ± 1.9	7.5 ± 1.9	0.3059
VAS^2 Pain: Regular	0.3 ± 1.0	0.2 ± 0.9	0.0036*
VAS Pain: Worse	1.2 ± 1.9	1.3 ± 2.0	0.2826
Combined ROM	272.2 ± 42.1	270.4 ± 34.4	0.5600
Radiographic Data			
AIA	35.9 ± 5.5	33.9 ± 4.9	<0.0001*
Under RAIL (# Hips, %)	1266/1374 (92.1%)	1565/1565 (100.0%)	<0.0001*
Radiolucency (# Hips, %)	0 (0.0%)	0 (0.0%)	1.000
Osteolysis (# Hips, %)	0 (0.0%)	0 (0.0%)	1.000

the wedge-fit approach (0.5% to <0.1%, p=0.03). Diagnoses were confirmed intraoperatively at revision surgery. With standard acetabular implantation techniques (Group 1), there was a 0.6% rate of revision due to early acetabular failures (before 2 years postoperatively); after the new bone preparation techniques, this reduced to 0.1% (p=0.03). The incidence of unexplained pain between 2 and 4 years declined significantly from 2.6% to 1.3% (p=0.006). Unrevised early cup shifts also reduced significantly from 1.1% to 0.4% (p=0.04).

While all patients were at least two years out from surgery, the rate of follow-up was significantly lower for Group 2 (Table 3). Of those that returned for their 2-year follow-up, mean Harris pain score and worse VAS pain score were similar, while regular VAS pain score was significantly higher for Group 1. UCLA score and combined range-of-motion were also similar between the two groups. There were no instances of radiolucency or osteolysis.

4. Discussion

Our data indicate that a wedge-fit acetabular preparation strategy promotes acetabular component stability and ensures a higher rate of stable bone ingrowth. We developed this wedge-fit strategy based on the hypothesis that failure of acetabular component ingrowth was due to inadequate initial fixation. The three prerequisites [19, 20] required to achieve bone ingrowth in uncemented implants include live and healthy bone, an adequate porous surface, and a tight initial fit that prevents micromotion of more than 100 μm. If these conditions are not met, failure of bone ingrowth can occur. In our experience, failure of acetabular bone ingrowth most often presents in one of two ways. Either the component suddenly spins out, or the patient presents with explained pain and normal early radiographs. Over time, the component moves on serial x-rays, at which point the surgeon makes the diagnosis. There may be a third group of bone ingrowth failure in which the patient presents unexplained pain without any x-ray changes over time. The senior author (TPG) has rarely found failure of acetabular component ingrowth to be the explanation for previously unexplained pain. Instead, unexplained pain likely comes from soft tissue problems, back pain, or other unrelated issues.

With the previous standard reaming technique (no apex relief), the surgeon had less control over the implant contact points. We believed that, in some cases, the implant bottomed out on the apex with relative loose fit around the periphery. With eccentric loading, toggling of the implant could cause micromotion resulting in fibrous rather than bone ingrowth. We hypothesized that if we tailored the reaming method by bone density and relieved the apex, we could prevent apex toggling and achieve a more reliable press-fit with improved bone ingrowth.

Although Group 2 had a lower mean preoperative function score, clinical outcomes were largely similar. While Harris pain score and worst VAS pain score were similar between the two groups, mean regular VAS pain score was lower for Group 2. All Group 2 patients met the RAIL; this was significantly higher than Group 1. Likewise, average AIA was lower for Group 2 even though mean component size was similar between both cohorts.

There are some notable limitations to this study. There were some minor demographic differences between the two groups; Group 2 cases were slightly older, on average, but we have never selected against patients based on age. Additionally, there were significantly fewer cases of osteoarthritis in Group 1 and more cases of posttrauma than in Group 2. However, proportions of high-risk diagnoses (dysplasia and osteonecrosis) were similar.

Next, the x-rays required to diagnose early cup shift were not part of our protocol until November 2007. Thus, we likely missed some cup shifts in Group 1. When we compare only cases after these x-rays, the rate of unrevised cup shift is even higher in Group 1, and the difference in rate of shift between Groups 1 and 2 becomes even greater (p=0.009).

Another limitation is the difference in rate of follow-up and postoperative time. Group 1 had a longer follow-up interval and had more patients return for follow-up. However, when prompted, many patients that never returned for follow-up reported great results and felt no need to return. Therefore, it is unlikely that there were enough missed complications in Group 2 to change the results.

Lastly, this study investigates the outcomes of the wedge-fit method on the Biomet Magnum-ReCap™ resurfacing system only. While it seems possible that many hemispherical, porous-coated metal cups would behave similarly with these techniques, we cannot be certain. Titanium shells typically used in THA may be more flexible than the cobalt-chrome Magnum resurfacing component we evaluated, but all metal cups are much stiffer than bone and therefore may act similarly. The roughness of the porous coating and any supplemental fixation, such as screws or spikes, would likely markedly alter the results.

Additionally, an experienced resurfacing surgeon performed these cases. Reports suggest that HRA requires a steep learning curve [21]. Therefore, we cannot guarantee another surgeon employing the same device and method would achieve comparable results.

It is not clear whether more rigid cobalt-chrome resurfacing components have a higher rate of ingrowth failure than THA cups. According to New Zealand registry data [22], failure before 90 days postoperatively due to loose acetabular component was <0.1% for cemented, uncemented, and hybrid cemented THAs. However, we define failure of ingrowth as a loose acetabular component before 2 years postoperatively, so this rate in the New Zealand registry is not comparable. Latteier *et al.* [23] published outcomes for MoM THA and reported a higher incidence of failure of ingrowth (2.6%) than our study sample but is comparable with other reports on HRA. Kim *et al.* [24] published a multicenter study on HRA with a significantly higher rate of failure ingrowth at 5% for the Conserve Plus® cobalt-chrome cementless acetabular components. This study comprised 5 surgeons, only one of which was an experienced HRA surgeon. We have experienced a much lower rate of overall failure and of ingrowth failure in HRA. A detailed analysis of the Conserve Plus by Amstutz *et al.* [25] identified femoral loosening as the main mode of failure, with 1.8% of cases failing due to loosening. It is unclear how many of these were early loosenings. This compares to our rate of ingrowth failure prior to the wedge-fit technique.

5. Conclusions

After implementing the wedge-fit acetabular bone preparation method, we observed a reduction in the rate of failure of acetabular component ingrowth (0.5% versus <0.1%), the rate of asymptomatic cup shifts (1.1% versus 0.4%), and the incidence of unexplained pain between 2 and 4 years of follow-up (2.6% versus 1.3%). We suggest that some cases of unexplained pain may be the result of fibrous ingrowth into the acetabular component. Unfortunately, there is currently no reliable way to diagnose fibrous ingrowth except by exploring and removing an acetabular component, which could lead to unnecessary removal of a well-fixed cup.

Abbreviations

HRA: Hip resurfacing arthroplasty
THA: Total hip arthroplasty
MoM: Metal-on-metal
AWRF: Adverse wear-related failure
OD: Outer diameter
AIA: Acetabular inclination angle.

Disclosure

The authors present a retrospective analysis of prospectively collected data, with patient information withheld. This type of study is exempt from IRB review based on 45 CFR 46, "Collection or Study of Existing Data", considering the HIPPA Privacy Rule (45 CFR 160 and 164a).

Acknowledgments

This study was funded internally in full by the primary surgeon and Midlands Orthopaedics & Neurosurgery. The research department staff is paid for by Midlands Orthopaedics & Neurosurgery surgeons.

References

[1] G. S. Matharu, H. G. Pandit, D. W. Murray, and R. B. Treacy, "The future role of metal-on-metal hip resurfacing," *International Orthopaedics*, vol. 39, no. 10, pp. 2031–2036, 2015.

[2] H. C. Amstutz and M. J. Le Duff, "Hip resurfacing: history, current status, and future," *Hip International*, vol. 25, no. 4, pp. 330–338, 2018.

[3] D. McMinn, R. Treacy, K. Lin, and P. Pynsent, "Metal on metal surface replacement of the hip: experience of the McMinn prothesis," *Clinical Orthopaedics and Related Research*, vol. 329, pp. S89–S98, 1996.

[4] S. Cutts and P. B. Carter, "Hip resurfacing: a technology reborn," *Postgraduate Medical Journal*, vol. 82, no. 974, pp. 802–805, 2006.

[5] E. J. Yue, M. E. Cabanela, G. P. Duffy, M. G. Heckman, and M. I. O'Connor, "Hip resurfacing arthroplasty: risk factors for failure over 25 years," *Clinical Orthopaedics and Related Research*, vol. 467, no. 4, pp. 992–999, 2009.

[6] A. Malviya, G. H. Stafford, R. J. F. Villar, and R. N. Villar, "Have the media influenced the use of hip resurfacing arthroplasty? a review of UK print media," *Annals of the Royal College of Surgeons of England*, vol. 94, no. 6, pp. 432–437, 2012.

[7] O. Panel and RDA, Metal-on-Metal Implant Systems.

[8] J. Kärrholm, H. Lindahl, H. Malchau et al., "The Swedish Hip Arthroplasty Register: Annual Report," Tech. Rep., The Swedish Hip Arthroplasty Register, 2016.

[9] S. E. Graves, D. Davidson, L. Ingerson et al., "The australian orthopaedic association national joint replacement registry," *Medical Journal of Australia*, vol. 180, pp. S31–S34, 2004.

[10] S. Williams, I. Leslie, G. Isaac, Z. Jin, E. Ingham, and J. Fisher, "Tribology and wear of metal-on-metal hip prostheses: influence of cup angle and head position," *The Journal of Bone and Joint Surgery-American Volume*, vol. 90, no. Suppl 3, pp. 111–117, 2008.

[11] M. D. Gaillard and T. P. Gross, "Metal-on-metal hip resurfacing in patients younger than 50 years: A retrospective analysis," *Journal of Orthopaedic Surgery and Research*, vol. 12, pp. 1–12, 2017.

[12] H. C. Amstutz, M. J. Le Duff, P. A. Campbell, and F. J. Dorey, "The effects of technique changes on aseptic loosening of the femoral component in hip resurfacing. results of 600 conserve plus with a 3 to 9 year follow-up," *The Journal of Arthroplasty*, vol. 22, no. 4, pp. 481–489, 2007.

[13] P. E. Beaulé, M. LeDuff, F. J. Dorey et al., "Fate of cementless acetabular components retained during revision total hip arthroplasty," *Journal of Bone and Joint Surgery*, vol. 85A, pp. 2288–2293, 2003.

[14] B. J. Bessette, F. Fassier, M. Tanzer, and C. E. Brooks, "Total hip arthroplasty in patients younger than 21 years: a minimum 10-year follow-up," *Canadian Journal of Surgery*, vol. 46, no. 4, pp. 257–262, 2003.

[15] H. C. Amstutz, S. M. Ma, R. H. Jinnah, and L. Mai, "Revision of aseptic loose total hip arthroplasties," *Clinical Orthopaedics and Related Research*, vol. 170, pp. 21–33, 1982.

[16] H. C. Amstutz and M. J. Le Duff, "Aseptic loosening of cobalt chromium monoblock sockets after hip resurfacing," *Hip International*, vol. 25, no. 5, pp. 466–470, 2018.

[17] G. Tsikandylakis, M. Mohaddes, P. Cnudde, A. Eskelinen, J. Kärrholm, and O. Rolfson, "Head size in primary total hip arthroplasty," *EFORT Open Reviews*, vol. 3, no. 5, pp. 225–231, 2018.

[18] W. Harris and W. J. Maloney, "Endosteal errosion in association with stable uncemented femoral components," *Journal of Bone and Joint Surgery*, vol. 72, pp. 1025–1034, 1990.

[19] H. Kienapfel, C. Sprey, A. Wilke, and P. Griss, "Implant fixation by bone ingrowth," *The Journal of Arthroplasty*, vol. 14, no. 3, pp. 355–368, 1999.

[20] F. Javed, H. B. Ahmed, R. Crespi, and G. E. Romanos, "Role of primary stability for successful osseointegration of dental implants: factors of influence and evaluation," *Interventional Medicine and Applied Science*, vol. 5, no. 4, pp. 162–167, 2013.

[21] R. M. Nunley, J. Zhu, P. J. Brooks et al., "The learning curve for adopting hip resurfacing among hip specialists," *Clinical Orthopaedics and Related Research*, vol. 468, no. 2, pp. 382–391, 2010.

[22] G. J. Hooper, A. G. Rothwell, M. Stringer, and C. Frampton, "Revision following cemented and uncemented primary total hip replacement: A seven-year analysis from the New Zealand joint registry," *The Journal of Bone & Joint Surgery (British Volume)*, vol. 91, no. 4, pp. 451–458, 2009.

[23] M. J. Latteier, K. R. Berend, A. V. Lombardi, A. F. Ajluni, B. E. Seng, and J. B. Adams, "Gender is a significant factor for failure of metal-on-metal total hip arthroplasty," *The Journal of Arthroplasty*, vol. 26, no. 6, pp. 19–23, 2011.

[24] P. R. Kim, P. E. Beaulé, G. Y. Laflamme, and M. Dunbar, "Causes of early failure in a multicenter clinical trial of hip resurfacing," *The Journal of Arthroplasty*, vol. 23, no. 6, pp. 44–49, 2008.

[25] H. C. Amstutz, P. E. Beaulé, F. J. Dorey, M. J. Le Duff, P. A. Campbell, and T. A. Gruen, "Metal-on-metal hybrid surface arthroplasty: two to six-year follow-up study," *The Journal of Bone and Joint Surgery-American Volume*, vol. 86A, no. 1, pp. 28–39, 2004.

24

Cumulative Incidence of Revision for a Balanced Knee System at a Mean 8-Year Follow-Up: A Retrospective Review of 500 Consecutive Total Knee Arthroplasties

Michael H. Bourne, Tony L. Miller, and E. Marc Mariani

Salt Lake Orthopaedic Clinic, St. Mark's Hospital, Salt Lake City, Utah, USA

Correspondence should be addressed to Michael H. Bourne; mhbourne@msn.com

Academic Editor: Allen L. Carl

Purpose. The primary purpose of this study was to evaluate mid-term survival of a Balanced Knee System in the first 500 total knee arthroplasty (TKA) cases using a fully cemented, posterior stabilized TKA at a high-volume private practice. *Patients and Methods.* In this IRB approved retrospective cohort study, data were extracted from a surgical registry at a high-volume orthopaedic practice for the first 500 total knee arthroplasty (TKA) cases performed using the Balanced Knee® System (BKS, Ortho Development®, Draper, Utah, USA). Procedures were performed between June 2000 and September 2003 by one of two orthopaedic surgeons. Follow-up was performed at 6 weeks, 6 months, 1 year, 5 years, and 10 years. 48 patients (9.6%) were considered lost to follow-up. A competing risk analysis was performed to evaluate the cumulative incidence of revision while accounting for the competing risk of death. In the model, failure was defined as revision of any BKS component. Those who failed prior to two years remained in the analysis. *Results.* The mean age of the population was 69 years (range: 40–94) and 73% were female. The cumulative incidence of revision of any component was approximately 1% at a mean 8-year follow-up (range: 0.11–14.1 years) when accounting for the competing risk of death. When considering all those lost to follow-up as failures, the cumulative incidence of failure at 8 years was approximately 10%. *Conclusion.* Based on the results of the current study, a posterior stabilized primary TKA, implanted using a flexion and extension gap balancing technique, had excellent survivorship and outcomes at a mean 8-year follow-up.

1. Introduction

Total knee arthroplasty (TKA) is one of the most common surgical procedures for restoring physical function and mitigating pain associated with arthritic knees, and the frequency of TKA is expected to rise [1, 2]. When performing this procedure, one common technique is gap balancing [3]. This technique involves a step-by-step approach to ensure equal flexion and extension gaps with equalization of soft tissue tension [3]. Proponents of this technique note that the equalization of soft tissue tension, as well as the creation of equal flexion and extension gaps, improves the function and longevity of TKA [4–8].

However, this technique presents with some limitations. In a recent review of surgical techniques for TKA, Sheth et al. [3] reported that the gap balancing technique could result in raising of the joint line, mid-flexion instability, irregularities in femoral rotation, and excessive flexion gap when performed in posterior stabilized TKA [9]. Given these potential pitfalls, continued postmarket clinical follow-up for gap balancing systems is needed.

The purpose of this study was to evaluate mid-term survival of a Balanced Knee System in the first 500 total knee arthroplasty (TKA) cases using a fully cemented, posterior stabilized TKA at a high-volume private practice. Additionally, we sought to evaluate the frequency of postoperative complications associated with the surgical procedure, the reasons for revision, radiographic outcomes, and differences in Knee Society Scores and arc of motion from pre- to last follow-up visits.

2. Materials and Methods

After obtaining approval from the institutional review board (IRB# 0114), data were extracted from a surgical registry at

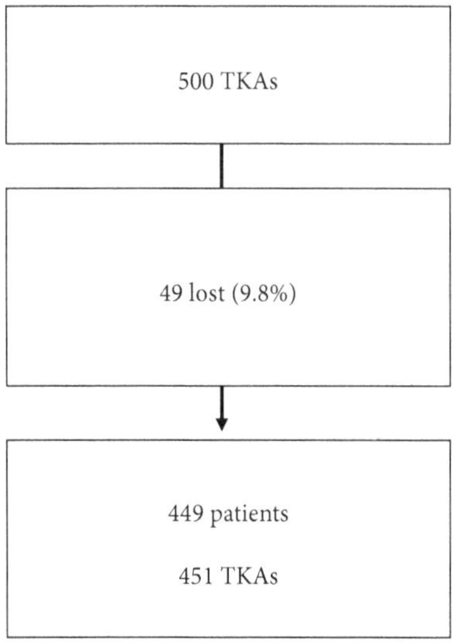

FIGURE 1: Flow diagram demonstrating patient attrition.

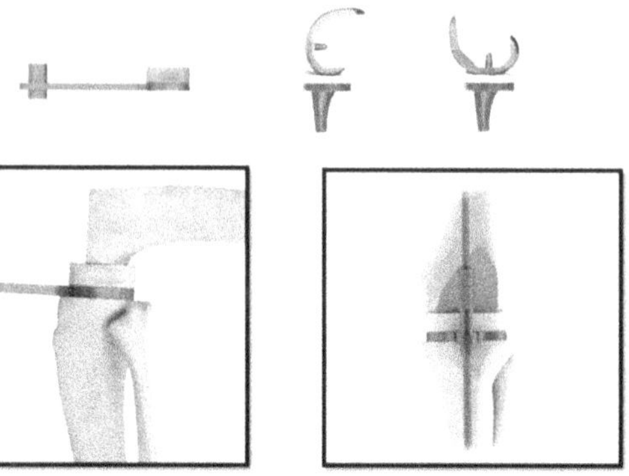

FIGURE 2: The spacer block system provided in the instrumentation of the Balanced Knee System used in this study.

a high-volume orthopaedic practice for the first 500 total knee arthroplasty (TKA) cases performed using the Balanced Knee® System (BKS, Ortho Development®, Draper, Utah, USA). Posterior stabilized, fully cemented implants were used in all knees. The procedures were performed between June 2000 and September 2003 by one of two high-volume, private practice, orthopaedic surgeons. Follow-up was performed during routine office visits or phone call follow-up at 6 weeks, 6 months, 1 year, 5 years, and 10 years. A minimum two-year follow-up was required for each patient in order to be included in the analysis. If patients did not have a minimum two-year follow-up, public death records were referenced to determine if a date of death was present. Patients without a minimum two-year follow-up, who had not experienced a known postoperative complication before, and without a confirmed death record were considered "lost to follow-up". Of the 500 TKAs, 48 patients (9.6%) were considered lost to follow-up (Figure 1).

2.1. Surgical Procedure. The surgical procedure was standardized between the two surgeons, both performing a total knee arthroplasty utilizing the medial retinacular approach, tourniquet control, and general anesthetic and femoral nerve block. Gap balancing was performed using both bony resection and soft tissue balancing. The bony portion of the balancing technique used an intramedullary guide on the femur with the distal cut at 5° valgus, and an extramedullary tibial guide was used with the proximal cut perpendicular to the longitudinal axis of the tibia in the coronal plane and following the normal tibial posterior slope of 3–5 degrees in the sagittal plane. A recent review of the literature suggests an ideal posterior slope of 0–7 degrees [10]. The distal femoral cut in conjunction with the proximal tibial resection determined the extension gap.

The anterior and posterior femoral resections were made in line with the epicondylar axis or perpendicular to Whiteside's line. The posterior femoral cut combined with the proximal tibial surface defined the flexion gap. Posterior femoral osteophytes as well as medial and lateral femoral and tibial osteophytes were resected. Soft tissue balancing was next performed followed by adjusted bony cuts to create symmetric rectangular flexion and extension gaps. A composite spacer block (replicating the total thickness of the tibial component plus the femoral component plus the polyethylene spacer) was utilized during the process to aid in the extent of soft tissue releases and additional boney cuts to ultimately create medial-lateral soft tissue balancing with equalization of the flexion and extension gaps (Figure 2). With this system, the spacer blocks increase by 1mm increments from 5 to 14 mm, with additional blocks of 16, 18, and 20 mm if needed. This allows for precise measuring of the flexion-extension gaps for placement of the appropriate tibial insert. The tibial inserts range in size from 7 to 14mm, also increasing by 1mm each, followed by 16,18, and 20mm inserts.

After the initial bone cuts and equalization of the soft tissues, if the flexion gap was tighter than the extension gap, the flexion gap was enlarged by downsizing the femoral component, as the additional bone removed in downsizing was taken from the posterior femoral condyles. In cases where the extension gap was tighter than the flexion gap, an appropriate amount of bone was taken from the distal femur. When gaps are equally too tight in both flexion and extension, additional tibial resection was performed to enlarge the flexion and extension gaps equally.

Only after the flexion and extension gaps were equalized and soft tissues balanced, were finishing cuts (notch and chamfers) completed on the femur. The center tibial component rotation is determined by aligning the center of the component facing the medial third of the tibial tubercle which usually aligns the anterior edge of the tibial component parallel with the anterior edge of the tibia. A trial reduction was then performed ensuring stability throughout a full range of motion.

Both surgeons utilized a layered closure of absorbable suture with a final subcuticular closure using a nonabsorbable suture. Patients averaged three days postoperative hospitalization with a return to home or an extended care facility.

Both physicians used Coumadin for deep vein thrombosis prophylaxis as well as perioperative intermittent compression boots and compression hose. Postoperative physical therapy and continuous passive motion machines were employed as part of the standard care-pathways.

2.2. Outcome Measures. Revisions and surgical complications were collected from the surgical database and verified by review of the electronic medical records. Additionally, manual chart review was performed on a random sample of 20% of the population (91/451) in order to verify the outcomes from the database. Of these, charts were unavailable for 7/451 (1.6%) knees. The findings from the review were consistent with the database results, and no further review was performed. A failure of the implant was defined as any post-arthroplasty removal of one or more implant, or polyethylene, components for any reason. A complication was defined as an untoward surgical or post-arthroplasty event that did not require removal of an implant component, but that was directly related to the arthroplasty procedure.

Hip to ankle radiographs were obtained prior to surgery to assess lower extremity alignment and after TKA to determine anatomical axis. Of the 406 postoperative X-rays, with minimum two-year follow-up, available for review, 344 (85%) were completed in a standing position, 35 (9%) were completed in a recumbent position, and 27 (7%) were missing this information. Radiographs were evaluated using the knee society roentgenographic rating system [11].

As part of routine care, the Knee Society Clinical Rating System (KS) was used [12]. The KS score is composed of both a knee score and a functional score. The scores are reported on a scale of 0–100 with higher scores indicating better outcomes. Lee et al. [13] have recently reported a minimal clinically important difference for the KS score at approximately 6 points for both the knee and functional scores with 95% confidence intervals of roughly 4–8 points.

Patient range of motion (ROM) was assessed in the office by the surgeon, using a standard goniometer with the patient in the supine position, and is reported as the arc of motion (complete extension to full flexion).

2.3. Statistical Analysis. Given the large proportion of patients expired (26%, 116/451) over the course of the study period, a competing risk analysis, using the methods of Fine & Gray, was performed to evaluate the cumulative incidence of revision while accounting for the competing risk of death [14, 15]. In the model, failure was defined as revision of any BKS component. A worst-case analysis was also performed where failure was defined as revision or lost to follow-up. As there was approximately 11% missing data for KSS and arc of motion outcome variables, imputations were performed using the multivariate imputation by chained equations (MICE) method of multiple multivariate imputation [16–18]. A simple linear generalized estimating equation (GEE) regression analysis with an independent correlation matrix was then performed to evaluate the difference between pre- and last follow-up visits in the KS knee score, KS functional score, and arc of motion. Model fit was assessed using the quasi-likelihood independence model criterion [19]. The minimum clinically important difference (MCID) was considered as a change of 6 points on the KS scores as described by Lee et al. [13]. Given the high mortality rate, and in order to better understand the survival free from death, a subanalysis was performed using a Kaplan–Meier analysis with death as failure. Additionally, the proportion of expired patients was dichotomized by age ≥80 vs <80 and evaluated using a chi-square analysis. Statistical analyses were performed using Stata/IC version 15.1 (College Station, Texas, USA). Significance was assessed at $p<0.05$.

TABLE 1: Patient Characteristics.

Characteristics	Results
Sex, n (%)	
Female	330 (73%)
Male	122 (27%)
Age, mean (range)	69 (40 – 94)
BMI, mean (range)	30.2 (17.5 – 60.4)
ASA Score, median (IQR)	2 (2 – 3)
Deceased, n (%)	116 (26%)
Primary Diagnosis, n (%)	
Osteoarthritis	428 (95%)
Post-traumatic arthritis	8 (2%)
Rheumatoid arthritis	11 (2%)
Avascular necrosis	1 (<1%)
Psoriatic Arthritis	2 (<1%)
Other	1 (<1%)
Missing	1 (<1%)

3. Results

The mean age of the population was 69 years (range: 40–94) with 73% being female (Table 1). Osteoarthritis was the primary diagnosis for 95% (428/451) of the cases (Table 1). The mean preoperative coronal alignment was 5° (range: 1°–16°).

The cumulative incidence of revision of any component was approximately 1% at a mean 8-year follow-up (range: 0.11–14.1 years) when accounting for the competing risk of death (Figure 3). Those who failed prior to two years remained in the analysis. When evaluating the worst-case scenario, considering all those lost to follow-up as failures, the cumulative incidence of failure at 8 years was approximately 10% (Figure 4). Finally, when reviewing only death as failure, the survivorship at 8 years was 77% (Figure 5).

There was a total of 28 complications for an incidence of 6%. Of the complication (Table 2), the majority consisted of adhesions (15/28, 53%), persistent pain (2/28, 7%), instability (2/28, 7%), and deep infections (2/28, 7%). All those with adhesions required a return to the operating theatre for manipulation under anesthesia (MUA). The median time to MUA was 6 weeks (IQR: 5–9 weeks). Nine patients (2%) required removal of one or more implant components over the entire follow-up period. The primary reasons for revision (Table 3) included persistent pain (2/9, 22%) and instability (2/9, 22%).

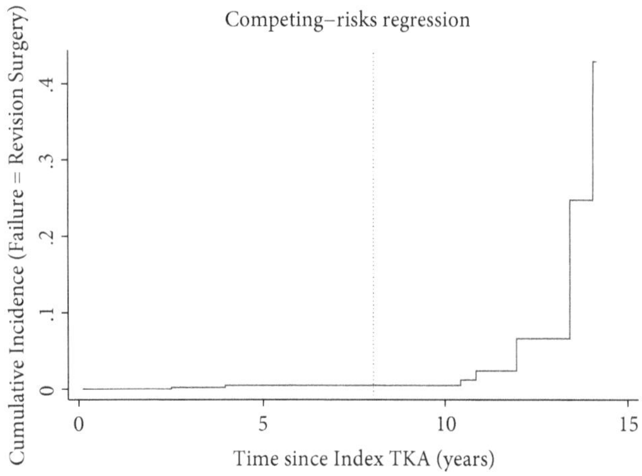

FIGURE 3: The cumulative incidence curve with failure defined as revision of any component.

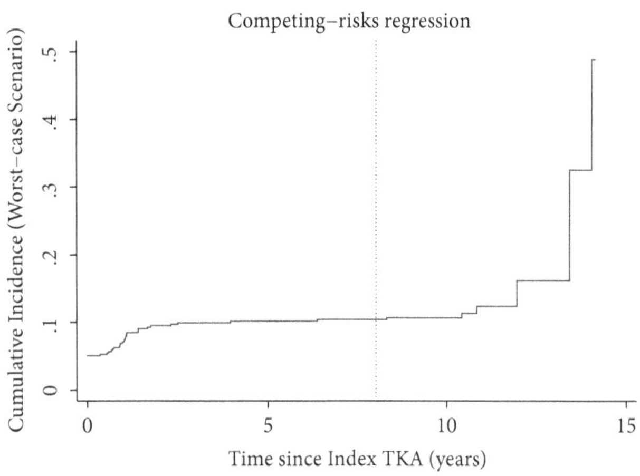

FIGURE 4: The cumulative incidence curve for the worst-case scenario with failure defined as revision of any component or lost to follow-up.

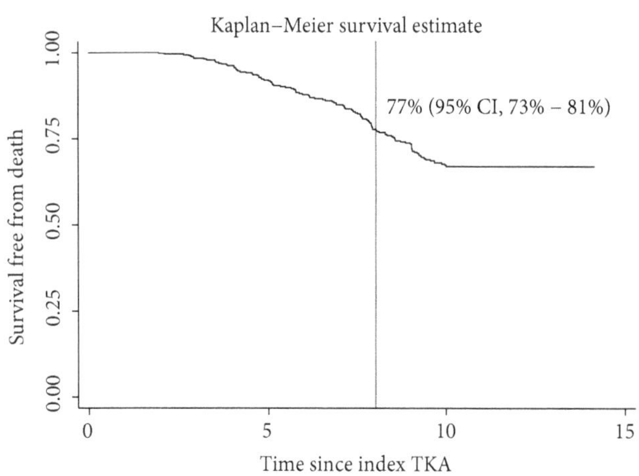

FIGURE 5: A Kaplan-Meier survival curve with death as failure.

TABLE 2: Postoperative complications.

Diagnosis	n (%)
Adhesions	15 (53%)
Persistent pain	2 (7%)
Instability	2 (7%)
Superficial infections	2 (7%)
Patellar fracture	2 (7%)
Deep infections	1 (4%)
Missing	1 (4%)
Patellar tendon rupture	1 (4%)
Tibial loosening	1 (4%)
Periprosthetic femur fracture	1 (4%)

TABLE 3: Reasons for Revision (removal of one or more implant components).

Diagnosis	n (%)
Persistent pain	2 (22%)
Instability	2 (22%)
Deep infection	1 (11%)
Tibial Loosening	1 (11%)
Periprosthetic fracture	1 (11%)
Patellar Tendon Rupture	1 (11%)
Unknown	1 (11%)

TABLE 4: Distribution of radiolucent lines.

Component	Patients with Radiolucencies, n (%)
Femoral: bone interface	18 (4.5%)
Femoral: cement/prosthesis	2 (<1%)
Patella: bone interface	0
Patella: cement/prosthesis	0
Tibia: bone interface (lateral)	2 (<1%)
Tibia: cement/prosthesis (lateral)	0
Tibia: bone interface (AP[a])	5 (1.2%)
Tibia: cement/prosthesis (AP[a])	3 (<1%)

a: anteroposterior.

Of the 451 TKAs, 406 had a minimum two-year radiograph available for review. The mean valgus angle was 5 degrees (95% CI, 4.6–5.1). There were 18 TKAs (4.5%) with femoral radiolucencies at the bone interface, 2 (<1%) at the tibial bone interface on lateral views, five (1.2%) with A/P tibial bone interface lucencies, and 3 (<1%) with A/P tibial cement/prosthesis lucencies (Table 4). There was no evidence of subsidence at the last follow-up. The majority of radiolucencies were found in the femoral bone interface zone 1 (Tables 5–7). The zone with the greatest width of radiolucent lines was the femoral bone interface in femoral zone 4 (Table 8), whereas the width of radiolucent lines in the tibia was greatest in the bone interface of tibial zone 1 (Table 9).

TABLE 5: Frequency of radiolucent lines in the femoral zones.

Radiolucent Zones	n (%)
Femoral Bone	
zone 1	14 (78%)
zone 2	0
zone 3	0
zone 4	6 (33%)
zone 5	0
zone 6	0
zone 7	0
Femoral cement/prosthesis	
zone 1	2 (100%)
zone 2	0
zone 3	0
zone 4	0
zone 5	0
zone 6	0
zone 7	0

TABLE 6: Frequency of radiolucent lines in the anteroposterior (AP) tibial zones.

Radiolucent Zones	n (%)
Tibia: bone interface (AP[a])	
zone 1	4 (80)
zone 2	1 (20)
zone 3	1 (20)
zone 4	1 (20)
zone 5	1 (20)
zone 6	1 (20)
zone 7	0
Tibial: cement/prosthesis (AP[a])	
zone 1	2 (67)
zone 2	2 (67)
zone 3	2 (67)
zone 4	2 (67)
zone 5	0
zone 6	0
zone 7	0

a: anteroposterior.

The KS knee scores improved from an adjusted mean value of 41.6 (95% CI 39.2–44.0) preoperatively to 80.8 (95% CI, 78.5–83.1) postoperatively (p<0.001). Similarly, the KS functional score improved from a preoperative adjusted mean score of 42.6 (95% CI, 40.4–44.9) to a postoperative score of 71.0 (95% CI, 68.8–73.3, p<0.001). Finally, the arc of motion improved from a preoperative adjust mean value of 110° (95% CI, 108°–111°) to a postoperative value of 122° (95% CI, 120°–123°, p<0.001).

3.1. Subanalysis. Given the 26% mortality, the subanalysis for 8-year survival free from death was 77% (Figure 5).

TABLE 7: Frequency of radiolucent lines in the Lateral Tibial zones.

Radiolucent Zones	n (%)
Tibia: bone interface (lateral)	
zone 1	1 (50%)
zone 2	0
zone 3	1 (50%)
Radiolucent Zones	n (%)
Tibia: bone interface (lateral)	
zone 1	1 (50%)
zone 2	0
zone 3	1 (50%)

When dichotomized by age, 15% (67/451) of knees were from octogenarians and a greater proportion of them expired during the study time period (p<0.001), where 8% (27/335) of TKA patients less than eighty and 34.5% (40/116) of TKA patients ≥80 expired. The mean time to death was 6.6 ± 2 years.

4. Discussion

The gap balancing technique for total knee arthroplasty has been shown to be an effective method of performing TKA resulting in excellent clinical outcomes [20–22]. The most important finding in this study was that this posterior stabilized implant, with the gap balancing technique for obtaining symmetrical flexion and extension gaps, resulted in excellent survivorship and good clinical outcomes at a mean 8-year follow-up after TKA.

This study is not without limitations including that of missing data, a large number of deceased patients, and a potential for individual scientific bias. As the missing data was relatively low, approximately 11%, statistical methods were employed to impute this data appropriately. The mortality in this population was rather high for a primary TKA population with our data showing 8-year survival free from death at 77% (Figure 5), whereas a recent report using the National Joint Registry of England and Wales showed 8-year survival free from death at approximately 89% following primary TKA [23]. To better understand our mortality rate, we performed a subgroup analysis dichotomizing age into those ≥80 (octogenarians) and those <80. Fifteen percent (67/451) of knees were from octogenarians and approximately 35% of them had expired during the review (p<0.001), compared to only 8% of those <80. Murphy et al. [24] demonstrated increased mortality in patients greater than 80 years. As such, the risk for increased mortality in this population is likely due to the older nature of this cohort. Regardless, a competing risks model was used in order to determine the cumulative incidence of failure while accounting for those who expired making them unable to be at risk for failure. Finally, the two surgeons (MHB, EMM) have significant financial relationships with the manufacturer of the BKS system and as such the results of this study should be reviewed with this in mind.

TABLE 8: The proportion of radiolucent line widths per femoral zone.

Component	None	<1 mm	1 -2 mm	>2 mm
Femoral: Bone interface, n=18				
zone 1	4	5	9	0
zone 4	12	6	0	0
Femoral: cement/prosthesis, n=2				
zone 1	2	0	0	0

Component	None	<1 mm	1 -2 mm	>2 mm
Femoral: Bone interface, n=18				
zone 1	4	5	9	0
zone 4	12	6	0	0
Femoral: cement/prosthesis, n=2				
zone 1	2	0	0	0

TABLE 9: The proportion of radiolucent line widths per tibial zone.

Component	None	<1 mm	1 -2 mm	>2 mm
Tibia: bone interface (AP[a]), n=5	1	1	3	0
zone 1	4	1	0	0
zone 2	4	1	0	0
zone 3	4	1	0	0
zone 4	4	1	0	0
zone 5	1	1	0	0
zone 6				
Tibia: bone cement/prosthesis (AP[a]), n=3	1	1	0	1
zone 1	1	1	0	1
zone 2	1	2	0	0
zone 3	1	2	0	0
zone 4	3	0	0	0
zone 5	3	0	0	0
zone 6				

a: anteroposterior.

Total knee arthroplasty has become one of the most reliable and durable procedures for restoring patient function. Excellent long-term results have been reported in the literature with survival rates ranging from 90 to 100 percent after 5–15 years, based upon failure definition [25–29]. The technique used with this system of gap balancing reliably provides a well-functioning TKA with results comparable to those previously reported in the literature [29]. Through a series of initial bone cuts, followed by soft tissue balancing, and then equalization of the flexion/extension gaps with final bone cuts, our cumulative incidence of failure was limited to 1%. Even with counting all patients lost to follow-up as knee failures (an extreme example), this TKA system demonstrated an acceptable cumulative incidence rate of failure (10%) at 8-year follow-up.

Of the 451 TKAs available for follow-up, 6% (n= 27) experience postoperative complications. The patellar fracture, the patellar tendon rupture, and the periprosthetic fracture all occurred postoperatively from traumatic falls. Both patients with "instability" did well with placement of a larger polyethylene spacer. The 15 patients (3.3%) with "adhesions" did well with a manipulation under anesthesia performed at a median of 5 weeks after the initial procedure. One patient underwent MUA 46 weeks after the index TKA due to continued adhesions and lack of compliance with his recovery pathway. This patient also struggled with mental health and was being treated for profound clinical depression. Unfortunately, he continued to ignore protocol and at last follow-up was still struggling with pain and lack of motion. The single case of tibial loosening was a 47-year-old male with evidence of polyethylene wear approximately 14 years after the primary TKA. At the time of revision surgery, a significant cyst was also noted on the femur and thus all components were revised.

Nonprogressive bone-cement lucencies were most commonly seen in femoral zone 1 and tibial zone 1. These were seen in the immediate postoperative X-rays. It is felt that these changes are seen merely as a result of the tangential cementing forces that occur with sliding the femoral component into place (zones 1 and 4 on the femoral side) as well as the often more sclerotic medial side (varus knees) with cementing of the tibial side. Again, these changes were seen early and had not progressed throughout follow-up.

Others have reported similar findings [30–32].

Regarding patient reported outcomes, our results are similar to prior reports where mean KS outcome scores at two- and five-year follow-up have ranged from 82.4 to 95.8 for the KS knee score and from 58.8 to 96.2 for the KS function score [33]. Both the KS knee score and functional scores achieved the MCID of approximately 6 points as reported by Lee et al. [13]. Finally, the arc of motion of a mean of 122 degrees postoperatively is also similar to that previously reported in the literature. While a functional ROM has been reported to be 105 degrees, we find that most patients will obtain between 120 and 130 degrees of flexion. Most flexion is limited by posterior soft tissue mass rather than limitations in the prosthesis. Slender patients will oftentimes exceed 140 degrees. Posterior stabilized knees allow for greater flexion through posterior femoral rollback than posterior cruciate retaining knees. The equalization of flexion/extension gaps along with soft tissue balancing also ensures the likelihood of an excellent resultant arc of motion.

5. Conclusion

Based on the results of the current study, a posterior stabilized primary TKA, implanted using a flexion and extension gap balancing technique, had excellent survivorship and outcomes at a mean 8-year follow-up. This technique allows all surgeons to obtain excellent results by following a step-by-step sequence that ensures equalization of the flexion/extension gaps as well as soft tissue balancing. Further studies are needed to evaluate the long-term survival of these implants.

References

[1] H. M. Kremers, D. R. Larson, C. S. Crowson et al., "Prevalence of total hip and knee replacement in the United States," *The Journal of Bone and Joint Surgery-American Volume*, vol. 97, no. 17, pp. 1386–1397, 2015.

[2] S. M. Kurtz, E. Lau, K. Ong, K. Zhao, M. Kelly, and K. J. Bozic, "Future young patient demand for primary and revision joint replacement: national projections from 2010 to 2030," *Clinical Orthopaedics and Related Research*, vol. 467, no. 10, pp. 2606–2612, 2009.

[3] N. P. Sheth, A. Husain, and C. L. Nelson, "Surgical techniques for total knee arthroplasty: measured resection, gap balancing, and hybrid," *Journal of the American Academy of Orthopaedic-Surgeons*, vol. 25, no. 7, pp. 499–508, 2017.

[4] B. K. Daines and D. A. Dennis, "Gap balancing vs. measured resection technique in total knee arthroplasty," *Clinics in Orthopedic Surgery*, vol. 6, no. 1, pp. 1–8, 2014.

[5] B. D. Springer, S. Parratte, and M. P. Abdel, "Measured resection versus gap balancing for total knee arthroplasty," *Clinical Orthopaedics and Related Research*, vol. 472, no. 7, pp. 2016–2022, 2016.

[6] D. A. Dennis, R. D. Komistek, R. H. Kim, and A. Sharma, "Gap balancing versus measured resection technique for total knee arthroplasty," *Clinical Orthopaedics and Related Research*, vol. 468, no. 1, pp. 102–107, 2010.

[7] D.-H. Lee, J.-H. Park, D.-I. Song, D. Padhy, W.-K. Jeong, and S.-B. Han, "Accuracy of soft tissue balancing in TKA: Comparison between navigation-assisted gap balancing and conventional measured resection," *Knee Surgery, Sports Traumatology, Arthroscopy*, vol. 18, no. 3, pp. 381–387, 2010.

[8] T. Matsumoto, H. Muratsu, S. Kubo et al., "Soft tissue balance using the tibia first gap technique with navigation system in cruciate-retaining total knee arthroplasty," *International Orthopaedics*, vol. 36, no. 5, pp. 975–980, 2012.

[9] T. L. Kinsey and O. M. Mahoney, "Balanced flexion and extension gaps are not always of equal size," *The Journal of Arthroplasty*, vol. 33, no. 4, pp. 1062.e1065–1068.e1065, 2018.

[10] K. Gromov, M. Korchi, M. G. Thomsen, H. Husted, and A. Troelsen, "What is the optimal alignment of the tibial and femoral components in knee arthroplasty?" *Acta Orthopaedica*, vol. 85, no. 5, pp. 480–487, 2014.

[11] F. C. Ewald, "The knee society total knee arthroplasty roentgenographic evaluation and scoring system," *Clinical Orthopaedics and Related Research*, vol. 248, pp. 9–12, 1989.

[12] J. N. Insall, L. D. Dorr, R. D. Scott, and W. N. Scott, "Rationale of the Knee Society clinical rating system," *Clinical Orthopaedics and Related Research*, vol. 248, pp. 13-14, 1989.

[13] W. C. Lee, Y. H. Kwan, H. C. Chong, and S. J. Yeo, "The minimal clinically important difference for Knee Society Clinical Rating System after total knee arthroplasty for primary osteoarthritis," *Knee Surgery, Sports Traumatology, Arthroscopy*, vol. 25, no. 11, pp. 3354–3359, 2017.

[14] P. C. Austin and J. P. Fine, "Practical recommendations for reporting Fine-Gray model analyses for competing risk data," *Statistics in Medicine*, vol. 36, no. 27, pp. 4391–4400, 2017.

[15] J. P. Fine and R. J. Gray, "A proportional hazards model for the subdistribution of a competing risk," *Journal of the American Statistical Association*, vol. 94, no. 446, pp. 496–509, 1999.

[16] S. Van Buuren, H. C. Boshuizen, and D. L. Knook, "Multiple imputation of missing blood pressure covariates in survival analysis," *Statistics in Medicine*, vol. 18, no. 6, pp. 681–694, 1999.

[17] P. Royston, "Multiple imputation of missing values," *The Stata Journal: Promoting Communications on Statistics and Stata*, vol. 4, no. 3, pp. 227–241, 2018.

[18] P. Royston, "Multiple imputation of missing values: Further update of ice, with an emphasis on categorical variables," *Stata Journal*, vol. 9, no. 3, pp. 466–477, 2009.

[19] J. Cui, "QIC program and model selection in GEE analyses," *The Stata Journal*, vol. 7, no. 2, pp. 209–220, 2007.

[20] F. Lavoie, "Spacer-based gap balancing in total knee arthroplasty: clinical success with a reproducible technique," *Journal of Knee Surgery*, vol. 30, no. 8, pp. 798–806, 2017.

[21] J. L. Churchill, A. Khlopas, A. A. Sultan, S. F. Harwin, and M. A. Mont, "Gap-balancing versus measured resection technique in total knee arthroplasty: a comparison study," *Journal of Knee Surgery*, vol. 31, no. 1, pp. 13–16, 2018.

[22] T. Huang, Y. Long, D. George, and W. Wang, "Meta-analysis of gap balancing versus measured resection techniques in total knee arthroplasty," *The Bone & Joint Journal*, vol. 99-B, no. 2, pp. 151–158, 2017.

[23] A. D. Liddle, A. Judge, H. Pandit, and D. W. Murray, "Adverse outcomes after total and unicompartmental knee replacement in 101330 matched patients: a study of data from the national joint registry for England and Wales," *The Lancet*, vol. 384, no. 9952, pp. 1437–1445, 2014.

[24] B. P. Murphy, M. M. Dowsey, T. Spelman, and P. F. Choong, "The impact of older age on patient outcomes following primary total knee arthroplasty," *The Bone & Joint Journal*, vol. 100-B, no. 11,

pp. 1463–1470, 2018.

[25] C. E. Scott, K. R. Bell, R. T. Ng, D. J. MacDonald, J. T. Patton, and R. Burnett, "Excellent 10-year patient-reported outcomes and survival in a single-radius, cruciate-retaining total knee arthroplasty," *Knee Surgery, Sports Traumatology, Arthroscopy*, vol. 27, no. 4, pp. 1106–1115, 2019.

[26] M. Sartawi, D. Zurakowski, and A. Rosenberg, "Implant survivorship and complication rates after total knee arthroplasty with a third-generation cemented system: 15-year follow-up," *American journal of orthopedics (Belle Mead, N.J.)*, vol. 47, no. 3, 2018.

[27] R. Stempin, K. Stempin, W. Kaczmarek, and J. Dutka, "Midterm results of cementless total knee arthroplasty: a retrospective case series," *The Open Orthopaedics Journal*, vol. 12, no. 1, pp. 196–202, 2018.

[28] R. C. Oliviu, A. Zazgyva, S. Septimiu, N. Örs, and P. T. Sorin, "Mid-term results of total knee replacement with single-radius versus multi-radius posterior-stabilized implants," *Acta Orthopaedica et Traumatologica Turcica*, vol. 50, no. 2, pp. 125–131, 2016.

[29] H. Hommel, D. Kunze, P. Hommel, and P. Fennema, "Small Improvements in postoperative outcome with gap balancing technique compared with measured resection in total knee arthroplasty," *The Open Orthopaedics Journal*, vol. 11, no. 1, pp. 1236–1244, 2017.

[30] Y. S. Jeon, J. S. Shin, J. H. Jung, and M. K. Kim, "Total knee arthroplasty using NexGen LPS-flex® improves clinical outcomes without early loosening: minimum 6-year follow-up results," *Journal of Orthopaedic Surgery and Research*, vol. 11, no. 1, article 83, 2016.

[31] C. P. Yang, K. Y. Hsu, Y. H. Chang, Y. S. Chan, H. N. Shih, and A. C. Chen, "Mid-term survivorship of cruciate-retaining versus posterior-stabilized total knee arthroplasty using modular mini-keel tibial implants," *Journal of Orthopaedic Surgery and Research*, vol. 13, no. 1, article 35, 2018.

[32] R. Fernandez-Fernandez and E. C. Rodriguez-Merchan, "Better survival of total knee replacement in patients older than 70 years: A prospective study with 8 to 12 years follow-up," *Archives of Bone and Joint Surgery*, vol. 3, no. 1, pp. 22–28, 2015.

[33] S. Li, X. Luo, P. Wang, H. Sun, K. Wang, and X. Sun, "Clinical outcomes of gap balancing vs measured resection in total knee arthroplasty: a systematic review and meta-analysis involving 2259 subjects," *The Journal of Arthroplasty*, vol. 33, no. 8, pp. 2684–2693, 2018.

25

Compensatory Function of the Subtalar Joint for Lower Extremity Malalignment

Kensei Yoshimoto, Masahiko Noguchi, Akifumi Yamada, and Yuki Nasu

Orthopaedic Foot and Ankle Center, Shiseikai Daini Hospital, 5-19-1 Kamisoshigaya, Setagaya-ku, Tokyo, 157-8550, Japan

Correspondence should be addressed to Masahiko Noguchi; mnfootor@yahoo.co.jp

Guest Editor: Yasushi Oshima

It is important to evaluate the subtalar joint and hip-knee-ankle alignment to understand lower extremity alignment. In this review, we focused on the compensatory changes in the subtalar joint alignment for the deformity of the knee and ankle joint, reviewing previous research. The subtalar joint alignment was compensatory valgus in patients with varus knee and ankle deformity, whereas it was uncertain whether the subtalar joint alignment was compensatory varus in patients with valgus knee and ankle deformity. The subtalar joint valgus alignment improved after total knee arthroplasty or high tibial osteotomy for varus knee deformity, even if the deformity was severe. In contrast, whether the subtalar joint alignment changed after the surgery for ankle or valgus knee deformity has not been considered. Further research on the compensatory function of the subtalar joint is needed.

1. Introduction

When treatment for lower extremity malalignment is needed, it is important to evaluate the lower extremity alignment correctly. Many studies assessed only the hip-knee-ankle alignment, such as the femorotibial alignment or the mechanical axis running from the center of the femoral head to that of the ankle [1–3]. However, weight-bearing on the lower extremity runs from the hip to the knee, ankle, and foot, and then to the ground. As calcaneus is in contact with the ground, it is necessary to evaluate the alignment of the subtalar joint in addition to the hip-knee-ankle alignment to correctly measure the lower extremity alignment [4].

Each joint of the lower extremity compensates the malalignment caused by deformities of the other joints [10, 11, 20]. In particular, recent studies have discussed the compensatory function of the subtalar joint [7, 13, 19]: several reports show that the subtalar joint compensates for the deformities of the knee and ankle joints [10, 12, 17, 18, 20], and the subtalar joint alignment which was 2°-6° valgus in healthy legs [21, 22] changed after surgery to correct these deformities [7, 14, 16]. When surgery for knee or ankle deformity is needed, it is helpful for surgical planning to understand the mechanism of subtalar joint compensation and how the subtalar joint alignment changes after surgery.

In this literature review, we discuss the compensatory function of the subtalar joint in patients with deformities of the lower extremity, reviewing previous research.

2. Radiographic Assessment of the Hindfoot Alignment

Several methods can be used for the radiographic imaging of the coronal plane alignment of the subtalar joint or hindfoot. Cobey [23] and Saltzman et al. [24] reported the hindfoot alignment view: subjects stood on a floor, and an X-ray beam with an inclination angle of 20° to the floor was directed from the posterior to the anterior side. A modified method was also reported, with a film cassette lying on the floor and the X-ray beam directed at it with an inclination angle of 45° [5, 25] (Figure 1(b)). In these methods, the hindfoot alignment was usually evaluated using the heel alignment distance (HD) as the distance between the contact point of the heel and the intersection of the extended tibial axis and the distal part of the calcaneus [7, 19, 24], and the heel alignment

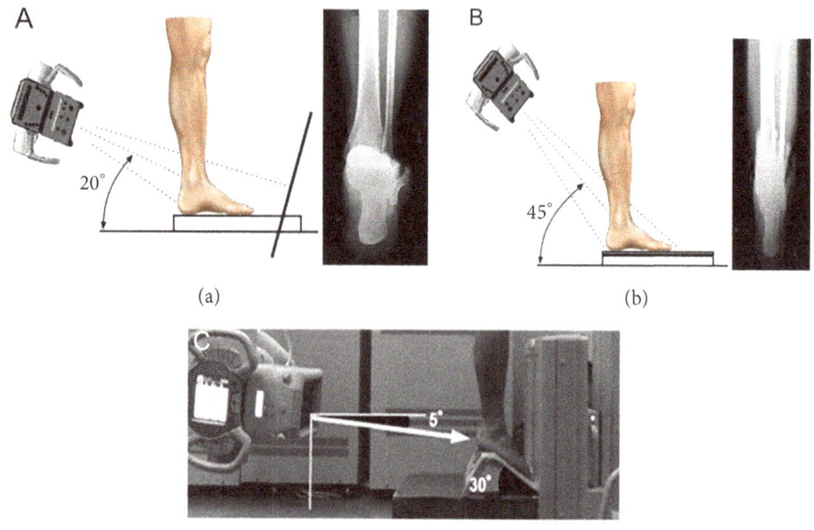

Figure 1: (a) The inclination angle of the beam is 20° to the floor. The film cassette is perpendicular to the central beam of the radiation source. (b) The film cassette is lying on the floor and the subject is standing on the film cassette. The inclination angle of the beam is 45° to the floor. (a) and (b) are reproduced from Reilingh et al. 2010 [5] [under the Creative Commons Attribution License/public domain]. (c) Participants stood on a radiolucent platform with equal weight on both feet. This platform was flat in the rear part and inclined by 30° in the front part, so that the midfoot and forefoot of participants were planter-flexed. The X-ray beam was oriented down 5° from the horizontal position. (c) is reproduced from Ikoma et al. 2013 [6] [under the Creative Commons Attribution License/public domain].

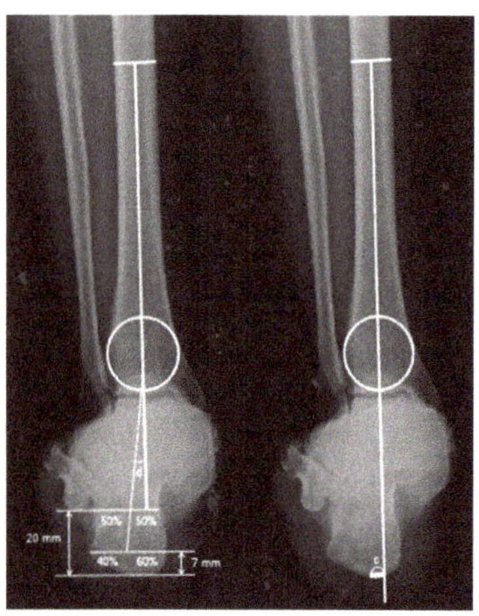

Figure 2: Heel alignment angle (HA) was defined as the angle (d) between the tibial axis and the calcaneal axis. Heel alignment distance (HD) was defined as the distance (c) between the contact point of the heel and the intersection of the extended tibial axis and the distal part of the calcaneus. Figure 2 is reproduced from Jeong et al. 2018 [7].

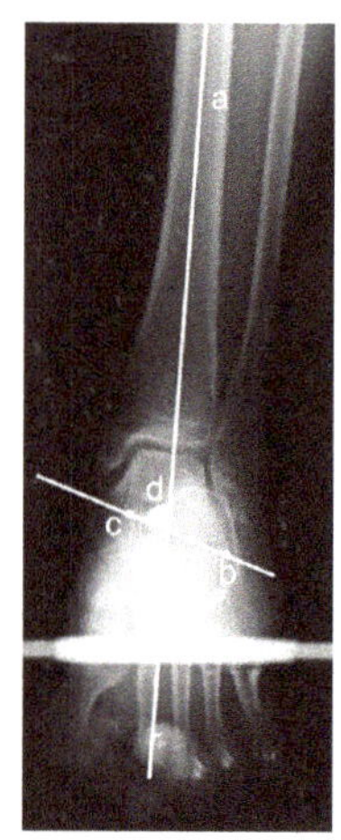

Figure 3: The measurement of the V-V angle. Line a indicates the long axis of the tibia. Point b indicates the lateral extremity of the calcaneus at the posterior surface of the talocalcaneal joint. Point c indicates the superior margin of the sustentaculum tali. Angle d is the V-V angle. Figure 3 is reproduced from Takenaka et al. 2015 [8] [under the Creative Commons Attribution License/public domain].

angle (HA) measured as the angle between the axis of the distal tibia and the axis of the calcaneus [11, 12, 15, 26, 27] (Figure 2). HA is also referred to as hindfoot alignment angle or tibiocalcaneal angle. On the other hand, Ikoma et al. [6] reported a different method, whereby subjects stood on a radiolucent platform, which was flat in the rear part and inclined by 30° in the front part. The X-ray beam was oriented down 5° from the horizontal position (Figure 1(c)).

This method assessed the hindfoot alignment using the V-V angle, measured as the angle between the axis of the line from the top of the sustentaculum tali to the lateral-inferior end of the posterior facet of the calcaneus and tibial axis (Figure 3). Moreover, the utility of weight-bearing computed tomography (CT) scans has also been recently suggested [28, 29]. In CT scans, the subtalar vertical angle (SVA) and

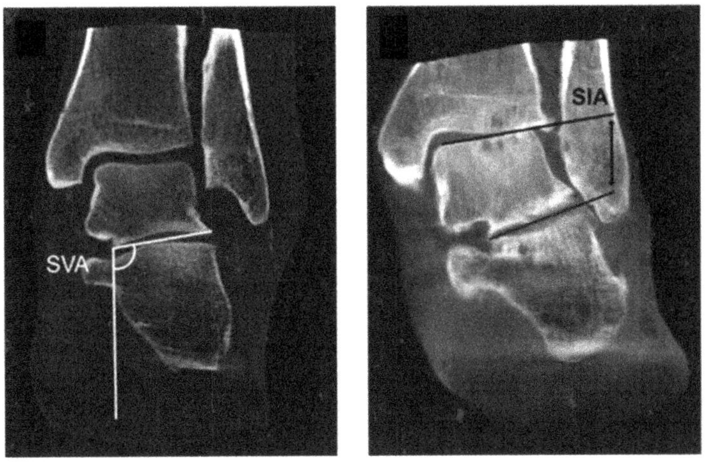

(a) (b)

Figure 4: (a) Corresponding weight-bearing computed tomography (CT) scan. The orientation of the subtalar joint to the ground was assessed using the subtalar vertical angle (SVA). (b) Corresponding weight-bearing CT scan. The subtalar inclination angle (SIA) was used to assess the inclination of the subtalar joint. Figure 4 is reproduced from Krahenbuhl et al. 2017 [9].

subtalar inclination angle (SIA) were measured for evaluating the subtalar joint alignment (Figure 4).

3. Compensatory Function of the Subtalar Joint for Deformity of the Knee

Norton et al. [12] showed that there was a significant correlation between knee and hindfoot alignment, and a moderately strong correlation in patients with knee deformity, and this correlation was remarkable with larger knee deformity (≥ 10°). The correlation coefficient between hindfoot angle and mechanical axis angle was -0.413 and was -0.536 for those with larger knee deformity. These results indicate that the hindfoot alignment was compensatory valgus in patients with varus knee osteoarthritis (OA) and was varus in patients with valgus knee OA. Several reports supported this hindfoot compensatory function in patients with varus knee OA [11, 14]. However, hindfoot compensation for valgus knee OA could not be found in the report by Mullaji et al. [11].

Nakada et al. [15] demonstrated the subtalar joint compensation for the deformity of knee joints with rheumatoid arthritis (RA). The positive correlation between the femorotibial angle (FTA) and the HA only existed in knees with a Larsen grade≥ 4 (r= 0.544), but not in knees with a Larsen grade≤ 3 (r= 0.180). In measurement of the FTA, a lesser value is considered as valgus knee and bigger as varus. In measurement of the HA, a lesser value is considered as varus hindfoot and bigger as valgus. This correlation was stronger in patients with less damaged subtalar joints (Larsen grade≤ 3) (r= 0.705).

4. Compensatory Function of the Subtalar Joint for Deformity of the Ankle

Several reports showed that the subtalar joint could compensate the varus ankle OA [9, 17–19]. The subtalar inclination angle (SIA) increased from Takakura Stages 1 to 3a [30] (2.9° ± 7.0° in Stage 1, 8.0° ±8.6° in Stage 2, and 11.5° ±5.7° in Stage 3a) compared to the control (1.5° ± 5.9°) and decreased at Stages 3b and 4 (4.0° ± 9.2° in Stage 3b and 3.0° ± 9.8° in Stage 4) [17]. This suggested that the subtalar joint was compensatory valgus in patients with early to intermediate Takakura stage but could not compensate in patients with the end stage. In contrast, Krahenbuhl et al. [9] found that the subtalar joint compensation for the varus ankle OA was independent of the stage of ankle joint osteoarthritis, extent of the talar tilt in the ankle joint mortise.

In patients with valgus ankle OA, the subtalar joint compensation might be small [9, 19]. Wang et al. [19] showed that only 38.6% of valgus ankles were compensated by subtalar joints (HA < -7.7°), whereas 53% of varus ankles were compensated (HA > -13.1°). Krahenbuhl et al. [9] could not find the subtalar joint compensation in patients with valgus ankle OA. In their study using weight-bearing CT scans, SVA and SIA measurement revealed that the subtalar joint was valgus synchronizing the valgus ankle deformity.

5. The Subtalar Joint Alignment after Surgery for the Knee Malalignment

Chandler et al. [10] first described that the hindfoot varus or valgus angle changed after the correction of knee deformity with total knee arthroplasty (TKA), showing that the hindfoot compensated the knee deformity. However, they did not clearly explain the correlation between them. Thereafter, several reports found that the compensatory subtalar valgus was corrected after TKA in patients with knee OA [7, 8, 11, 13, 14, 31]. Hara et al. [31] and Takenaka et al. [8] evaluated the subtalar joint alignment using the V-V angle, which averaged a normal value of 76.0° [6] and showed significant improvement in the subtalar joint alignment in patients with subtalar valgus (V-V angle ≥ 76.0°) from 80.5° ± 3.1° to 78.6° ± 3.7° three weeks after TKA and further improved to 77.1° ± 2.7° one year after TKA. However, in patients with subtalar varus (V-V angle < 76.0°), the preoperative V-V angle (72.7° ± 2.6°) did not improve three weeks and one year after TKA (72.3° ± 3.3°, and 73.5° ± 3.0°, respectively). In another report from Cho et al. [14], greater improvements of hindfoot valgus were found in patients with a severe varus deformity of the knee joint (varus ≥ 10°). Greater improvement of the mechanical axis angle from 13.9° ± 3.7° varus to 2.6° ± 3.5° varus in these patients might result in a greater improvement of hindfoot valgus from 6.5° ± 3.8° valgus to 2.5° ± 4.1° valgus. Similar results were observed by Jeong et al. [7], who found a correlation between the pre-postoperative variance in the mechanical axis angle and the ground-talar dome angle, HA and HD (r = 0.7, -0.348 and -0.418, respectively). Okamoto et al. [13] focused on the American Orthopaedic Foot and Ankle Society (AOFAS) ankle–hindfoot scale in addition to the hindfoot alignment after TKA. They also evaluated calcaneal pitch and naviculocuboid overlap in plane weight-bearing lateral foot radiograph as the index of hindfoot alignment. They found that calcaneal pitch, naviculocuboid overlap, and AOFAS ankle–hindfoot scale with moderate varus deformity of the knee (≤ 6° varus) improved after TKA, but those with severe varus deformity of the knee (> 6°) did not improve after TKA.

In contrast, only one report assessed the subtalar joint alignment after TKA in patients with valgus knee OA [11]. They showed that the subtalar joint was valgus before TKA and remained valgus after TKA. However, because their study included quite a small number (n= 12) of patients with valgus OA, further studies with larger sample sizes are needed.

The change of the subtalar joint alignment after tibial osteotomy for knee malalignment was also assessed. Choi et al. [16] evaluated the hindfoot alignment after high tibial osteotomy. They found that the preoperative degree of hindfoot valgus deviation (7.8° valgus) decreased progressively 3 months, 6 months, and 12 months after HTO (4.0°, 3.4°, and 2.3° valgus, respectively).

6. The Subtalar Joint Alignment after Surgery for the Ankle Malalignment

There is only one report by Choi et al. [16] which evaluated the hindfoot alignment after surgery for ankle OA. They evaluated the hindfoot alignment after low tibial osteotomy (LTO) [32] for ankle OA. They included patients with severe ankle OA averaged Takakura stage of 3.2 [30], and preoperative mild hindfoot varus deviation (1.0° varus) was seen. After LTO, the hindfoot alignment was changed to valgus deviation without any compensatory mechanism 3 months, 6 months, and 12 months after LTO (4.8°, 4.7°, and 4.8° valgus, respectively).

7. Discussion

The subtalar joint alignment was compensatory valgus for varus knee deformity, but this compensatory function remains controversial in the valgus knee deformity (Table 1) [11, 12, 15]. On the other hand, the subtalar joint could compensate for early stage varus ankle OA, but not for end-stage varus ankle OA and valgus ankle OA [9, 17–19]. If the subtalar joint was destroyed, the subtalar joint compensation for deformity in the knee and ankle joints might not occur [15, 19]. Lee et al. [18] reported that patients with a well-preserved subtalar range of motion may better compensate varus ankle OA. These results may indicate that the destroyed subtalar joint was rigid and did not have enough joint movement to compensate for the deformity of the knee and ankle. Nakada et al. [15] assessed the subtalar compensatory alignment for the knee deformity in patients with RA. They found that the subtalar joint could compensate the knee deformity, and this compensation was stronger in patients with less damaged subtalar joints (Larsen grade≤ 3). The subtalar joint without severe destruction could compensate both the varus and valgus deformity of the knee in patients with RA. However, the destructed subtalar joint could not compensate the knee deformity and became varus or valgus synchronizing to the varus or valgus knee deformity.

Surgical procedures such as TKA or HTO for the varus knee OA could also improve the subtalar compensatory malalignment (Table 1) [7, 8, 11, 13, 14, 16]. In particular, greater improvements of hindfoot valgus occurred in patients with a severe varus deformity of the knee joint [14], and the variation of correction of varus knee alignment was significantly correlated with that of valgus subtalar alignment after TKA [7]. In contrast, Okamoto et al. [13] found that subtalar valgus did not improve in severe knee OA. However, they evaluated the subtalar alignment using calcaneal pitch and naviculocuboid overlap in a plane weight-bearing lateral foot radiograph. It was unclear whether these sagittal alignment parameters directly reflected the coronal subtalar joint varus or valgus alignment. Takenaka et al. [8] found that the subtalar joint alignment did not improve after TKA in the subtalar joint varus group. The preoperative subtalar joint varus could indicate that the subtalar joint lost the ability to compensate and result in rigid varus. Therefore, the subtalar joint remained varus after TKA. Although correction of varus knee OA could improve the subtalar valgus alignment, it was unclear whether correction of valgus knee OA could also influence the subtalar joint alignment. Further study is desirable to pursue these additional research gaps.

The influence of surgery for the ankle deformity to the subtalar joint was only evaluated in one study (Table 1) [16] and was quite unclear. They showed that the hindfoot alignment was varus in patients with advanced ankle OA and changed to valgus after LTO. Because the ability of subtalar joint compensation might be lost in advanced ankle OA [17, 18], hindfoot alignment became valgus after LTO, synchronizing to the correction of ankle alignment. Further assessments for change of the subtalar joint alignment at several stages of ankle OA after LTO, total ankle arthroplasty, and ankle arthrodesis could reveal the compensation mechanism of the subtalar joint.

TABLE 1: Review of studies which assessed the subtalar joint compensation for the knee or the ankle deformity.

	Total number	Reasons for deformation	Surgical procedure	Evaluation of subtalar alignment	Findings
Chandler et al. [10]	86	Varus and valgus knee OA	TKA	plane radiographs	The subtalar joint compensated the deformity of the knee. There was no correlation between the knee and subtalar joint alignment.
Mullaji et al. [11]	165	Varus and valgus knee OA	TKA	plane radiographs	The hindfoot valgus decreased after TKA. 87% of the subtalar joint continued to have valgus alignment even after TKA.
Norton et al. [12]	401	Varus and valgus knee OA	-	plane radiographs	Most of the compensation to angular deformity at the knee occurred in the subtalar joint. There was a correlation between knee and hindfoot deformities in patients with a larger knee deformity ($\geq 10^{\circ}$).
Takenaka et al. [8]	71	Varus knee OA	TKA	plane radiographs	The subtalar joint alignment improved 3 weeks after TKA in the subtalar joint valgus group, and further improvement was noted 1 year following TKA. The subtalar joint alignment did not improve after TKA in the subtalar joint varus group.
Okamoto et al. [13]	75	Varus knee OA	TKA	plane radiographs	Calcaneal pitch, naviculocuboid overlap and hindfoot pain with moderate varus deformity of knee ($\leq 6^{\circ}$ varus) improved after TKA, but those with severe varus deformity of knee ($> 6^{\circ}$) did not improve after TKA.
Cho et al. [14]	195	Varus knee OA	TKA	plane radiographs	Greater improvements of hindfoot valgus occurred in patients with a severe varus deformity of the knee joint ($\geq 10^{\circ}$) after TKA. There was no further improvement in hindfoot alignment between 6 weeks and 2 years post-operatively.

Table 1: Continued.

	Total number	Reasons for deformation	Surgical procedure	Evaluation of subtalar alignment	Findings
Jeong et al. [7]	375	Varus knee OA	TKA	plane radiographs	The variation of correction of varus knee alignment was significantly correlated with that of the valgus ankle and subtalar alignment after TKA.
Nakada et al. [15]	205	Knee RA with varus and valgus deformity	-	plane radiographs	Correlation exists between the knee and hindfoot alignments only in knees with a Larsen grade ≥ 4. This correlation was stronger in patients with less damaged subtalar joints (Larsen grade ≤ 3).
Choi et al. [16]	38 for HTO 46 for LTO	Varus knee and ankle OA	HTO and LTO	plane radiographs	Hindfoot alignment was valgus in patients with advanced arthritis of the knee, but mild hindfoot varus deviation was seen in patients with advanced arthritis of the ankle. Preoperative hindfoot valgus deviation was decreased after HTO, whereas the hindfoot alignment was changed to valgus deviation synchronizing to the ankle alignment after LTO.
Hayashi et al. [17]	133	Varus ankle OA	-	plane radiographs	The subtalar joint compensates varus deformity of the ankle at the intermediate stage ankle OA, but not at the end stage.
Lee et al. [18]	154	Varus ankle OA	-	plane radiographs	Hindfoot alignment was valgus in many ankles in stage II and IIIA, and the mean value was varus in stage IIIB and IV.
Wang et al. [19]	233	Varus and valgus ankle OA	-	plane radiographs	Compensation of the subtalar joint was identified in 39% of valgus ankle OA and 53% of varus ankle OA. The patients with no or mild degenerative changes of the subtalar joint may compensate the ankle malalignment
Krahenbuhl et al. [9]	88	Varus and valgus ankle OA	-	computed tomography	Compensation of the subtalar joint for the ankle deformity could only be verified for varus ankle osteoarthritis and not for valgus ankle osteoarthritis. Subtalar joint alignment had no influence on the stage of ankle osteoarthritis, extent of the tibiotalar tilt and stage of subtalar joint osteoarthritis.

OA: osteoarthritis, TKA: total knee arthroplasty, HTO: high tibial osteotomy, LTO: low tibial osteotomy

References

[1] Y. Tashiro, S. Matsuda, K. Okazaki, H. Mizu-uchi, U. Kuwashima, and Y. Iwamoto, "The coronal alignment after medial unicompartmental knee arthroplasty can be predicted: usefulness of full-length valgus stress radiography for evaluating correctability," *Knee Surgery, Sports Traumatology, Arthroscopy*, vol. 22, no. 12, pp. 3142–3149, 2014.

[2] J. De Muylder, J. Victor, O. Cornu, L. Kaminski, and E. Thienpont, "Total knee arthroplasty in patients with substantial deformities using primary knee components," *Knee Surgery, Sports Traumatology, Arthroscopy*, vol. 23, no. 12, pp. 3653–3659, 2015.

[3] S. Kawahara, S. Matsuda, K. Okazaki et al., "Relationship between the tibial anteroposterior axis and the surgical epicondylar axis in varus and valgus knees," *Knee Surgery, Sports Traumatology, Arthroscopy*, vol. 20, no. 10, pp. 2077–2081, 2012.

[4] J.-M. Guichet, A. Javed, J. Russell, and M. Saleh, "Effect of the foot on the mechanical alignment of the lower limbs," *Clinical Orthopaedics and Related Research*, vol. 415, pp. 193–201, 2003.

[5] M. L. Reilingh, L. Beimers, G. J. M. Tuijthof, S. A. S. Stufkens, M. Maas, and C. N. Van Dijk, "Measuring hindfoot alignment radiographically: The long axial view is more reliable than the hindfoot alignment view," *Skeletal Radiology*, vol. 39, no. 11, pp. 1103–1108, 2010.

[6] K. Ikoma, M. Noguchi, K. Nagasawa et al., "A new radiographic view of the hindfoot," *Journal of Foot and Ankle Research*, vol. 13, no. 6(1), article 48, 2013.

[7] B. O. Jeong, T. Y. Kim, J. H. Baek, H. Jung, and S. H. Song, "Following the correction of varus deformity of the knee through total knee arthroplasty, significant compensatory changes occur not only at the ankle and subtalar joint, but also at the foot," *Knee Surgery, Sports Traumatology, Arthroscopy*, vol. 26, no. 11, pp. 3230–3237, 2018.

[8] T. Takenaka, K. Ikoma, S. Ohashi et al., "Hindfoot alignment at one year after total knee arthroplasty," *Knee Surgery, Sports Traumatology, Arthroscopy*, vol. 24, no. 8, pp. 2442–2446, 2016.

[9] N. Krähenbühl, L. Siegler, M. Deforth, L. Zwicky, B. Hintermann, and M. Knupp, "Subtalar joint alignment in ankle osteoarthritis," *Journal of Foot and Ankle Surgery*, vol. S1268-7731(17)31298-5, 2017.

[10] J. T. Chandler and J. T. Moskal, "Evaluation of knee and hindfoot alignment before and after total knee arthroplasty: A prospective analysis," *The Journal of Arthroplasty*, vol. 19, no. 2, pp. 211–216, 2004.

[11] A. Mullaji and G. M. Shetty, "Persistent hindfoot valgus causes lateral deviation of weightbearing axis after total knee arthroplasty," *Clinical Orthopaedics and Related Research*, vol. 469, no. 4, pp. 1154–1160, 2011.

[12] A. A. Norton, J. J. Callaghan, A. Amendola et al., "Correlation of knee and hindfoot deformities in advanced knee OA: compensatory hindfoot alignment and where it occurs," *Clinical Orthopaedics and Related Research*, vol. 473, no. 1, pp. 166–174, 2015.

[13] Y. Okamoto, S. Otsuki, T. Jotoku, M. Nakajima, and M. Neo, "Clinical usefulness of hindfoot assessment for total knee arthroplasty: persistent post-operative hindfoot pain and alignment in pre-existing severe knee deformity," *Knee Surgery, Sports Traumatology, Arthroscopy*, vol. 25, pp. 2632–2639, 2017.

[14] W.-S. Cho, H.-S. Cho, and S.-E. Byun, "Changes in hindfoot alignment after total knee arthroplasty in knee osteoarthritic patients with varus deformity," *Knee Surgery, Sports Traumatology, Arthroscopy*, vol. 25, no. 11, pp. 3596–3604, 2017.

[15] I. Nakada, I. Nakamura, T. Juji, K. Ito, and T. Matsumoto, "Correlation between knee and hindfoot alignment in patients with rheumatoid arthritis: The effects of subtalar joint destruction," *Modern Rheumatology*, vol. 25, no. 5, pp. 689–693, 2015.

[16] J. Y. Choi, S. J. Song, S. J. Kim, S. H. Kim, J. S. Park, and J. S. Suh, "Changes in hindfoot alignment after high or low tibial osteotomy," *Foot & Ankle International*, vol. 39, pp. 1097–1105, 2018.

[17] K. Hayashi, Y. Tanaka, T. Kumai, K. Sugimoto, and Y. Takakura, "Correlation of compensatory alignment of the subtalar joint to the progression of primary osteoarthritis of the ankle," *Foot & Ankle International*, vol. 29, no. 4, pp. 400–406, 2008.

[18] W.-C. Lee, J.-S. Moon, H. S. Lee, and K. Lee, "Alignment of ankle and hindfoot in early stage ankle osteoarthritis," *Foot & Ankle International*, vol. 32, no. 7, pp. 693–699, 2011.

[19] B. Wang, C. L. Saltzman, O. Chalayon, and A. Barg, "Does the subtalar joint compensate for ankle malalignment in end-stage ankle arthritis?" *Clinical Orthopaedics and Related Research*, vol. 473, no. 1, pp. 318–325, 2015.

[20] S. S. Desai, G. M. Shetty, H.-R. Song, S. H. Lee, T. Y. Kim, and C. Y. Hur, "Effect of foot deformity on conventional mechanical axis deviation and ground mechanical axis deviation during single leg stance and two leg stance in genu varum," *The Knee*, vol. 14, no. 6, pp. 452–457, 2007.

[21] W. W. Strash and P. Berardo, "Radiographic assessment of the hindfoot and ankle," *Clinics in Podiatric Medicine and Surgery*, vol. 21, no. 3, pp. 295–304, 2004.

[22] H. J. Haight, D. L. Dahm, J. Smith, and D. A. Krause, "Measuring standing hindfoot alignment: Reliability of goniometric and visual measurements," *Archives of Physical Medicine and Rehabilitation*, vol. 86, no. 3, pp. 571–575, 2005.

[23] J. C. Cobey, "Posterior roentgenogram of the foot," *Clinical Orthopaedics and Related Research*, pp. 202–207, 1976.

[24] C. L. Saltzman and G. Y. El-Khoury, "The hindfoot alignment view," *Foot & Ankle International*, vol. 16, no. 9, pp. 572–576, 1995.

[25] B. M. Lamm, R. W. Mendicino, A. R. Catanzariti, and H. J. Hillstrom, "Static rearfoot alignment: A comparison of clinical and radiographic measures," *Journal of the American Podiatric Medical Association*, vol. 95, no. 1, pp. 26–33, 2005.

[26] S. E. Seltzer, B. N. Weissman, E. M. Braunstein, D. F. Adams, and W. H. Thomas, "Computed tomography of the hindfoot," *Journal of Computer Assisted Tomography*, vol. 8, no. 3, pp. 488–497, 1984.

[27] F. M. Buck, A. Hoffmann, N. Mamisch-Saupe, N. Espinosa, D. Resnick, and J. Hodler, "Hindfoot alignment measurements: Rotation-stability of measurement techniques on hindfoot alignment view and long axial view radiographs," *American Journal of Roentgenology*, vol. 197, no. 3, pp. 578–582, 2011.

[28] S. J. Ellis, T. Deyer, B. R. Williams et al., "Assessment of lateral hindfoot pain in acquired flatfoot deformity using weightbearing multiplanar imaging," *Foot & Ankle International*, vol. 31, no. 5, pp. 361–371, 2010.

[29] N. Krähenbühl, M. Tschuck, L. Bolliger, B. Hintermann, and M. Knupp, "Orientation of the subtalar joint: measurement and reliability using weightbearing CT scans," *Foot & Ankle International*, vol. 37, no. 1, pp. 109–114, 2016.

[30] Y. Takakura, Y. Tanaka, T. Kumai, and S. Tamai, "Low tibial osteotomy for osteoarthritis of the ankle. Results of a new

operation in 18 patients," *The Journal of Bone & Joint Surgery (British Volume)*, vol. 77, no. 1, pp. 50–54, 1995.

[31] Y. Hara, K. Ikoma, Y. Arai, S. Ohashi, M. Maki, and T. Kubo, "Alteration of hindfoot alignment after total knee arthroplasty using a novel hindfoot alignment view," *The Journal of Arthroplasty*, vol. 30, no. 1, pp. 126–129, 2015.

[32] K. W. Nha, S. H. Lee, I. J. Rhyu et al., "Safe zone for medial open-wedge supramalleolar osteotomy of the ankle: a cadaveric study," *Foot & Ankle International*, vol. 37, no. 1, pp. 102–108, 2016.

26

A Dynamic Model of Hip Joint Biomechanics: The Contribution of Soft Tissues

Joseph F. Fetto

The Brooklyn Hospital Medical Center, Brooklyn, NY 11201, USA

Correspondence should be addressed to Joseph F. Fetto; jfetto@tbh.org

Guest Editor: Nobuyoshi Watanabe

Before recent advances in computer modeling technology, it has been nearly impossible to define the contribution of soft tissue structures when constructing models of the body, and in particular the lower extremity. For almost 100 years, the design and fixation of femoral components for total hip arthroplasty (THA), whether cemented or press fit, have been predicated on the Koch model of hip biomechanics. A more comprehensive model, which includes the dynamic contribution of soft tissues, has expanded the Koch's static model. This new model has led to a more complete representation of reality and has become the basis for the inclusion of a new stem design element (a lateral flare), a new concept of implant fixation (rest fit), and consequent significant increase in bone preservation and implant stability.

1. Introduction

It has been long recognized that soft tissues, such as ligaments and muscle-tendon units, are important stabilizing structures of articulations. However, the exact magnitude and character of their contribution have been the subject of much controversy. Historically, paradoxes have been recognized in the articulations of the lower extremity which have dramatized this issue. For example, if osteoarthritis (OA) is considered to be a "wear and tear" process, the incidence of OA in the joints of the lower extremity should be proportional to load/unit area (L/A) over time. Since the hip, knee, and ankle are exposed to an identical number of cycles of load and carry approximately the same body mass, the relative incidence of OA in each of these articulations, over time, should be proportional to their relative size. However, it has been universally recognized that the knee, the largest of these articulations, is the most frequently undergoing arthroplasty; and the ankle appears, unless its architecture has been disrupted, virtually immune to OA over a lifetime of use. Implicit in this reality is the conclusion that OA is more than a L/A phenomenon.

In its most basic form OA is the consequence of compromise of the integrity of the surface layer of the articular cartilage. This leads to a loss of the unique hydrostatic, frictionless nature of intact articular movement. Stability of an articulation protects an articular surface from excessive frictional wear. As such the incidence of OA will be inversely proportional to the stability of a given articulation, with stability being provided by a combination of geometry and soft tissue stabilizers crossing a given joint.

In this manner, it is predictable that the incidence of OA occurring in the geometrically unstable knee joint consisting of two large round condyles of the distal femur resting on a flat tibial plateau knee joint will be greater over time than that in the very geometrically stable ankle, where the talus is keystoned into the mortise of the ankle.

In addition to bony geometry, articulations are also stabilized by the soft tissues crossing that joint. For each plane of movement, these soft tissue structures can be subdivided into couples composed of a static (ligamentous) component and a dynamic (muscle-tendon) component. In this fashion it is apparent that the knee is much more dependent upon soft tissues for stability than is the ankle. It further explains why the relatively smaller ankle becomes so rapidly compromised and arthritic following unrepaired disruption of the syndesmosis ligament.

This importance of soft tissue stabilizers and their consequence for the loading of the lower extremity articulations have been of great consequence in the understanding and treatment of many conditions of the hip joint. In 1917, John Koch published his model of hip biomechanics [1]. It was to become accepted as the definitive model of the hip and lower extremity, for the next century. This model became the basis for the design of femoral implants employed in millions of hip arthroplasty surgeries performed around the world. Although intuitively attractive, this static model was plagued with many internal contractions and paradoxes.

It correctly assumed that the body's center of gravity (COG) was located in the midline of the body, 1 cm anterior to the first sacral segment. From this point the effect of gravity on the lower extremity was represented by a vertically oriented, downward directed vector. From these assumptions, it was proposed that during *unilateral stance* the weight of the body (B) would create both a compressive and varus load on points along the entire lower extremity. It further suggested that the magnitude of this varus deforming force acting at any point along the lower extremity could be calculated by multiplying the vector force created by gravity (body's weight) by its perpendicular medial displacement from that point along the lower limb (b), or B x b. It further hypothesized that this destabilizing torque must be counterbalanced by an equally strong valgus torque in order to maintain a stable equilibrium state during the gait cycle.

When Koch applied this analysis to the hip joint, he assumed the counterbalancing valgus torque would be supplied by isometric contraction of an abductor muscle (A), specifically the gluteus medius. He further assumed that the average length of the body's lever arm (b) from the center of the hip's rotation was approximately twice that of the length of the abductor's insertion on the lateral aspect of the greater trochanter to the center of hip rotation (a), b = 2a.

From these assumptions, Koch wrote the equation for hip stability as B x b = A x a. And since b = 2a, he concluded that the gluteus medius must generate twice the weight of the body force, 2 x B, in order to maintain a stable equilibrium during unilateral stance. (Figure 1).

However, a more critical examination of Koch's assumptions must be undertaken before accepting his model as an accurate depiction of reality and in particular events occurring during gait.

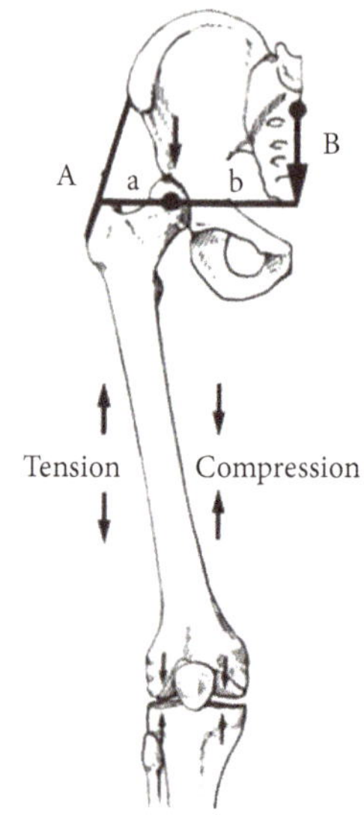

FIGURE 1: The Koch model of hip biomechanics (1) is static cadaveric model, (2) demonstrates his hypothesis of hip loading, and (3) requires the gluteus medius to exert a force twice that of the body's weight in order to maintain equilibrium during single stance.

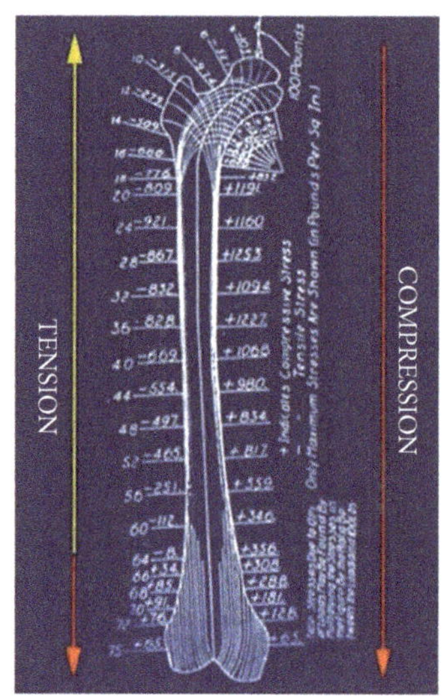

FIGURE 2: Koch's "quantification" of forces within the femur [1]. According to the Koch Model, during unilateral stance, (1) most of the lateral cortex experiences tensile loading and (2) the distal 1/3 of the lateral cortex and entire medial cortex experiences compression.

2. History of Hip Biomechanics

To begin with, Koch's model is static, unlike the conditions that occur during gait, where the body's center of gravity usually remains medial to the supporting foot in a dynamic equilibrium. Secondly, Koch limits the source of resistance to the body's varus load to a single structure, the gluteus medius. These two factors have dramatic consequences for conclusions drawn from the Koch model. The most important of them is the conclusion that, below the insertion point of the gluteus medius, the entire lateral aspect of the lower extremity experiences a tensile load. Koch went so far, in his original article, as to attempting to qualify the loads experienced by the femur during unilateral support. He used positive integers to represent compressive forces and negative integers to designate areas of tensile loading (Figure 2). Intuitively, it can be understood that he labeled the entire medial aspect of the femur as experiencing compressive loading. However, curiously he does not explain how the lateral femur experiences tension along its lateral proximal 2/3's but coverts to compression along the lateral distal 1/3 of its length. It may be assumed that Koch was attempting to keep his model consistent with the reality, and contemporary belief, that there is compression within the lateral compartment of the knee. It was believed, at that time, to be the explanation for the presence of a lateral meniscus within the knee's

TABLE 1: Importance of an intact ITB to amputee function.

	Iliotibial band	Gluteus medius	Trendelenburg sign	Energy expenditure
BKA	Intact	+	–	−10%
AKA	Transected	+	+	−40 ~ −70%

lateral compartment. An element intended to buttress against compressive loading.

The static model raised additional paradoxes. For example, at birth the neck-shaft angle of the femur is similar to that of a quadruped, approximately 160-165 degrees. As one assumes, in bipedal gait, by the age of four, the neck-shaft angle reduces to its final value of 130-135 degrees and remains so throughout the remainder of a lifetime. This has been explained as being the result of the upright posture placing a varus load on the young plastic bone. However it is interesting, that in spite of significant time spent in an upright posture and with increasing body mass, the femoral neck-shaft angle remains relatively unchanged throughout the remainder of growth and development of the femur.

It is further interesting to note that in neuromuscular conditions involving spasticity, the valgus deformity of the femoral neck is often corrected with a varus osteotomy. However, if insufficient soft tissue releases are performed at the time of the osteotomy, the valgus deformity will reoccur over time in spite of bipedal stance.

Another paradox of the Koch model occurs among lower extremity amputees. It has been found that below knee amputees (BKA) do not usually exhibit a positive Trendelenburg gait pattern. They only lose about 10% of their metabolic efficiency and with today's technological and material advancements can function at near normal levels of performance, while above knee amputees always exhibit a positive Trendelenburg gait pattern and lose 40-70% of their metabolic efficiency. Yet both the BKA and the AKA have intact abductor, gluteus medius, and musculature. The question is an obvious one. What is lost in an AKA that creates such a significant compromise of the gluteus medius' ability to provide stability against the varus load of the body during gait? (Table 1)

These clinical paradoxes suggest an explanation for why femoral components whose designs are based on the static, flawed, or at least incomplete Koch model of hip loading have provided unintended consequences. They have been plagued with outcomes which have included loss of proximal femoral bone mass termed "stress shielding"; diaphyseal hypertrophy; thigh pain; subsidence due to "poor bone quality"; loosening; and fracture on insertion.

Bone, as all connective tissues, responds to its environment. It hypertrophies and atrophies in response to demand. Also, the quality of bone reflects the type of load it experiences: cortical bone appears in areas of compression and cancellous bone in areas of tensile loading, i.e., apophyses and points of tendon attachment. It would appear that, rather than "reconstruct" damaged hip anatomy, femoral component designs and various methods for their fixation, based on the Koch model, have created nonphysiologic patterns of loading within the femur following hip replacement surgery (Figures 3(a) and 3(b)).

Over the past 150 years, there have been many theories proposed as models of hip biomechanics [2–7]. In efforts to avoid the paradoxes raised by the Koch model, each proposed the inclusion of additional structures to complement and supplement the action of the gluteus medius. However, due to a lack of the necessary means of investigation to prove their theory, all of these alternative models have been unable to displace the accepted model of Koch. This situation changed in the later 20th and early 21st century with the introduction of technological advances such as electromyograhic (EMG) studies, Finite Element Analysis (FEA), and radiologic techniques such as radio-stereotactic analysis (RSA) and DEXA analysis of bone density.

Electromyographic studies of Inman [8] directly challenged the conclusion of the Koch model. He demonstrated that the gluteus medius was most active just before and just after the midstance phase of gait. This implied that some additional factor was acting at midstance phase of gait to reduce the demand on the abductor musculature. The question was, How is this accomplished and what structure(s) is responsible?

3. Articular Cartilage

Unrelated was the observation that although the knee, hip, and ankle joint go through an equal number of load cycles throughout life and carry a similar load, it remains a fact that the smallest of these joints, the ankle, appears to be the most resistant to mechanical wear and development of osteoarthrosis requiring replacement. An explanation for this phenomenon can be deduced from an understanding of the ultrastructure of articular cartilage.

Articular cartilage is the soft covering at the end of bones and is present in all joints. It is the product of chondrocytes and is an avascular tissue, dependent upon the passive and active diffusion of nutrients and water through a porous surface layer. Chondrocytes produce two critical components of articular cartilage. They are collagen and proteoglycan. Collagen fibers are formed by long linear cross-linked triple helix molecules, specifically designed to resist tensile loading. It is paradoxical that they would be crucial to the integrity of articular cartilage, which is specifically intended to function in a compression environment. The key to the understanding of this paradox is the orientation of the collagen fibers within the cartilage cap. They are parallel at the surface forming a "skin" and dive from the surface into the hyaline cartilage to anchor themselves perpendicularly into the subchondral bone. As such they form an arcade in which the fibers have a

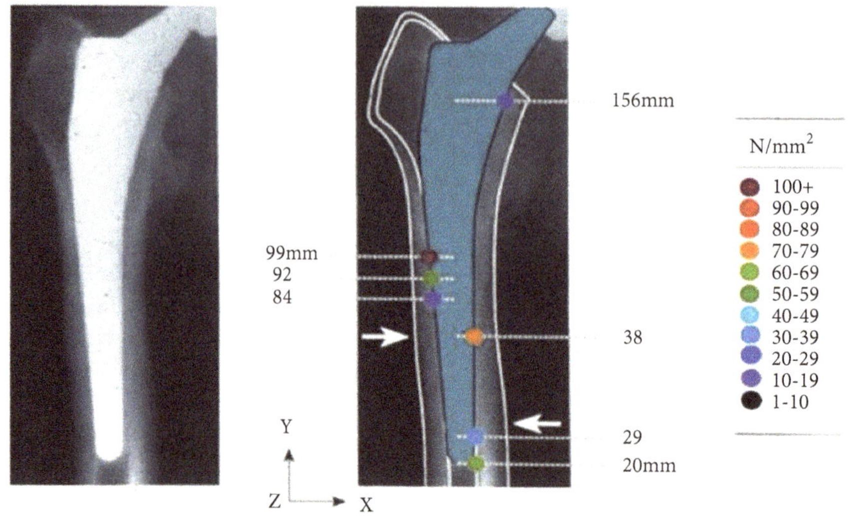

(a) Traditional press fit loading of the femur showing diaphyseal hypertrophy and proximal stress shielding

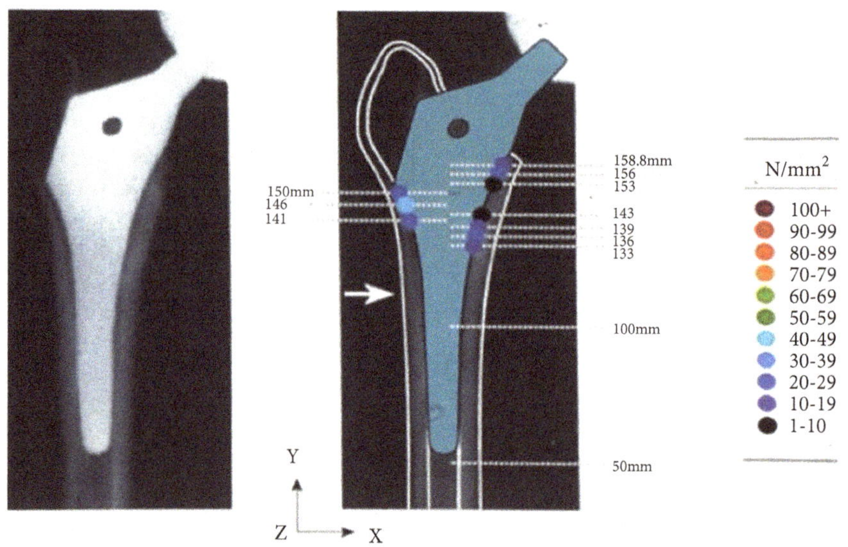

(b) Proximal femoral loading with a stem design based on the dynamic model of the hip showing bone preservation and no abnormal diaphyseal bone formation

FIGURE 3: 2-year stress distribution within the femur as a consequence of stem design.

specified orientation. Their orientation is such that as water is drawn into the cartilage tissue by the hydrophilic nature of the proteoglycan molecules, the surface layer of the cartilage structure is tethered to the subchondral bone by the collagen fibers, as it is pushed outward analogous to that of the surface of a stuffed pillow. The integrity of this structure then allows, when a compressive load is applied, water to exude from the cartilage to create a frictionless hydrostatic bearing between the surfaces of any joint. Thus, unless anything occurs to compromise the integrity of the hyaline cartilage surface layer, the cartilage cap is virtually immune to wear over time. From this description it is easy to understand how the demise of articular cartilage and resultant arthrosis can come about: proteolytic enzymatic action from bacteria of synovial inflammation; macrotrauma such as fracture; metabolic abnormalities affecting collagen or proteoglycan synthesis such as vitamin C deficiency and mucopolysaccharidoses; or most importantly microtrauma caused by excessive frictional wear. This last causative etiology is the direct result of joint instability.

Joint stability is a function of two factors: articular geometry and soft tissue integrity. In terms of geometry, it is easy to describe the three major joints of the lower extremity as being either inherently geometrically stable or unstable. The ankle, although the smallest of these three joints, has an extremely stable mortise structure with very limited degrees of freedom, particularly in the dorsiflexed position during weight bearing. As such it suffers minimal frictional wear throughout a lifetime unless the integrity of the mortise is compromised by either a fracture or more subtly disruption of the syndesmosis ligament. In either event, translational movement increases across the articular surfaces and demise of the ankle is rapid. With regard to soft tissues contributing to the stability of a joint, they can be divided into static and dynamic structures. Each plane of movement is stabilized by a couple comprised of a dynamic and a static entity. The dynamic structure is a muscle-tendon unit and the static stabilizer is a ligament. Muscles can adjust their length in response to demand. Ligaments however cannot. Hence since ligaments are critically important at extremes of motion and are lax at mid-range, all ligaments are composed of two parts: one taut in extension, the reciprocal part taut in flexion.

Because joint stability is critical to the preservation of the integrity and functionality of articular cartilage, and the knee joint is an inherently geometrically unstable articulation, it is easy therefore to understand and predict the knee's greater susceptibility to becoming arthritic over time.

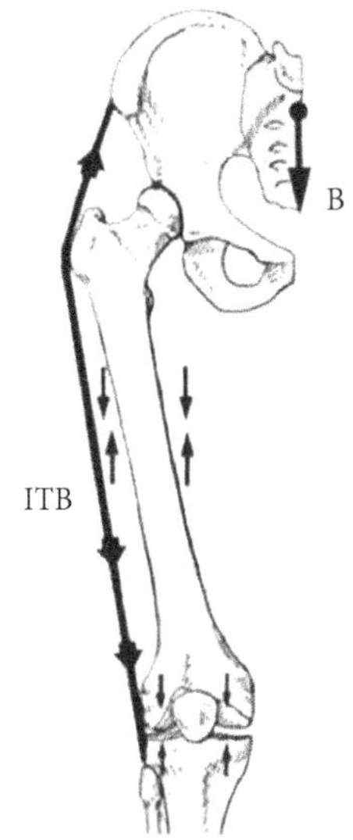

FIGURE 4: Compression band effect of the ITB. As a "tension band" lateral to the femur, the ITB neutralizes tensile loads and creates compression loading along the lateral aspect of the femur during unilateral stance phase of gait. This explains the presence and distribution of cortical bone in the lateral femur and is consistent with Wolff's Law.

4. The ITB Dynamic Tension Band Effect on the Hip Joint Biomechanics

Applying this type of analysis to the hip joint, it is possible to characterize the hip as being more geometrically stable than the knee but less so than the ankle. This is particularly true in the sagittal plane. In this plane the geometry of the hip provides no resistance against the varus deforming force which occurs during midstance phase of gait. The hip therefore must rely on a dynamic stabilizer such as the gluteus medius and some static stabilizer as well in order to maintain equilibrium at this phase of the gait cycle.

Cadaveric studies, in which a weight was suspended from the midline of the sacrum while soft tissue structures were divided into various combinations and permutations, demonstrated that the iliotibial band (ITB) is that static stabilizer of the hip against varus loads [9].

From this observation, it was concluded that the ITB should be included in the analysis of hip biomechanics to produce a more complete, dynamic, and accurate model of hip stability. The inclusion of the ITB served to resolve many of the paradoxes raised by the previous static model. It resolved the seeming contradiction of the gluteus medius being less active at the midstance phase of gait. At that point of the gait cycle the ITB apparently serves as a tension band to relieve the metabolic demand and reduce electrical activity of the gluteus medius (Figure 4). It also provides an explanation for the poorer functioning of an AKA relative to that of a BKA, where loss of the distal attachment of the ITB in an AKA compromises the function of the ITB as a static stabilizer of the hip joint. It further gives rationale to the surgical technique of tenodesis of the ITB and lateral soft tissue structures to the distal femur in the performance of an above-the-knee amputation. This would be similar to the technique of wrapping the posterior calf musculature around the distal end of a below-the-knee amputation.

This more dynamic model, which includes the ITB as a tension band, provides an explanation for the presence of cortical bone along the lateral aspect of the femur as being a predictable consequence of compression loading (Figure 4). Extending this concept to the knee, it is also possible to predict the actual relative magnitudes of compressive loads in the medial and lateral compartments of that joint, which are 60% and 40%, respectively. Similarly, it explains, as Wolff's Law [9] predicts, the relative growth and dimensions of the medial and lateral femoral condyles being the consequence of the lateral stabilizing and tension band effect of the ITB, LCL, biceps femoris, and popliteus creating gradually increasing compressive loads across the distal femoral growth plate.

5. Femoral Component Design

Returning to femoral component design, it becomes possible, with this expansion of the Koch model to a dynamic model of the hip, to explain the shortcomings of component designs predicated on the 1917 model. Those previous designs treated the femur as a static element. Their placement and stability were analogous to that of a nail in a piece of wood, with the stability of the implant depending on a combination of friction and hoop-stress displacement. Their survival is totally dependent upon the quality of the host bone into which the component is being "pressed". The risk was for subsidence with the choice of an undersized component, insertion into "poor quality bone", or femoral fracture on insertion due to excessive force.

In contrast to traditional means of achieving implant stability whether cemented or noncemented, the dynamic ITB model suggests an alternative method of achieving long term implant survival and superior outcomes for THR. The dynamic ITB model predicts that the lateral femur distal to the greater trochanter experiences compressive loading. Therefore it becomes reasonable to utilize the lateral

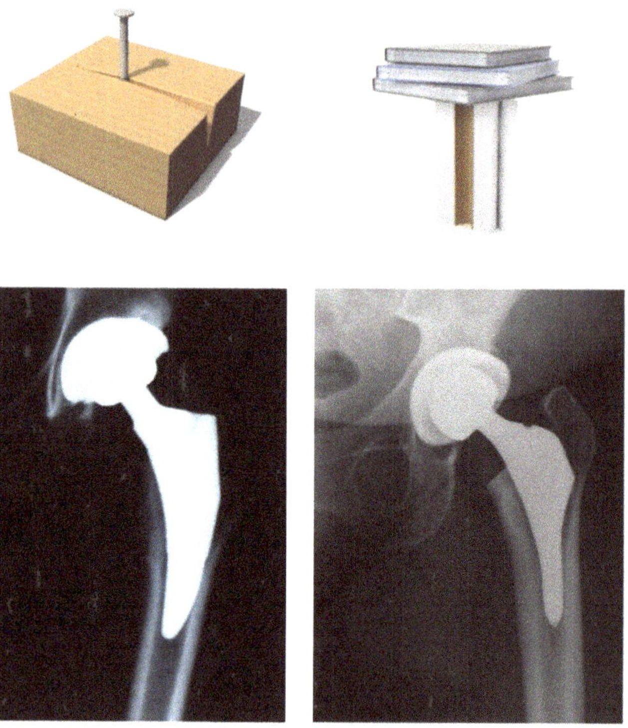

(a) (b)

FIGURE 5: Press fit (a) vs rest fit (b).

endosteal surface of the proximal femur as an additional area to support the femoral component. In this way the entire circumference of the femur would be utilized as a pedestal upon which the body, as well as a femoral component, will be supported. The requirement for the design of a femoral component to achieve this "rest fit" would be to extend the lateral dimension of the component so as to engage the endosteal surface of the femur in the region of Gruen zone 1. This lateral expansion, or "lateral flare", would create an internal collar which would provide the means to transfer load to the entire proximal perimeter of the femur (Gruen zones 1 and 7). As such the component could rest on the entire femur, distributing load both medially and laterally in a more physiologic fashion (Figure 5). This design concept predicts the means to preserve proximal bone stock and avoid transfer of nonphysiologic loading into more distal Gruen zones 2,3,4,5, and 6. It also negates the belief that a long stem design element is required to achieve fixation. Rather the stem portion of a component could simply serve as an alignment device and not a load bearing structure. It would also predict that stem length may be safely reduced without compromising stability or longevity of the construct.

6. Merit of the Lateral Flare and Rest Fit Fixation

The validity of these predictions was evaluated by several means: FEA, in vitro laboratory testing, and finally prospective DEXA and subsidence clinical studies. These published results have shown that, unlike prior stem designs which demonstrate stress shielding, diaphyseal hypertrophy, thigh pain, subsidence, and occasional fracture on insertion, the "lateral flare" stem design has minimized these adverse outcomes. Lateral flare stems have demonstrated preservation of >95% bone stock in proximal Gruen zones 1 and 7; less than 0.5 mm subsidence; no fracture on insertion of the stem when employing a "rest fit" rather than press fit insertion technique; and no thigh pain [10–13].

7. Conclusion

In conclusion, over the past 30 years the application of recent technological advances through laboratory and clinical investigations has led to an expansion of the static Koch model of 1917 to create a more accurate and complete understanding of hip biomechanics. This has produced a more valid dynamic model of the hip. The consequences of this expansion has led to a better explanation of the growth and development of the femur, the functional differences between BKA and AKA patients, suggestions for improved surgical techniques in various clinical situations, and the addition of an important design element to femoral components, specifically the "lateral flare". More importantly this new understanding of hip biomechanics has advanced femoral fixation from a static "nail in a piece of wood" press fit technique to an improved means of femoral fixation termed a "rest fit", which has demonstrated improved outcomes in total hip arthroplasty.

References

[1] J. C. Koch, "The laws of bone architecture," *American Journal of Anatomy*, vol. 21, no. 2, pp. 177–298, 1917.

[2] J. H. Maissiat, "Etude de physique animale," Tech. Rep., Bethune et Plon, Paris, France, 1843.

[3] W. Oberlander, ""Spontaneous" fracture of the femur following damage to the ilio-tibial tract," *Zeitschrift für Orthopädie und ihre Grenzgebiete*, vol. 113, pp. 46–51, 1975.

[4] F. Pauwels, *Biomechanics of the Normal and Diseased Hip: Theoretical Foundation, Technique and Results of Treatment: An Atlas*, Springer, New York, NY, USA, 1976.

[5] E. F. Rybicki, F. A. Simonen, and E. B. Weis Jr., "On the mathematical analysis of stress in the human femur," *Journal of Biomechanics*, vol. 5, no. 2, pp. 203–215, 1972.

[6] F. G. St Clair strange, *The Hip*, Heinemann, London, UK, 1965.

[7] W. Thomsen, "Zur static and mechanic der gesunden und geluntenhuffe: uber die bedeutung des tractus ilio-tibialis," *Zeitschrift für Orthopädie und ihre Grenzgebiete*, vol. 80, p. 41, 1934.

[8] V. T. Inman, "Functional aspects of the abductor muscles of the hip," *The Journal of Bone & Joint Surgery*, vol. 29, no. 3, pp. 607–619, 1947.

[9] J. Wolff, *The Law of Bone Remodeling*, Springer, New York, NY, USA, 1986.

[10] A. Leali, J. Fetto, H. Insler, and D. Elfenbein, "The effect of a lateral flare feature on implant stability," *International Orthopaedics*, vol. 26, no. 3, pp. 166–169, 2002.

[11] A. Leali and J. F. Fetto, "Preservation of femoral bone mass after total hip replacements with a lateral flare stem," *International Orthopaedics*, vol. 28, no. 3, pp. 151–154, 2004.

[12] A. Leali and J. Fetto, "Promising mid-term results of total hip arthroplasties using an uncemented lateral-flare hip prosthesis: a clinical and radiographic study," *International Orthopaedics (SICOT)*, vol. 31, no. 6, pp. 845–849, 2006.

[13] A. Leali, J. Fetto, and H. Insler, "Favorable mid-term results of total hip arthoplasties with a lateral flare uncemented stem," *Clinical Orthopaedics and Related Research*, vol. 11, pp. 2–7, 2006.

27

Proximal Humerus Reconstruction after Tumor Resection: An Overview of Surgical Management

Antonio D'Arienzo, Edoardo Ipponi, Alfio Damiano Ruinato, Silvia De Franco, Simone Colangeli, Lorenzo Andreani, and Rodolfo Capanna

Department of Orthopaedic and Trauma Surgery, University of Pisa, Pisa, Italy

Correspondence should be addressed to Edoardo Ipponi; edward.ippo@gmail.com

Academic Editor: Francesco Liuzza

Proximal humerus is one of the anatomical sites that are most frequently involved by bone and soft tissue malignant tumors. Alone or in association with adjuvant treatments, surgery represents the main therapeutic option to treat and eradicate these diseases. Once the first-line option, in the last decades, amputation lost its role as treatment of choice for the large majority of cases in favor of the modern limb sparing surgery that promises to preserve anatomy and—as much as possible—upper limb functionality. Currently, the main approaches used to replace proximal humerus after a wide resection in oncologic surgery can be summarized in biological reconstructions (allografts and autografts), prosthetic reconstructions (anatomic endoprostheses, total reverse shoulder prostheses), and graft-prosthetic composite reconstructions. The purpose of this overview is to present nowadays surgical options for proximal humerus reconstruction in oncological patients, with their respective advantages and disadvantages.

1. Introduction

Proximal humerus is the fourth most common localization for primary bone tumors, the first between the bones of the upper limb, representing the site of 10%–15% among all osteosarcomas and 10% among Ewing sarcomas [1, 2]. In addition, humerus is the second bone for metastatic involvement [3]. Shoulder as a whole is also the third anatomical site for incidence of soft tissue sarcomas in mankind, with deltoid muscle and supraspinatus fossa to be the most frequently involved sites [4, 5].

The combined incidence of bone and soft tissue sarcomas of the shoulder is about 0.25 per 100000 individuals [5, 6].

Surgical approach to tumors of the proximal humerus, just as much as the neoplasms involving other areas of the musculoskeletal system, requires preoperative work-up; shoulder function, neurological and vascular status, alongside with patient's general health must be accurately assessed.

If once amputations and arthrodesis were considered the approach of choice after massive resections, through the decades, the progress of modern surgery provided new and better opportunities to orthopaedic oncologists. Advances in oncology, imaging, and surgical technologies led the way to safer and more accurate resections, increasing the chances to achieve free-of-disease surgical margins and therefore making local recurrence a less frequent event in the postoperative phase. The reconstructive phase likewise saw the flourishing of several different approaches to restore—as much as possible—the preexisting shape and functionality of the shoulder. Osteoarticular allografts, bone autografts, prostheses, and graft-prothesis composites represent the current treatment of choice for proximal humerus reconstruction. All the aforementioned solutions guarantee the static repair of the shoulder in association with atleast partial restoration of its articularity. Overall, the objectives of oncological surgery for the treatment of proximal humerus neoplasms can be resumed in (a) removal of the tumoral mass with wide margins in order to reduce the risk of local recurrence, (b) limb sparing, and (c) restitution of the arm's length and shape in association with a shoulder mobility that could allow restitution of patient's activities of daily living, all making sure to maintain low the risk of local or systemic complications [7–18].

So far, consensus about the best reconstructive technique is far from being established [19–22]. The most suitable approach can vary depending on patients' age, clinical picture (considering comorbidities as well as life expectancy), functional demands, and the eventual sacrifice of rotators cuff, deltoid muscle, or axillary nerve through the procedure [22–28].

The aim of our study is to review the surgical management of tumors affecting the proximal humerus and evaluate the correct indications for every reconstructive option, in consideration of their advantages and disadvantages.

2. Options for Surgical Reconstruction

Upper limb sparing surgery often needs wide bone and soft tissue resections in order to achieve wide disease-free surgical margins. The tissue loss, if not treated properly, could impair both the shoulder and the arm from a static and a dynamic point of view. Arm's length and shape, as well as the articular ROM (range of motion) of the shoulder, are crucial for the functionality of the upper limb, which in turn is pivotal to restore patients' autonomy and therefore increase their postoperative quality of life.

According to the most recent advances in orthopaedic oncology, reconstruction of the proximal humerus can be performed with—among the others—autografts, allografts, implanted prostheses, or prosthetic-biological composites [13, 18, 23, 24, 28–35].

Despite the increasing interest on the topic and the spread of reports in literature, the choice between the various approaches to reconstruct proximal humerus remains controversial, with studies that come down for or against the various options available at the moment [9, 16, 35–37].

In the following sections, we are going to expose different reconstructive techniques, evaluating their pros and cons in association with their functional results and complications rate, all to offer the readers a state-of-the-art overview about the modern surgical opportunities to recreate functional proximal humerus after wide resection.

2.1. Graft Reconstructions. Homologous and heterologous transplants of bone tissue as a concept have its roots at the dawn of civilization. In the Old Testament, Adam's rib is used to create Eve, while in the Greek mythology, Haephestus manufactures an ivory shoulder for Tantalus' son, Pelops [38]. However, it was not until the 1970s, with the evolution in cooling techniques and a detailed comprehension of the pivotal role played by vascularization that allografts and autografts established themselves as reliable reconstructive options in orthopaedic surgery.

To this date, the use of both allografts and autografts as reconstructive options after the resection of proximal humerus has been largely described in literature. Although the results are often encouraging, it is important to point their advantages and the disadvantages, in order to make sure they represent the best therapeutic option for the single patient.

2.1.1. Allografts. In particular, young and active patients with few comorbidities are the most suited to be treated with an allograft; their long life expectancy, in association with good healing capacities, justify the use of bone grafts considering the high chances of osteointegration as well as the possibility to provide them a life-long restoration of the shoulder [39]. Unlike prosthesis, grafts do not have default duration, and if the treatment is successful, revision surgery might not be necessary even after decades. Mourikis et al. in 2007 had an implant survival rate of 67% 16 years after surgery [40]. Aponte-Tinao et al. in 2013 reported a rate of 65% after 10 years [32].

Graft functionality often gets better as the years go by, and osteointegration is perfected, as opposed to prosthetic reconstructions that undergo unavoidable wear after many years of use. Prosthesis are also burdened by the risk of dislocation [13, 30, 41–47], aseptic loosening [29, 48, 49], and infection [48], a threat that in grafts is partially mitigated by the presence in loco of the patient's immune system and the absence of large metal segments ideal for the deposit of bacteria's biofilm [50].

Another intraoperative advantage in favor of allografts is attributable to the fact that modern cryoconservation technologies allow maintaining viable articular chondrocytes, so that the graft articular surface may include a living chondral surface for the reconstructed shoulder joint, providing a lower risk of postoperative osteoarthrosis [9, 10]. Finally, grafts can ensure sites for the reattachment of rotator cuff, deltoid, and pectoralis muscles respecting patient's own anatomy in a fashion that could never be performed with prosthesis [26]. For these reasons, in many cases, allograft reconstruction is a valid option and can represent the first choice of treatment [23, 28, 30, 40, 51–55].

On the other hand, allografts are not exempt from defects. Their use presupposes a rapid and successful colonization of atleast a part of the bone scaffold by the living cells of the receiving patient; in case it does not happen, the whole procedure would be destined to failure. Such an eventuality is more likely to happen in patients with advanced age, metabolic, or neurovascular disorders (such as type 2 diabetes); all factors negatively affect patient's healing capacity. In oncologic patients such as the ones subject of our discussion, pre and postoperative treatment with local radiotherapy or even systemic chemotherapy may also represent an obstacle to a proper osteointegration [38, 39]. Inhibition and death of the cells that surround the graft, alongside with alterations of the local homeostatic balance, make the allograft colonization harder to achieve and even more complicated, in case of postoperative irradiation which would make the implanted bone scaffold even less suitable for eventual settlers. Another concern associated with the use of allografts is their relatively high risk of postoperative complications. Unfortunately, the use of osteoarticular allografts has been often associated with high rates of local complications such as chondrolysis, subchondral collapse, and implant fractures [9, 13, 18, 23, 24, 28–35, 40, 51, 54, 55]. These adverse events often require revision surgery, leading to a significant decrease in terms of implant [30]. Aponte-Tinao et al. [32], albeit praising the good overall results of this technique, described among their shoulder graft reconstructions a risk of failure that amounted to 23%. Comparable rates were shown also by DeGroot et al. (22%) [51], Jamshidi et al. (22%) [52], and Ogink et al. (23%) [53]; others had even higher rates, such as Mourikis et al. (33%) [40], Yao et al. (38%) [54], or Potter et al. (29%) [30]. Potter et al. pointed an overall success lower than the ones achieved by the same authors using other reconstructive approaches. In fact, allografts, compared to endoprostheses and allograft-prosthetic composites, had more complications and required almost twice as much reinterventions. Potter, as well as van de Sande et al. [23], therefore preferred other methods to allografts precisely as a consequence of their lower complication rate. Other studies such as the one by Rödl et al. [28], for their part, showed complication rates remarkably lower (Table 1).

Implant fractures are among the most feared major complications that might occur after graft surgery (8–53%), being one of the main reasons for its failures [23, 28, 30, 40, 54]. In their population, Bus et al. [56] found that proximal humerus implants in particular had a significantly higher incidence of fractures compared to other anatomical districts. Literature suggests that the addition of cement inside the graft's intramedullary canal might be a strategy to prevent this eventuality. DeGroot et al. [51] and Jamshidi et al. [52] indicated how cement-augmented allografts seem to be associated with a lower rate of diaphysal and metaphysal fractures in comparison to nonaugmented allografts. This strategy could theoretically be an effective and inexpensive solution to decrease both the risk of fractures and infections, although operators should always keep in mind the risks associated with the use of PMMA [57].

Literature reports postoperative functional (MSTS) scores that range between 21.3 and 25.5 as represented in Table 1. Rödl et al. [28] obtained a mean MSTS score of 22.2, a solid value, but nevertheless lower than the ones boasted by prostheses (23.7) and autografts (24.6). Potter et al. [30] treated 17 patients with osteoarticular allografts getting a mean MSTS score of 21.3, a result that was slightly better than the one of endoprostheses (20.7) but worse than the APC's group (23.7).

2.1.2. Autografts. Autologous bone grafting involves bone segments obtained from the patient himself in donor sites that can be near or far from the recipient one. Bone tissue can be picked up from nonessential bones, whose sacrifice would not cause major repercussions on patient's quality of life. Among these, not only fibula is most frequently used and described in literature but also other donor sites can be used for the purpose, such as ribs or the neighboring scapula and clavicle [14, 27–29, 58–70].

Harvested bones require continuous blood supply to survive in the receiving area. Their vascularization must thus be preserved, if the donor site is adjacent to the shoulder, or restored anastomosing the vascular peduncle of the graft with local vessels, if the tissue is taken from a far region.

In comparison to allografts, autografts do not only serve as a scaffold that receives the nearby osteoblasts (osteoconduction) but also have a greater tendency to stimulate the osteoprogenitor cells of the nearby tissues to differentiate into osteoblasts and begin new bone formation (osteoinduction).

Moreover, consisting in vital and metabolically active bone tissue, autologous grafts bring their own osteogenesis potential to the receiving site, giving their contribution to the local bone growth and postoperative healing. This is supposed to translate in better fusion rates, mechanical strength, and infection resistance.

These factors theoretically mean that allografts have the best osteointegrative potential among the other reconstructive approaches available today and may represent the treatment of choice especially for young patients with long life expectancy [71–75]. Patients still in the process of growing, in particular, could benefit from the inclusion of an open growth plate inside the implant, allowing graft's growth in length and miming the structural evolution of the native bone in the following years [76–78]. Another positive factor is the fact that, since the donor and the receiving patient are the same individual, there is no risk of graft-versus-host-disease.

At the same time, however, this approach is not free of disadvantages. The stock of bones suitable to replace proximal humerus in terms of size and shape is limited, and their removal always deprives the donor site of one of its natural elements [78]. In practice, in order to harvest, an allograft is necessary to extend the surgical access (if the graft is taken close to the receiving site) or even to create a second access centered on the bone of choice; in either case, the result is lengthening of surgical time, with consequential increasement in blood loss and higher complications risk also due to anesthetic procedures [28]. Unlike allografts, it is also hard to obtain a vascularized bone graft provided with an articular surface covered with living chondral tissue, which would represent an advantage to restore properly the distal side of shoulder articulation. For these reasons, autografts are at times considered unattractive to reconstruct proximal humerus after major resections.

We report a summary of the autograft techniques mostly described in literature as follows.

(1) Free Vascularized Fibula Graft (FVFG). Fibula is one of the most suitable donor bones to replace proximal humerus. Free vascularized fibular graft (FVFG) was first described in 1975 by Taylor et al. [79] and since that moment emerged as a reliable option for a large variety of reconstructions, including large defects of the upper and lower extremities. Its popularity can be attributed to the fibula's favorable anatomy, being long and straight, providing up to 26 cm of bone and having a dependable dual endosteal and periosteal blood supply [80]. These features make the FVFG particularly suitable to replace long bones such as humerus, even after a wide resection. Relatively low donor site morbidity was

Table 1: Summary data for allograft studies.

Study	Resection (cm)	Reconstruction	N	Age (y)	F-U (m)	Hardware issues	Graft resorptions	Fractures	Infections	PSA	Failures	MSTS score
DeGroot et al. [51]	12	Osteoarticular allograft	32	30	64	3% (1)	0	37% (11)	1	16% (5)	22% (7)	22.4
Jamshidi et al. [52]	15	Osteoarticular allograft	32	27	46	0	11% (4)	8% (3)	8% (3)	6% (2)	22% (8)	25.5
Mourikis et al. [40]	—	Osteoarticular allograft	32	42*	192*	0	0	19% (6)	13% (4)	16% (5)	33% (10)	—
Ogink et al. [53]	14	Osteoarticular allograft	32	47	—	6% (3)	2% (1)	28% (13)	4% (2)	13% (6)	23% (11)	—
Potter et al. [30]	15	Osteoarticular allograft	32	36	24	0%	0%	53% (9)	12% (2)	6% (1)	29% (5)	21.3
Rödl et al. [28]	16	Osteoarticular allograft	32	20	59*	0	0	18% (3)	0	6% (1)	12% (2)	22.2
van de Sande et al. [23]	15	Osteoarticular allograft	32	34	228	0	0	23% (3)	8% (1)	15% (2)	—	22.8
Yao et al. [54]	23	Osteoarticular allograft/TBIR	32	19	62	0	77% (10)	38% (5)	8% (1)	23% (3)	38% (5)	—

N, patients' number; F-U, follow-up; PSA, pseudoarthrosis (nonunion/severe union delay). *Data referring to the whole population of the study, in which allografts are only a subpopulation.

another point of interest [58, 81]. In pediatric patients, surgeons may include proximal fibula and its growing plate inside the implant, so that the graft conserves its growing potential and will allow the lengthening of the recreated humerus in the future [64] (Figure 1). Although the large variety of patients does not show signs of local complications in the donor site, particular attention should be given to the postoperative knee stability. To avoid this issue and increase articular firmness, we recommend fixing the detached lateral collateral ligament (LCL) and biceps tendons to the lateral surface of the tibial plateau with suture anchors.

In 1999, Wada et al. [14] used a free vascularized fibular graft as a functional spacer to replace proximal humerus, practicing a sling procedure to preserve passive scapulohumeral mobility. 8 patients with a mean age of 27 years (10–47) were treated using the contralateral or ipsilateral fibula whose proximal pole was fixed to the proximal trump of the humerus with a dynamic compression plate. Fibular head was suspended and connected to the remaining part of the scapula by the tendons of the tendon grafts and transient stainless steel wires. In some cases, a latissimus dorsi flap was required to create adequate muscle coverage. The population treated had good functional outcomes (MSTS 23.7, 79%), and no functional problem was observed eventhough 5 of the 8 patients had radiographical signs of absorption, collapse, or fracture of the fibular head. Manfrini et al. [64] and Bilgin [63] obtained comparable results, respectively, in 2011 and 2012 (Table 2).

FVFG can also be used as a bone substrate to perform arthrodesis [61, 62]. In orthopaedic oncology, shoulder arthrodesis (with fibular graft alone or associated with allografts) is currently indicated for patients with brachial plexus injury, rotators cuff, and deltoid muscle dysfunction or in case of failed prosthetic arthroplasty [81]. This approach was widely accepted as a salvage procedure, especially if the resection of the proximal humerus was larger than 6 cm [63]. Surgical procedure may involve the use of one [82] or two plates, with this latter addition that is supposed to improve fixation strength and reliability [83, 84]. Wang et al. [33] reported that patients with extensive proximal humeral bone loss and abductor muscle sacrifice treated by arthrodesis had superior function and strength compared with others who had prosthesis or allograft-prosthesis composites (APCs). A further advantage of the autografts, in comparison to prosthetic reconstructions, is due to the progressive degradation these later suffer over the time, whereas biologic reconstructions strengthen over the years as bone hypertrophy occurs [63].

Bilgin [63] and Fuchs et al. [85] reported good functional outcomes (MSTS scores, respectively, 23 and 22.7) despite the severe loss of shoulder articularity. Unfortunately, these solid results were atleast partially overshadowed by a high risk of postoperative complications that often made necessary a revision surgery. In 2005, Fuchs et al. [85] had a failure rate of 43%, mainly attributable to nonunions, fractures, or infections. Slightly better results were obtained by Bilgin in 2012 [63] who used double-barrel grafts in some patients to reduce their risk of postoperative fracture. In summary, reconstructions that involve free vascularized fibular grafts (FVFGs) can restore the humeral length and provide active bone healing, at the price of a complex long-lasting surgical procedure and a relatively high risk of postoperative complications.

(2) Scapular Pillar Graft. Scapular pillar bone graft was first described by Gilbert and Teot in 1981 [86]. Their innovative study led the way to its wider use in the following decades for the treatment of humeral bone losses, especially in young tumoral patients with long life expectancy and medium-to-high functional requests [67, 87–89]. The technique, presented in detail by Le Reun et al. in 2019 [89], consists in the use of the lateral border of the scapula as an autologous vascularized bone graft to bridge the defect

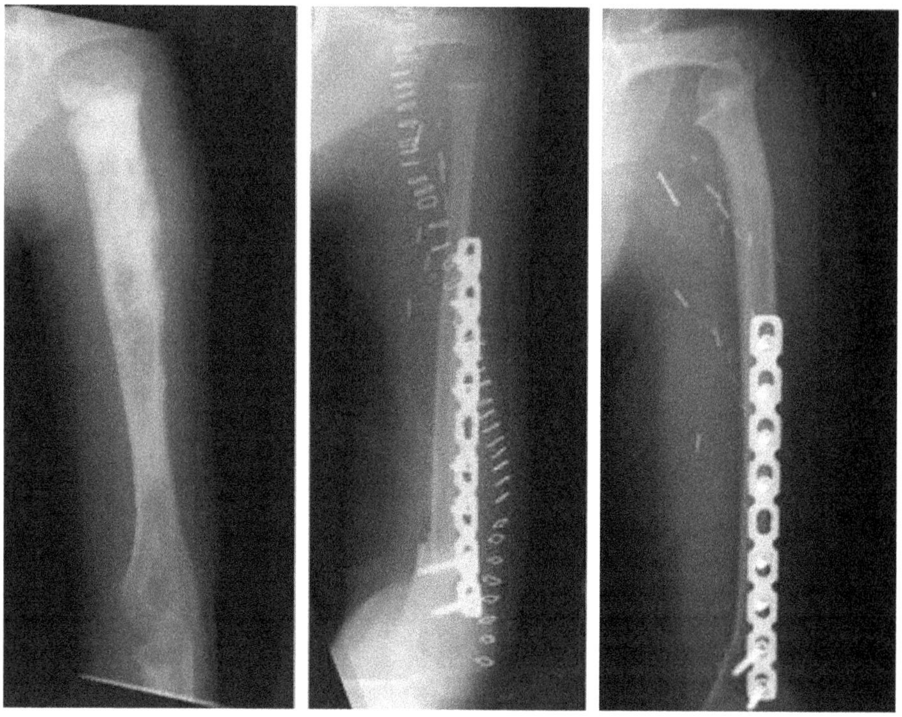

FIGURE 1: A FVFG (free vascularized fibular graft) is used to replace proximal humerus in a young growing patient who underwent massive resection to treat a malignant bone tumor. The proximal growing plate of the fibula allowed the autograft to increase its length, mimicking the growth of the native proximal humerus.

resulting from the humerus resection. Scapular pillar must be resected involving also the inferior portion of the glenoid, being careful to preserve the circumflex scapular vessels that supply blood to the bone segment of interest. Once the graft has been mobilized, the operator should rotate it laterally, using the inferior pole of the glenoid as a pivot. With a useful width of at least 2 cm and a length up to 15 cm, this vascularized graft can be solidarized to the distal humerus and to the remaining scapula performing an arthrodesis. The base of the scapular pillar itself is the best anchoring point for the scapular end [89, 90]. Compared to most frequently described vascularized fibular graft, the use of scapular pillar allows a faster procedure and does not require a second surgical field nor microsurgical anastomoses, avoiding complications such as vascular occlusions. On the other hand, the major limitation to its use might be the length of the graft that makes this surgery compatible only with resections shorter than 15 cm, according to Le Reun et al. [89] and Amin and Ebeid [66]. Therefore, this technique is primarily used to replace small defects, even though Padiolleau et al. [67] proposed the combination with free autologous grafts from other body sites (the iliac crest, fibula, tibia, or coronoid process) to increase reconstruction's length and stability. Moreover, this approach is contraindicated for cases with large metastasis of kidney cancer, since they might require preoperative embolization and consequentially could reduce the feasibility of local vascularized grafts. In terms of functional outcomes, Amin and Ebeid [66] testifies a mean MSTS score of 22.5 (75%) in their population of 16 patients, and Padiolleau et al. [67] had a mean value of 21.3 (71%) out of their 12 cases (Table 2). These results are comparable with the ones obtained using other procedures, and no major complications were found in either study.

(3) Clavicula Pro Humero (CPH). Described for the first time by Sulamaa in 1963 to treat patients suffering of phocomelia, this technique was imported for the use in cancer patients at the beginning of the 1990s with the work of Sulamaa and Winkelmann [11, 91]. Surgery is performed cutting the clavicle at its medial third and returning it through a lateral pivot point represented by the acromioclavicular joint. Once verticalized, the graft can be synthetized to what remains of the native humerus directly or through an interposed graft in case the length of clavicula alone would not be enough to fulfill the bone gap. This technique does not require a second operative field nor microsurgical skills as the native blood supply is maintained through the thoracoacromial trunk. Clavicula pro humero allows the maintenance of upper limb length and good restoration of shoulder stability and mobility. Clavicle graft also provides reconstruction with growth potential due to the presence of the lateral growth plate of the clavicle, eventhough the lengthening could not match one of the contralateral humeri. For these features, this reconstructive approach can be considered a reasonable option in pediatric patients [68, 69]. On the downside, this procedure is complex and time consuming compared to allograft surgery. Kitagawa et al. showed that patients treated with CPH had a higher revision rate compared to the ones treated with prosthetic arthroplasty or osteoarticular

allograft arthroplasty [27]. The main failure reasons in studies were graft fractures and infections. Rödl et al. in 2002 reported relatively good functional outcomes (mean MSTS score 23, 77%) but still with a high rate of postoperative complications and failures [28] (Table 2). Weighting in the balance advantages and disadvantages, clavicula pro humero can be viewed as an alternative in patients who cannot undergo prosthesis reconstructions because of their bone size and age or in countries where tumor prostheses are not available.

3. Prosthetic Reconstructions

Transversal studies testified that prosthetic reconstructions, compared to biological reconstructions, had fewer complications and a higher overall implant survival without this negatively influencing the postoperative functional outcomes [51, 92].

Advantages of prostheses are not only the relatively low complication rates but also the quick recovery of articular stability and upper limb movement [28, 36]. Newest designs brought further improvements in implants' complications-free survivorship [93] and fewer implant-associated complications [28, 47, 94, 95].

3.1. Anatomical Endoprostheses. Modern days' humeral endoprostheses sink their roots in the surgical and technical advances brought by Charles Sumner Neer II between the 1950s and the 70s. According to Neer, shoulder hemi-arthroplasty was intended to ease local pain, preserve the normal anatomy of the site, and meanwhile provide sufficient functionality to the involved upper limb [96].

Following this line of fought, modern humeral megaprostheses can be substantially considered as articular spacers whose purposes are to ensure the respect of shoulder's anatomical overview and give back an articular mobility that, with the help of the elbow and wrist, could allow patients to carry out basic activities, such as bring the fork to their mouth, brush their teeth, or touch their hair [1, 28, 36, 47, 97–99].

Nowadays, many endoprosthetic systems are available on the market, and the most varied implants have been described in literature from the modular to the custom-made devices, with both cemented or uncemented fixation concepts (Figure 2) [13, 36, 41, 94, 100, 101].

From a functional point of view, the mean MSTS scores reported in literature ranged between 18 and 25 out of 30 (Table 3). Though the 25 reported by Angelini et al. [43] in 2017 was encouraging, the evaluation of endoprostheses' functional results remains controversial [47, 100]. Although these implants represent a good platform for the functionality of the elbow and the hand below, their stability is not always perfect and shoulder's active range of motion is limited, with above shoulder activities that are often precluded [41, 43, 61, 107–112]. These limitations reflect the loss of the rotators cuff and almost total impossibility to properly reattach tendons and articular capsule to nonbiological prosthesis. In order to alleviate these criticalities, oncologic surgeons proposed alternative solutions to increase articular stability. Asavamongkolkul et al. [13] covered their custom-made endoprostheses with Dacron aortic grafts (DACs) that were sutured to the labrum and secured around the endoprostheses to make shoulders more stable and prevent subluxations or dislocations. van de Sande et al. [23] and Raiss et al. [41] described the use of trevira tubes to cover prostheses and provide reattach sites to the surrounding soft tissues. The tube was fixed on the interior to the prosthesis and outside with the remaining parts of the capsule, tendons, and muscles to better link the implant to the nearby structures.

Due to their mediocre functional outcomes, articular shoulder endoprostheses are not to be considered among the most suitable approaches for young high-demanding patients. On the contrary, these reconstructions represent reliable options for patients of older age, with lower functional requests, and/or suffering of systemic diseases. For cases with diabetes, high infective risks, or other systemic healing deficiencies, for whom grafts might represent a gamble due to their high risk of implant failure, prostheses pose as reliable solutions. Metastatic patients, for example, could benefit from the implant of an endoprosthesis since it could give early unrestricted motion of the elbow, wrist, and hand, quickly eases the pain, and limits postoperative immobilization [102]. In addition, surgical times are relatively short (which implies lesser blood loss and systemic stress), and the implant longevity should not represent a problem, since it is likely to exceed patient's life expectancy [30].

As mentioned before, the risk of complications is relatively low, but not even this technique is completely free of risks. Mechanical issues and even failures are possible; eventhough ruptures are extremely rare, dislocation and subluxation are described as the main complications of megaprostheses, involving up to 20% of the cases in literature [23, 41, 47, 94, 95, 104].

Infections remain another serious concern, with a reported risk that varies widely, ranging from 2% to 40% [13, 93, 97, 113–123]. These eventualities, for how much uncommon, are factors surgeons should focus on before deciding for a prosthetic reconstruction.

3.2. Reverse Total Shoulder Prostheses. Reverse total prostheses are implants in which the articular components switch; the socket is placed in the proximal humerus and the prosthetic ball is set on the glenoid (Figure 3). This design has been conceived to improve articular strength, stability, and range of motion, meanwhile keeping low the risks of dislocation and aseptic loosening.

For oncologic patients with proximal humerus resections, especially for those who lost their rotator cuff but maintained deltoid insertion and axillary nerve, reverse shoulder arthroplasty represents a reliable treatment that can generally lead to better functional results compared to hemiendoprosthesis. Mean MSTS scores described in literature ranged between 18 and 25.7 out of 30, with results that are on average higher than the ones obtained with endoprostheses. In comparison to these later, reverse total

Table 2: Summary data for autograft studies.

Study	Resection (cm)	Graft type	N	Age (y)	F-U (m)	Hardware issues	Fractures	Infections	PSA	Failures	MSTS score
Kumar et al. [61]	14	(Arthrodesis) FVFG	4	24	51	4% (1)	0	4% (1)	0	0	—
Mimata et al. [62]	—	(Arthrodesis) FVFG	5	21	75	0	40% (2)	0	0	0	21.4
Bilgin [63]	—	FVFG	9	38	60	22% (2)	11% (1)	11% (1)	0	0	24
Manfrini et al. [64]	13	FVFG	11	5	110	0	64% (7)	9% (1)			22.9
Wada et al. [14]	20	FVFG	8	27	70	0	0	0	12% (1)	12% (1)	23.7
Li et al. [65]	—	Allograft + FVGF	6	16	19	0	0	0	0	0	28
Liu et al. [29]	—	TBIR + FVFG	16	32	62	0	6% (1)	0	25% (4)	25% (4)	19
Amin and Ebeid [66]	14	Scapular pillar autograft	16	21	36	0	0	0	12% (2)	12% (2)	22.5
Padiolleau et al. [67]	12	Scapular pillar autograft	12	36	59	0	0	0	25% (3)	25% (3)	21.3
Barbier et al. [68]	9	CPH autograft	7	8–18	40	14% (1)	29% (2)	0	71% (5)	71% (5)	21.7
Calvert et al. [69]	14	CPH autograft	4	6	43	0	0	0	50% (2)	50% (2)	26-27
Kitagawa et al. [27]	—	CPH autograft	7	29	18	0	0	0	0	0	21.5
Rödl et al. [28]	—	CPH autograft	15	18	59	0	22% (4)	22% (4)	22% (4)	22% (4)	24.6
Tsukushi et al. [70]	—	CPH autograft	7	36	26	14% (1)	0	0	0	0	20.7

N, patients' number; F-U, follow-up; PSA, pseudoarthrosis (nonunion/severe union delay); FVFG, free vascularized fibular graft; CPH, clavicula pro humero.

shoulder prostheses also provide better flexion and abduction. In fact, the functionality allowed by reverse shoulder prostheses does not limit to morphological support to the elbow and wrist but extents to active shoulder flexion and abduction generally above the 90 degrees, greatly increasing patients' possibilities in terms of daily living activities [17, 44, 46, 104, 124]. As described by De Wilde et al. in 2005, patients with proximal humerus and rotators cuff resection treated with reverse shoulder arthroplasty rely on the deltoid muscle to generate active shoulder function; therefore, surgeons must focus on optimizing the deltoid moment arm and muscular elongation to get better clinical results [17]. Boileau et al. also testified promising functional results in nononcological patients when reverse shoulder arthroplasty was used in combination with a modified latissimus dorsi and teres major tendon transfer. Cases showed an improvement of mean active elevation and external rotation range that could encourage a similar use in oncological field [125]. Another possible variation capable of increasing shoulder stability is the addition of synthetic tubes to surround the reverse prostheses, similar to what above described in the prior subchapter [23, 41, 46, 47, 126].

Reverse shoulder total prostheses should be performed mainly in case both deltoid and axillary nerves are preserved, in order to maximize the aforementioned good outcomes in terms of postoperative functionality.

The overall complication rate in literature amounted between 0 and 40%. The most common were scapular notching (mean risk between 0 and 30%) [44, 46, 104, 106], articular instability or dislocations (0–30%) [44–46, 49, 104], and aseptic loosening (0–13.3%) [49, 106]. Infective risk was low, since no study reported infection rates higher than 6.7% [45, 47, 49]. Depending on the study, the total failure risk was between 0% and 36% (Table 3). These percentages elect reversed shoulder arthroplasty as a relatively safe option for patients whose tumor and consequential resection damaged the rotators cuff but saved deltoid muscle and axillary nerve. Before choosing this surgical approach, anyway, surgeons should consider that prostheses for their own nature have limited durability. Eventhough modern conception devices can remain functional for decades, still they are not everlasting and their mechanical properties might not stand the test of time as well as grafts could. Young patients with long life expectancy could possibly run into of prosthesis decay; therefore, revision surgery would be necessary. On the contrary, device durability should represent nothing but a minor concern for midlife patients or cases with limited life expectancy.

4. Allograft-Prosthesis Composite (APC) Reconstructions

In orthopaedic oncology, surgical treatment of proximal humerus often leads to wide resections of both bones and soft tissues. Removal of joint capsule, rotator cuff muscles, or deltoid could be necessary in order to achieve a radical excision of neoplastic tissue. This could compromise shoulder stability after reconstruction, especially because of

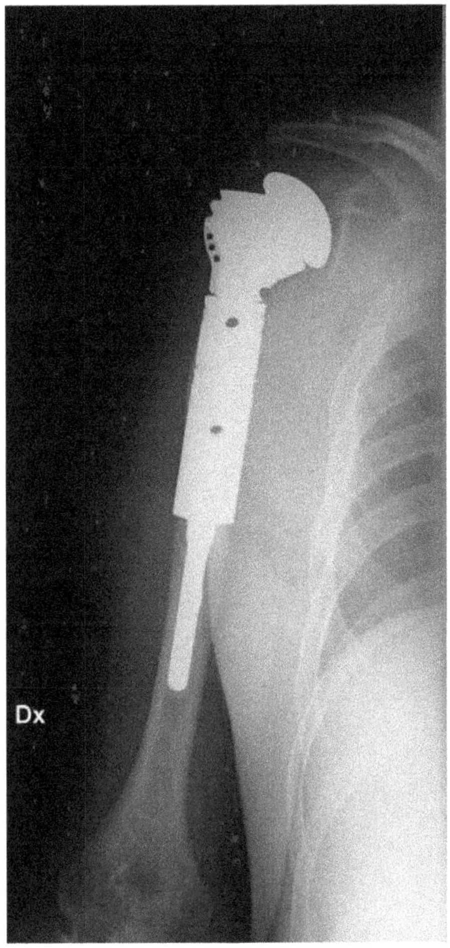

FIGURE 2: Anatomic megaprosthesis of proximal humerus implanted in our institution after massive bone resection due to resection of a malignant bone tumor.

the intrinsic instability of the joint without the stabilizers complex [34].

Endoprosthesis and allograft, as described in previous chapters, are two of the most dominant reconstructive options for proximal humerus to this date. However, in the postoperative medium-term follow-up, both these techniques count several major complications that make revision surgery inevitable. Endoprostheses cannot always provide a valid reattachment for rotator cuff tendons, threating joint stability and ending in an increased risk of dislocation and subluxation.

Compared to endoprostheses, allografts have a number of advantages: restoration of bone stock and soft tissues attachment guarantee better stability, wider shoulder range of motion, and consequently improved functional outcomes. Nevertheless, reconstruction with allografts as well leads to major complications such as bone resorption, fracture of the graft, and nonunion at bone-graft interface frequently described in literature [127].

Humeral reconstruction can also be performed matching biological and prosthetic approaches that meet allograft-prosthesis composite reconstructions (APC). This method was first described in 1991 by Gitelis to overcome the considerable risk of allografts alone to suffer fractures and implant failures. The association of allografts with prostheses theoretically allows matching the structural advantages from both reconstructions. Allograft's possibility to anchor surrounding soft tissues and therefore increase articular stability is combined with prostheses' durability; a more rigid construct is created and lower risk of fractures, subchondral collapses, and dislocations are achieved [128].

Almost all the testimonies of APCs in the oncologic field are case series of patients who underwent intraarticular resections 1A or 1B according to the Malawer classification.

After an intraarticular 1A resection of proximal humerus, an allograft-reverse prosthesis composite should be taken into consideration, remembering that this reconstruction requires good bone stock on the glenoid, integrity of the axillary nerve, and preserved deltoid function to guarantee satisfactory functional outcomes [128]. Surgical procedure assumes the use of an appositely prepared frozen allograft to replace proximal humerus and accommodate the prosthetic stem; the proximal part of the prosthesis is cemented to the graft and the distal stem is inserted in the native bone canal, either cemented or press-fitted. Cementation of the distal stem end is recommended especially in elderly people with low bone quality; according to Lozano-Calderón and Chen [128], cement augmentation of the

Table 3: Summary data for prosthetic studies.

Study	Resection (cm)	Prosthesis type	N	Age (y)	F-U (m)	Aseptic loosening	Nerve injury	Instability	Infections	Scapular notching	Reinterventions	Failure	MSTS score	Active ROM
Angelini et al. [43]	11.0	EndoPT (M)	33	46	94	2% (1)	0	15% (8)	4% (2)	—	35% (19)	22% (12)	25	—
Asavamongkolkul et al. [13]	—	EndoPT (CM/M)	33	33	81*	3% (2)*	0	10% (6)*	3% (2)*	—	20%*	7% (4)*	22.8	—
Cannon et al. [100]	14	EndoPT (CM/M)	83	55	30	0	0	6% (5)	2% (2)	—	1% (1)	1% (1)	18.9	Flex42° Abd41°
Fuhrmann et al. [102]	—	EndoPT (M)	21	57	47	0	0	0	5% (1)	—	9% (2)	0%	18	—
Kiss et al. [42]	—	EndoPT (M)	36	42	56*	0	6% (2)	25% (9)	3% (1)	—	6% (2)	6% (2)	19.7	—
Liu et al. [29]	11	EndoPT (CM)	25	30	55	36% (9)	0	0	0	—	36% (9)	36% (9)	19.1	—
Manfrini et al. [48]	15.3	EndoPT (M)	25	10	53	12% (3)	0	0	12% (3)	—	24% (6)	16% (4)	20.9	—
Raiss et al. [41]	13	EndoPT (M)	39	60	38	3% (1)	0	10.2% (4)	5% (2)	—	12% (5)	10% (4)	19	Flex34° Abd33°
Rödl et al. [28]	17	EndoPT (M)	19	37	59	0	0	0	0	—	0	0	23.6	—
Potter et al. [30]	13.6	EndoPT (M)	16	54	34	0	0	19% (3)	0	—	25% (4)	25% (4)	20.7	—
van de Sande et al. [23]	9.6	EndoPT (M)	14	45	120*	0	0	7% (1)	0	—	7% (1)	7% (1)	23.1	—
Wei et al. [103]	20.6	EndoPT (M)	20	24	40	10% (2)	15% (3)	5% (1)	0	—	5% (1)	5% (1)	21.5	—
Bonnevialle et al. [44]	10.5	Reverse shoulder (P)	10	55	42	0	10% (1)	30% (3)	0	30% (3)	20% (2)	10% (1)	20.2	Flex122°
De Wilde et al. [17]	—	Reverse shoulder (P)	4	42	38	0	0	0	0	0	0	0	27–29	Flex169° Abd172°
De Wilde et al. [104]	—	Reverse shoulder (P)	14	45	92	1	0	2	1	29% (4)	14% (2)	14% (2)	—	Abd157°
Griffiths et al. [45]	—	Reverse shoulder (P)	42	46	71	0	0	26% (14)	5% (2)	0	9% (4)	0%	21.7	—
Guven et al. [46]	10.2	Reverse shoulder (P)	10	49	18	0	0	20% (2)	0	20% (2)	20% (2)	0%	23.4	Flex96° Abd88°
Hu et al. [105]	11.8	Reverse shoulder (P)	7	35	24	0	0	0	0	0	0	0	25.7	Flex133 Abd137
Kaa et al. [49]	11	Reverse shoulder (P)	15	42	46	13% (2)	0	7% (1)	7% (1)	0	27% (4)	20% (3)	23	Flex98° Abd78°
Maclean et al. [106]	9.3	Reverse shoulder (P)	8	49	43	12% (1)	12% (1)	0	0	12% (1)	0%	0%	18	Flex71° Abd62°
Streitbuerger et al. [47]	15.1	Reverse shoulder (P)	18	42	34	0	0	22% (4)	6% (1)	0	6% (1)	6% (1)	25.1	Flex84° Abd80°

N, patients' number; F-U, follow-up. *Data referring to the whole population of the study, in which prostheses are only a subpopulation.

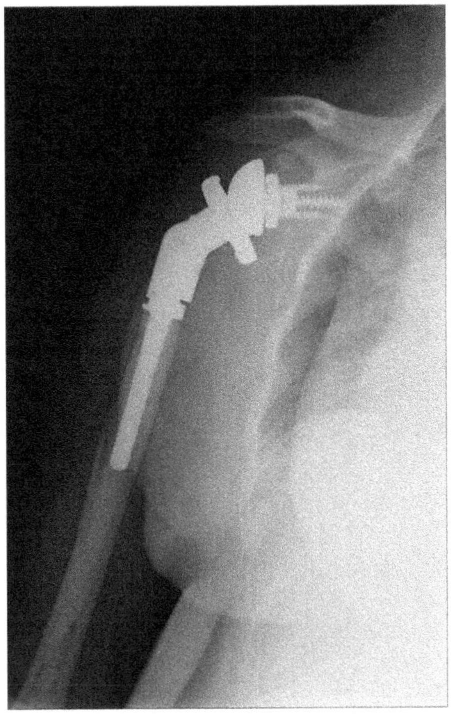

FIGURE 3: Reverse shoulder megaprosthesis implanted in our institution after massive bone resection due to resection of a malignant bone tumor.

proximal stem in the graft increases rigidity of the construct and reduces the risk of allograft fracture [128]. Stem could be press-fitted in younger patients to compound osteointegration of the stem in the host bone and at the bone-graft interface. Moreover, uncemented stems could reduce the risk of implant aseptic loosening in a long-term scenario. The employment of a long prosthetic stem provides stability to the graft-bone interface, which could be additionally increased with fixation plates. At the end of bone reconstruction, correct reattachment of soft tissues to the graft must be made; in particular, capsule repair along with reinsertion of rotator cuff and deltoid tendon are essential for the recovery of shoulder functionality [34, 128, 129].

Abdeen and Healey [34] presented the largest series of patients undergone intraarticular or extraarticular resection, with 36 cases and a mean follow-up of 5 years. They underlined the importance of deltoid preservation to restore a good range of motion: patients in whom a partial or complete deltoid resection had been necessary, the sacrifice translated in unsatisfying abduction and forward flexion. However, this aspect did not significantly influence the MSTS score in the medium-term follow-up that has been lowered in the extraarticular resection instead [34].

In literature, medium-term results were generally satisfactory in terms of pain, shoulder range of motion, and quality of life, if compared with preoperative ones. Average MSTS scores, when calculated, were always higher than 18 (60%) with good outcomes on patients' emotional and acceptance points of view (Table 4).

As always, in orthopaedic practice, a surgical technique must be evaluated, weighing in the balance its functional results together with the risks it poses.

The most frequent complication detected by authors was delayed union or nonunion at the graft-bone interface. Nonunion rate does not seems to be significantly conditioned by the choice of cementation or press-fitting of the prosthetic stem into the host bone and even the employment of fixation plates to increase composite stability and rotation control cannot entirely prevent nonunions. El Beaino et al. [130] collected a series of 21 cases with a median follow-up of 97 months. In seven patients, a plate at the junction was positioned; three of them (43%) had delayed union. In parallel, the same complication occurred in 7 of the 14 patients (50%) without plates at the junction. All patients had received primary grafting at the interface. Black et al. [25] reported six cases of allograft-endoprosthesis composite, all treated with exclusively grafting at the interface, without plating. Only one of six developed nonunion at the junction that required surgical revision with new grafting and stabilisation with a plate. Nonunions were the main cause of implant revision, generally requiring new grafting at the allograft-host bone junction and sometimes the application of additional plates. Resolution of nonunion was always achieved after surgery, as testified by postoperative radiographical and clinical evidences of bone healing, with adequate bone callus and pain relief.

Also, shoulder dislocations or subluxations were not infrequent, similar to what was observed for prosthetic reconstructions alone. El Beaino et al. [130] described 12

Table 4: Summary data for APC studies.

Study	Malawer classification	Reconstruction type	Ce.	N°	Age (y)	F-U (m)	Aseptic loosening	Fractures	Instability	Infections	PSA	Total failures	MSTS score
Abdeen and Healey [34]	—	Allograft + EndoPT	No	36	—	60	8% (3)	0	3% (1)	0	11% (4)	19% (7)	Lower in extra articular resection
Black et al. [25]	1A	Allograft + EndoPT	Yes	6	41	55	0	0	0	0	17% (1)	33% (2)	69% (21)
El Beaino et al. [130]	1A	Allograft − EndoPT	Yes	21	41	97	14% (3)	5% (1)	57% (12) (1 rev.)	5% (1)	48% (10)	10% at 5 y FU	78% (23)
King et al. [129]	1A	Allograft + RSR	Yes	2	31	51	0	0	0	0	100% (2)	100% (2)	—
Lazerges et al. [131]	1A	Allograft + RSR	Yes	6	66	71	0	0	17% (1)	0	17% (1)	17% (1)	73% (22)
Moran and Stalley [127]	1B	Allograft + EndoPT	No	11	22	70	0	0	36% (4) (3 rev.)	0	18% (2)	54% (6)	66% (20)
Ruggieri et al. [26]	1A	Allograft + resurface	Yes	14	35	25	0	21% (3)	0	7% (1) (rev.)	0	21% (3)	77% (23)
Sanchez-Sotelo et al. [132]	—	Allograft ± RSR	Yes	26	62	48	0	8% (2)	4% (1)	4% (1)	11% (3)	23% (6)	—
Potter et al. [30]	—	Allograft + EndoPT	Yes	16	56	24	0	6% (1)	19% (3)	13% (2)	6% (1)	6% (1)	79% (24)
van de Sande et al. [23]	IA	Allograft + EndoPT	Yes	10	34	204	0	20% (2)	40% (4)	20% (2)	30% (3)	30% (3)	72% (22)

Ce, cement; *N*, patients' number; F-U, follow-up; PSA, pseudoarthrosis (nonunion/severe union delay).

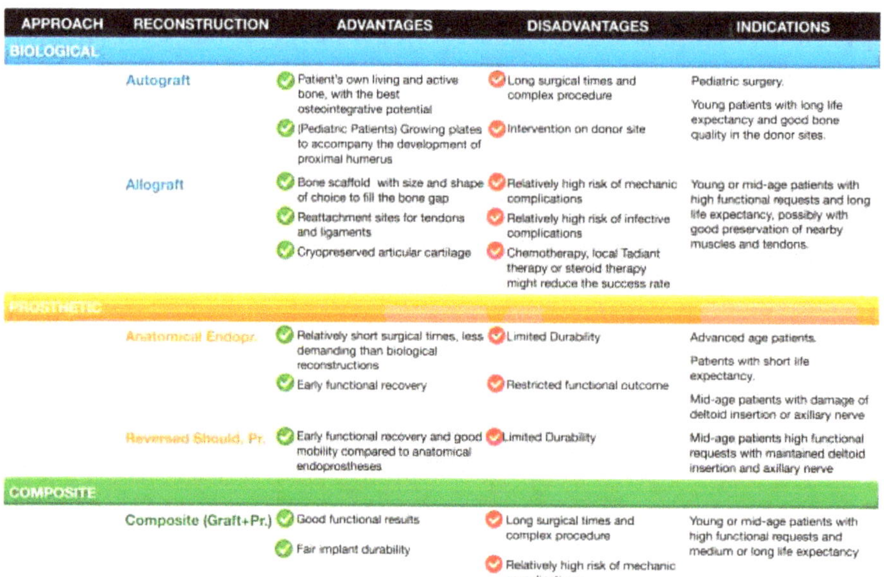

Figure 4: Schematic summary of the main advantages and disadvantages, with consequential indications, for the main reconstructive approaches to proximal humerus in oncologic surgery.

cases of shoulder subdislocations, although revision surgery was necessary in one patient only.

Aseptic loosening, infection, and fracture rates were low, but when they occurred, revision surgery was always required.

No cases of resorption of the graft have been described in literature to this date; this might establish APCs as a suitable solution to overcome one of the biggest problems associated with the use of allografts alone [127].

All in all, proximal humerus reconstruction with allograft prosthesis composite is a valid option of treatment in oncologic patients that required wide bone resections. Their overall good functional results, associated with a better implant longevity compared to allografts alone, made the allograft-prosthetic composites (APCs), a relevant technique especially for younger patients with primary bone tumors and absence of systemic involvement [30]. Surgery is longer and more complex compared to allograft or prosthesis placement, and unfortunately,

APCs are not lacking in complications neither. Nevertheless, they present advantages of both prosthetic and biological reconstructive approaches and can lead to a reduction of the classic complications that come along when using one of the two other techniques alone.

5. Conclusion

The choice of the most appropriate surgical treatment should result from an accurate overview covering not only resection extent but also patient' systemic and local clinical picture, life expectancy, and functional requests.

Although a unique line of thinking is yet to be established, modern literature suggests that biologic reconstructions are indicated mainly for young patients with long life expectancy and high functional requests. In fact, the osteointegration and mechanic performances promised by grafts could lead to great functional results through the long life of the implant. On the other hand, prosthetic reconstructions represent a reliable option especially for patients with medium or short life expectancy who could be allowed anyway to maintain decent upper limb functionality with a reasonable recovery time. A summary of advantages and disadvantages for each reconstructive strategy and the suggested indications in light of the aforementioned literature evidences and our own experience is shown in Figure 4.

Modern surgery provides a large variety of reconstructive solutions for proximal humerus after tumor resection, each one with its advantages and disadvantages; it is up to the surgeon to consider what patient needs and choose the technique that better suits the individual.

References

[1] J. C. Wittig, J. Bickels, K. L. Kellar-Graney, F. H. Kim, and M. M. Malawer, "Osteosarcoma of the proximal humerus: long-term results with limb-sparing surgery," *Clinical Orthopaedics and Related Research*, vol. 397, pp. 156–176, 2002.

[2] S. S. Bielack, B. Kempf-Bielack, G. Delling et al., "Prognostic factors in high-grade osteosarcoma of the extremities or trunk: an analysis of 1,702 patients treated on neoadjuvant cooperative osteosarcoma study group protocols," *Journal of Clinical Oncology*, vol. 20, no. 3, pp. 776–790, 2002.

[3] A. Piccioli, G. Maccauro, B. Rossi, L. Scaramuzzo, F. Frenos, and R. Capanna, "Surgical treatment of pathologic fractures of humerus," *Injury*, vol. 41, no. 11, pp. 1112–1116, 2010.

[4] D. C. Dahlin, *Bone Tumors: General Aspects and Data on 6221 Cases*, Charles C Thomas, Springfield, IL, USA, 3rd edition, 1978.

[5] W. F. Enneking, *Musculoskeletal Tumor Surgery*, Churchill Livingstone, New York, NY, USA, 1983.

[6] D. C. Dahlin and J. C. Ivins, "Benign chondroblastoma. A study of 125 cases," *Cancer*, vol. 30, no. 2, pp. 401–413, 1972.

[7] M. M. Malawer, P. H. Sugarbaker, M. Lampert, A. R. Baker, and N. L. Gerber, "The Tikhoff-Linberg procedure: report of ten patients and presentation of a modified technique for tumors of the proximal humerus," *Surgery*, vol. 97, no. 5, pp. 518–528, 1985.

[8] F. Sirveaux, "Reconstruction techniques after proximal humerus tumour resection," *Orthopaedics & Traumatology: Surgery & Research*, vol. 105, no. 1, pp. S153–S164, 2019.

[9] M. C. Gebhardt, Y. F. Roth, and H. J. Mankin, "Osteoarticular allografts for reconstruction in the proximal part of the humerus after excision of a musculoskeletal tumor," *The Journal of Bone & Joint Surgery*, vol. 72, no. 3, pp. 334–345, 1990.

[10] M. C. Gebhardt, D. I. Flugstad, D. S. Springfield, and H. J. Mankin, "The use of bone allografts for limb salvage in high-grade extremity osteosarcoma," *Clinical Orthopaedics and Related Research*, vol. 270, no. 270, pp. 181–196, 1991.

[11] W. W. Winkelmann, "Clavicula pro humero—a new surgical method for malignant tumors of the proximal humerus," *Zeitschrift fur Orthopadie und Ihre Grenzgebiete*, vol. 130, pp. 197–201, 1992.

[12] M. I. O'Connor, F. H. Sim, and E. Y. Chao, "Limb salvage for neoplasms of the shoulder girdle. Intermediate reconstructive and functional results," *Journal of Bone and Joint Surgery*, vol. 78, pp. 1872–1888, 1996.

[13] A. Asavamongkolkul, J. J. Eckardt, F. R. Eilber et al., "Endoprosthetic reconstruction for malignant upper extremity tumors," *Clinical Orthopaedics and Related Research*, vol. 360, pp. 207–220, 1999.

[14] T. Wada, M. Usui, K. Isu, S. Yamawaki, and S. Ishii, "Reconstruction and limb salvage after resection for malignant bone tumour of the proximal humerus. A sling procedure using a free vascularised bular graft," *The Journal of Bone and Joint Surgery. British Volume*, vol. 81-B, no. 5, pp. 808–813, 1999.

[15] J. C. Wittig, J. Bickels, F. Wodajo, K. L. Kellar-Graney, and M. M. Malawer, "Constrained total scapula reconstruction after resection of a high-grade sarcoma," *Clinical Orthopaedics and Related Research*, vol. 397, pp. 143–155, 2002.

[16] M. M. Malawer and L. B. Chou, "Prosthetic survival and clinical results with use of large-segment replacements in the treatment of high-grade bone sarcomas," *The Journal of Bone & Joint Surgery*, vol. 77, no. 8, pp. 1154–1165, 1995.

[17] L. F. De Wilde, F. S. Plasschaert, E. A. Audenaert, and R. C. Verdonk, "Functional recovery after a reverse prosthesis for reconstruction of the proximal humerus in tumor surgery," *Clinical Orthopaedics & Related Research*, vol. 430, pp. 156–162, 2005.

[18] Q. Yang, J. Li, Z. Yang, X. Li, and Z. Li, "Limb sparing surgery for bone tumours of the shoulder girdle: the oncological and functional results," *International Orthopaedics*, vol. 34, no. 6, pp. 869–875, 2010.

[19] V. Cladière-Nassif, C. Bourdet, V. Audard, A. Babinet, P. Anract, and D. Biau, "Is it safe to preserve the deltoid when resecting the proximal humerus for a primary malignant bone tumour? A comparative study," *Bone & Joint Journal*, vol. 99-B, no. 9, pp. 1244–1249, 2017 Sep.

[20] M. Malawer and J. Wittig, "Proximal humerus resection. The Tikhoff-Linberg procedure and its modifications," in *Musculoskeletal Cancer Surgery*, M. M. Walamer and P. H. Sugarbaker, Eds., pp. 519–552, Kluwer Academic Publishers, New York, NY, USA, 2004.

[21] P. Anract and B. Tomeno, "Résections—reconstructions pour tumeurs osseuse malignes du membre supérieur," *EMC Techniques Chirurgicales—Orthopédie Traumatologie*, vol. 44, 97 pages, 2005.

[22] M. Kassab, V. Dumaine, A. Babinet, M. Ouaknine, B. Tomeno, and P. Anract, "Les reconstructions après

résection tumorale de l'extrémité supérieure de l'humérus," *Revue de Chirurgie Orthopédique et Réparatrice de l'Appareil Moteur*, vol. 91, no. 1, pp. 15–23, 2005.

[23] M. A. J. van de Sande, P. D. S. Dijkstra, and A. H. M. Taminiau, "Proximal humerus reconstruction after tumour resection: biological versus endoprosthetic reconstruction," *International Orthopaedics*, vol. 35, no. 9, pp. 1375–1380, 2011.

[24] A. Abdeen, B. H. Hoang, E. A. Athanasian, C. D. Morris, P. J. Boland, and J. H. Healey, "Allograft-prosthesis composite reconstruction of the proximal part of the humerus. Functional outcome and survivorship," *The Journal of Bone and Joint Surgery-American Volume*, vol. 91, no. 10, pp. 2406–2415, 2009.

[25] A. W. Black, R. M. Szabo, and R. M. Titelman, "Treatment of malignant tumors of the proximal humerus with allograft-prosthesis composite reconstruction," *Journal of Shoulder and Elbow Surgery*, vol. 16, no. 5, pp. 525–533, 2007.

[26] P. Ruggieri, A. F. Mavrogenis, G. Guerra, and M. Mercuri, "Preliminary results after reconstruction of bony defects of the proximal humerus with an allograft-resurfacing composite," *The Journal of Bone and Joint Surgery. British Volume*, vol. 93-B, no. 8, pp. 1098–1103, 2011.

[27] Y. Kitagawa, D. Thai, and P. Choong, "Reconstructions of the shoulder following tumour resection," *Journal of Orthopaedic Surgery*, vol. 15, no. 2, pp. 201–206, 2007.

[28] R. W. Rödl, G. Gosheger, C. Gebert, N. Lindner, T. Ozaki, and W. Winkelmann, "Reconstruction of the proximal humerus after wide resection of tumours," *The Journal of Bone and Joint Surgery. British Volume*, vol. 84-B, no. 7, pp. 1004–1008, 2002.

[29] T. Liu, Q. Zhang, X. Guo et al., "Treatment and outcome of malignant bone tumors of the proximal humerus: biological versus endoprosthetic reconstruction," *BMC Musculoskeletal Disorders*, vol. 15, p. 69, 2014.

[30] B. K. Potter, S. C. Adams, J. D. Pitcher Jr., T. I. Malinin, and H. T. Temple, "Proximal humerus reconstructions for tumors," *Clinical Orthopaedics and Related Research*, vol. 467, no. 4, pp. 1035–1041, 2009.

[31] M. El-Sherbiny, "Reconstruction of the proximal humerus after wide resection of tumors: comparison of three reconstructive options," *Journal of the Egyptian National Cancer Institute*, vol. 20, no. 4, pp. 369–378, 2008.

[32] L. A. Aponte-Tinao, M. A. Ayerza, D. L. Muscolo, and G. L. Farfalli, "Allograft reconstruction for the treatment of musculoskeletal tumors of the upper extremity," *Sarcoma* vol. 2013, Article ID 925413, 6 pages, 2013.

[33] J. Wang, J. Shen, and I. C. Dickinson, "Functional outcome of arthrodesis with a vascularized fibular graft and a rotational latissimus dorsi flap after proximal humerus sarcoma resection," *Annals of Surgical Oncology*, vol. 18, no. 7, pp. 1852–1859, 2011.

[34] A. Abdeen and J. H. Healey, "Allograft-prosthesis composite reconstruction of the proximal part of the humerus: surgical technique," *Journal of Bone and Joint Surgery*, vol. 92, pp. 188–196, 2010.

[35] P. J. Getty and T. D. Peabody, "Complications and functional outcomes of reconstruction with an osteoarticular allograft after intra-articular resection of the proximal aspect of the humerus," *The Journal of Bone and Joint Surgery-American Volume*, vol. 81, no. 8, pp. 1138–1146, 1999.

[36] N. Mayilvahanan, M. Paraskumar, A. Sivaseelam, and S. Natarajan, "Custom mega-prosthetic replacement for proximal humeral tumours," *International Orthopaedics*, vol. 30, no. 3, pp. 158–162, 2006.

[37] K. H. Shin, H. J. Park, J. H. Yoo, and S. B. Hahn, "Reconstructive surgery in primary malignant and aggressive benign bone tumor of the proximal humerus," *Yonsei Medical Journal*, vol. 41, no. 3, pp. 304–311, 2000.

[38] J. Older, "Introduction: history and research on bone transplantation," in *Bone Implant grafting*Springer-Verlag, London, UK, 1992.

[39] R. A. Horowitz, M. D. Leventis, M. D. Rohrer, and H. S. Prasad, "Bone grafting: history, rationale, and selection of materials and techniques," *Compendium of Continuing Education in Dentistry*, vol. 35, no. 4, pp. 1–6, 2014.

[40] A. Mourikis, H. J. Mankin, F. J. Hornicek, and K. A. Raskin, "Treatment of proximal humeral chondrosarcoma with resection and allograft," *Journal of Shoulder and Elbow Surgery*, vol. 16, no. 5, pp. 519–524, 2007.

[41] P. Raiss, S. Kinkel, U. Sauter, T. Bruckner, and B. Lehner, "Replacement of the proximal humerus with MUTARS tumor endoprostheses," *European Journal of Surgical Oncology (EJSO)*, vol. 36, no. 4, pp. 371–377, 2010.

[42] J. Kiss, G. Sztrinkai, I. Antal, J. Kiss, and M. Szendrői, "Functional results and quality of life after shoulder girdle resections in musculoskeletal tumors," *Journal of Shoulder and Elbow Surgery*, vol. 16, no. 3, pp. 273–279, 2007.

[43] A. Angelini, A. F. Mavrogenis, G. Trovarelli et al., "Extra-articular shoulder resections: outcomes of 54 patients," *Journal of Shoulder and Elbow Surgery*, vol. 26, no. 11, pp. e337–e345, 2017.

[44] N. Bonnevialle, P. Mansat, J. Lebon, J.-M. Laffosse, and P. Bonnevialle, "Reverse shoulder arthroplasty for malignant tumors of proximal humerus," *Journal of Shoulder and Elbow Surgery*, vol. 24, no. 1, pp. 36–44, 2015.

[45] D. Griffiths, P. D. Gikas, C. Jowett et al., "Proximal humeral replacement using a fixed-fulcrum endoprosthesis," *The Journal of Bone and Joint Surgery. British Volume*, vol. 93-B, no. 3, pp. 399–403, 2011.

[46] M. F. Guven, L. Aslan, H. Botanlioglu, G. Kaynak, H. Kesmezacar, and M. Babacan, "Functional outcome of reverse shoulder tumor prosthesis in the treatment of proximal humerus tumors," *Journal of Shoulder and Elbow Surgery*, vol. 25, no. 1, pp. e1–e6, 2016.

[47] A. Streitbuerger, M. Henrichs, G. Gosheger et al., "Improvement of the shoulder function after large segment resection of the proximal humerus with the use of an inverse tumour prosthesis," *International Orthopaedics*, vol. 39, no. 2, pp. 355–361, 2015.

[48] M. Manfrini, S. Bindiganavile, F. Say et al., "Is there benefit to free over pedicled vascularized grafts in augmenting tibial intercalary allograft constructs?," *Clinical Orthopaedics & Related Research*, vol. 475, no. 5, pp. 1322–1337, 2017.

[49] A. K. S. Kaa, P. H. Jørgensen, J. O. Søjbjerg, and H. V. Johannsen, "Reverse shoulder replacement after resection of the proximal humerus for bone tumours," *The Bone & Joint Journal*, vol. 95-B, no. 11, pp. 1551–1555, 2013.

[50] S. Veerachamy, T. Yarlagadda, G. Manivasagam, and P. K. Yarlagadda, "Bacterial adherence and biofilm formation on medical implants: a review," in *Proceedings of the Institution of Mechanical Engineers, Part H: Journal of Engineering in Medicine*, vol. 228, no. 10, pp. 1083–1099, 2014.

[51] H. DeGroot, D. Donati, M. Di Liddo, E. Gozzi, and M. Mercuri, "The use of cement in osteoarticular allografts for proximal humeral bone tumors," *Clinical Orthopaedics and Related Research*, vol. 427, pp. 190–197, 2004.

[52] K. Jamshidi, F. Najd-Mazhar, F. Abolghasemzadeh Ahangar, and A. Mirzaei, "The effect of cement augmentation and anteromedial plating on proximal humerus allograft reconstruction," *Journal of Orthopaedic Science*, vol. 22, no. 1, pp. 69–74, 2017.

[53] P. T. Ogink, F. R. Teunissen, J. R. Massier, K. A. Raskin, J. H. Schwab, and S. A. Lozano-Calderon, "Allograft reconstruction of the humerus: complications and revision surgery," *Journal of Surgical Oncology*, vol. 119, no. 3, pp. 329–335, 2019.

[54] W. Yao, Q. Cai, J. Wang, and J. Hou, "Mid- to long-term effects of two different biological reconstruction techniques for the treatment of humerus osteosarcoma involving caput humeri," *World Journal of Surgical Oncology*, vol. 18, no. 1, p. 23, 2020.

[55] V. P. Kumar and K. Satku, "Osteoarticular allografts for reconstruction in the proximal part of the humerus after excision of a musculoskeletal tumor," *The Journal of Bone & Joint Surgery*, vol. 74, no. 1, p. 152, 1992.

[56] M. P. A. Bus, M. A. J. van de Sande, A. H. M. Taminiau, and P. D. S. Dijkstra, "Is there still a role for osteoarticular allograft reconstruction in musculoskeletal tumour surgery? A long-term follow-up study of 38 patients and systematic review of the literature," *The Bone & Joint Journal*, vol. 99-B, no. 4, pp. 522–530, 2017.

[57] R. S. Leão, J. R. S. Maior, C. A. A. Lemos et al., "Complications with PMMA compared with other materials used in cranioplasty: a systematic review and meta-analysis," *Brazilian Oral Research*, vol. 32, p. e31, 2018.

[58] M. J. Landau, I. Badash, C. Yin, R. K. Alluri, and K. M. Patel, "Free vascularized fibula grafting in the operative treatment of malignant bone tumors of the upper extremity: a systematic review of outcomes and complications," *Journal of Surgical Oncology*, vol. 117, no. 7, pp. 1432–1439, 2018.

[59] C. Gebert, A. Hillmann, A. Schwappach et al., "Free vascularized fibular grafting for reconstruction after tumor resection in the upper extremity," *Journal of Surgical Oncology*, vol. 94, no. 2, pp. 114–127, 2006.

[60] A. J. Weiland, H. E. Kleinert, J. E. Kutz, and R. K. Daniel, "Free vascularized bone grafts in surgery of the upper extremity," *The Journal of Hand Surgery*, vol. 4, no. 2, pp. 129–144, 1979.

[61] V. P. Kumar, S. K. Satku, A. K. Mitra, and R. W. H. Pho, "Function following limb salvage for primary tumors of the shoulder girdle: 10 patients followed 4 (1–11) years," *Acta Orthopaedica Scandinavica*, vol. 65, no. 1, pp. 55–61, 1994.

[62] Y. Mimata, J. Nishida, K. Sato, Y. Suzuki, and M. Doita, "Glenohumeral arthrodesis for malignant tumor of the shoulder girdle," *Journal of Shoulder and Elbow Surgery* vol. 24, no. 2, pp. 174–178, 2015.

[63] S. S. Bilgin, "Reconstruction of proximal humeral defectş with shoulder arthrodesis using free vascularized fibular graft," *The Journal of Bone & Joint Surgery*, vol. 94, no. 13, p. e94, 2012.

[64] M. Manfrini, A. Tiwari, J. Ham, M. Colangeli, and M. Mercuri, "Evolution of surgical treatment for sarcomas of proximal humerus in children: retrospective review at a single institute over 30 years," *Journal of Pediatric Orthopaedics*, vol. 31, no. 1, pp. 56–64, 2011.

[65] J. Li, Z. Wang, Z. Guo, Y. Wu, G. Chen, and G. Pei, "Precise resection and biological reconstruction for patients with bone sarcomas in the proximal humerus," *Journal of Reconstructive Microsurgery*, vol. 28, no. 6, pp. 419–425, 2012.

[66] S. N. Amin and W. A. Ebeid, "Shoulder reconstruction after tumor resection by pedicled scapular crest graft," *Clinical Orthopaedics and Related Research*, vol. 397, pp. 133–142, 2002.

[67] G. Padiolleau, J. B. Marchand, G. A. Odri, A. Hamel, and F. Gouin, "Scapulo-humeral arthrodesis using a pedicled scapular pillar graft following resection of the proximal humerus," *Orthopaedics & Traumatology: Surgery & Research*, vol. 100, no. 2, pp. 177–181, 2014.

[68] D. Barbier, B. De Billy, P. Gicquel, S. Bourelle, and P. Journeau, "Is the clavicula pro humero technique of value for reconstruction after resection of the proximal humerus in children?," *Clinical Orthopaedics & Related Research*, vol. 475, no. 10, pp. 2550–2561, 2017.

[69] G. T. Calvert, J. Wright, J. Agarwal, K. B. Jones, and L. R. Randall, "Is claviculo pro humeri of value for limb salvage of pediatric proximal humerus sarcomas?," *Clinical Orthopaedics & Related Research*, vol. 473, no. 3, pp. 877–882, 2015.

[70] S. Tsukushi, Y. Nishida, M. Takahashi, and N. Ishiguro, "Clavicula pro humero reconstruction after wide resection of the proximal humerus," *Clinical Orthopaedics & Related Research*, vol. 447, pp. 132–137, 2006.

[71] K. M. Zekry, N. Yamamoto, K. Hayashi et al., "Reconstruction of intercalary bone defect after resection of malignant bone tumor," *Journal of Orthopaedic Surgery (Hong Kong)*, vol. 27, no. 1, 2019.

[72] A. M. Jakoi, J. A. Iorio, and P. J. Cahill, "Autologous bone graft harvesting: a review of grafts and surgical techniques," *Musculoskeletal Surgery*, vol. 99, no. 3, pp. 171–178, 2015.

[73] M. J. Hubble, "Bone grafts," *Surgical Technology International*, vol. 10, pp. 261–265, 2002.

[74] E. Nkenke and F. W. Neukam, "Autogenous bone harvesting and grafting in advanced jaw resorption: morbidity, resorption and implant survival," *European Journal of Oral Implantology*, vol. 7, no. 2, pp. S203–S217, 2014.

[75] S. Stevenson, "Biology of bone grafts," *Orthopedic Clinics of North America*, vol. 30, no. 4, pp. 543–552, 1999.

[76] L. Zhang, Y. Fan, Y. Zhang, X. Chen, and Y. Liu, "Comparison of sartorius muscle-pedicle and circumflex iliac deep bone flap grafts in the treatment of early non-traumatic osteonecrosis of femoral head in young adults," *Acta Orthopaedica et Traumatologica Turcica*, vol. 53, no. 4, pp. 255–259, 2019.

[77] R. H. Gross, "The use of bone grafts and bone graft substitutes in pediatric orthopaedics: an overview," *Journal of Pediatric Orthopaedics*, vol. 32, no. 1, pp. 100–105, 2012.

[78] C. N. Steiger, P. Journeau, and P. Lascombes, "The role of the periosteal sleeve in the reconstruction of bone defects using a non-vascularised fibula graft in the pediatric population," *Orthopaedics & Traumatology: Surgery & Research*, vol. 103, no. 7, pp. 1115–1120, 2017.

[79] G. I. Taylor, G. D. H. Miller, and F. J. Ham, "The free vascularized bone graft. A clinical extension of microvascular techniques," *Plastic and Reconstructive Surgery*, vol. 55, no. 5, pp. 533–544, 1975.

[80] N. F. Jones, W. M. Swartz, D. C. Mears, J. B. Jupiter, and A. Grossman, "The "double barrel" free vascularized fibular bone graft," *Plastic and Reconstructive Surgery*, vol. 81, no. 3, pp. 378–385, 1988.

[81] W. C. Eward, V. Kontogeorgakos, L. S. Levin, and B. E. Brigman, "Free vascularized fibular graft reconstruction

of large skeletal defects after tumor resection," *Clinical Orthopaedics & Related Research*, vol. 468, no. 2, pp. 590–598, 2010.

[82] J. J. Scalise and J. P. Iannotti, "Glenohumeral arthrodesis after failed prosthetic shoulder arthroplasty," *The Journal of Bone and Joint Surgery-American Volume*, vol. 90, no. 1, pp. 70–77, 2008.

[83] G. Leblebicioglu, "Reliability of vascularized fibula in maintaining arthrodesis following extra-articular wide excisions of malignant musculoskeletal tumors," *Saudi Medical Journal*, vol. 27, no. 8, pp. 1204–1211, 2006.

[84] D. J. Clare, M. A. Wirth, G. I. Groh, and C. A. Rockwood Jr., "Shoulder arthrodesis," *The Journal of Bone and Joint Surgery-American Volume*, vol. 83, no. 4, pp. 593–600, 2001.

[85] B. Fuchs, M. I. O'Connor, D. J. Padgett, K. R. Kaufman, and F. H. Sim, "Arthrodesis of the shoulder after tumor resection," *Clinical Orthopaedics and Related Research*, vol. 436, no. 436, pp. 202–207, 2005.

[86] A. Gilbert and L. Teot, "The free scapular flap," *Plastic and Reconstructive Surgery*, vol. 69, no. 4, pp. 601–604, 1982.

[87] H. Seghrouchni, D. Martin, V. Pistre, and J. Baudet, "Composite scapular flap for recon- struction of complex humeral tissue loss: a case report," *Revue de Chirurgie Orthopedique et Reparatrice de l'Appareil Moteur*, vol. 89, pp. 158–162, 2003.

[88] V. Pinsolle, R. Tessier, V. Casoli, D. Martin, and J. Baudet, "The pedicled vascularised scapular bone flap for proximal humerus reconstruction and short humeral stump lengthening," *Journal of Plastic, Reconstructive & Aesthetic Surgery*, vol. 60, no. 9, pp. 1019–1024, 2007.

[89] O. Le Reun, G. A. Odri, V. Crenn, L.-R. Le Nail, F. Gouin, and M. Ropars, "Shoulder arthrodesis using a vascularized scapular pillar graft: cadaver study and surgical technique," *Orthopaedics & Traumatology: Surgery & Research*, vol. 105, no. 5, pp. 831–837, 2019.

[90] H. Asfazadourian, F. Teboul, and C. Oberlin, "Techniques d'arthrodèse de l'épaule," *EMC Techniques Chirurgicales—Orthopédie-Traumatologie*, vol. 15, pp. 44–287, 2001.

[91] M. Sulamaa, "Upper extremity phocomelia: a contribution to its operative treatment," *Clinical Pediatrics*, vol. 2, no. 5, pp. 251–257, 1963.

[92] G. R. Gupta, A. W. Yasko, V. O. Lewis et al., "Risk of local recurrence after deltoid-sparing resection for osteosarcoma of the proximal humerus," *Cancer*, vol. 115, no. 16, pp. 3767–3773, 2009.

[93] S. Sharma, R. E. Turcotte, M. H. Isler, and C. Wong, "Experience with cemented large segment endoprostheses for tumors," *Clinical Orthopaedics & Related Research*, vol. 459, pp. 54–59, 2007.

[94] D. Kumar, R. J. Grimer, A. Abudu, S. R. Carter, and R. M. Tillman, "Endoprosthetic replacement of the proximal humerus," *The Journal of Bone and Joint Surgery. British Volume*, vol. 85-B, no. 5, pp. 717–722, 2003.

[95] P. T. Funovics and M. Dominkus, "Modulare Tumorprothesen des Humerus," *Der Orthopäde*, vol. 39, no. 10, pp. 968–979, 2010.

[96] S. Zilber, "Shoulder arthroplasty: historical considerations," *The Open Orthopaedics Journal*, vol. 11, no. 1, pp. 1100–1107, 2017.

[97] G. Gosheger, C. Gebert, H. Ahrens, A. Streitbuerger, W. Winkelmann, and J. Hardes, "Endoprosthetic reconstruction in 250 patients with sarcoma," *Clinical Orthopaedics and Related Research*, vol. 450, pp. 164–171, 2006.

[98] F. Mittermayer, P. Krepler, M. Dominkus et al., "Long-term followup of uncemented tumor endoprostheses for the lower extremity," *Clinical Orthopaedics and Related Research*, vol. 388, pp. 167–177, 2001.

[99] M. Sluga, R. Windhager, S. Lang, H. Heinzl, S. Bielack, and R. Kotz, "Local and systemic control after ablative and limb sparing surgery in patients with osteosarcoma," *Clinical Orthopaedics and Related Research*, vol. 358, pp. 120–127, 1999.

[100] C. P. Cannon, G. U. Paraliticci, P. P. Lin et al., "Functional outcome following endoprosthetic reconstruction of the proximal humerus," *Journal of Shoulder & Elbow Surgery*, vol. 18, no. 5, pp. 705–710, 2009.

[101] A. Ross, J. Wilson, and J. Scales, "Endoprosthetic replacement of the proximal humerus," *The Journal of Bone and Joint Surgery. British Volume*, vol. 69-B, no. 4, pp. 656–661, 1987.

[102] R. x. e. A. Fuhrmann, A. Roth, and R. A. Venbrocks, "Salvage of the upper extremity in cases of tumorous destruction of the proximal humerus," *Journal of Cancer Research and Clinical Oncology*, vol. 126, no. 6, pp. 337–344, 2000.

[103] R. Wei, W. Guo, R. Yang, X. Tang, Y. Yang, and T. Ji, "Plate-prosthesis composite reconstruction after large segmental resection of proximal humeral tumors: a retrospective comparative study," *Medicine*, vol. 98, no. 22, Article ID e15787, 2019.

[104] L. De Wilde, P. Boileau, and H. Van der Bracht, "Does reverse shoulder arthroplasty for tumors of the proximal humerus reduce impairment?" *Clinical Orthopaedics & Related Research*, vol. 469, no. 9, pp. 2489–2495, 2011.

[105] H. Hu, W. Liu, Q. Zeng et al., "The personalized shoulder reconstruction assisted by 3D printing technology after resection of the proximal humerus tumours," *Cancer Management and Research*, vol. 11, pp. 10665–10673, 2019.

[106] S. Maclean, S. S. Malik, S. Evans, J. Gregory, and L. Jeys, "Reverse shoulder endoprosthesis for pathologic lesions of the proximal humerus: a minimum 3-year follow-up," *Journal of Shoulder and Elbow Surgery*, vol. 26, no. 11, pp. 1990–1994, 2017.

[107] R. Capanna, J. R. van Horn, R. Biagini, P. Ruggieri, A. Ferruzzi, and M. Campanacci, "The Tikhoff-Linberg procedure for bone tumors of the proximal humerus: the classical "extensive" technique versus a modified "transglenoid" resection," *Archives of Orthopaedic and Trauma Surgery*, vol. 109, no. 2, pp. 63–67, 1990.

[108] J. J. Creighton, C. A. Peimer, E. R. Mindell, D. C. Boone, C. P. Karakousis, and H. O. Douglass, "Primary malignant tumors of the upper extremity: retrospective analysis of one hundred twenty-six cases," *The Journal of Hand Surgery*, vol. 10, no. 6, pp. 805–814, 1985.

[109] S. B. Hahn, N. H. Kim, and N. H. Choi, "Treatment of bone tumors around the shoulder joint by the Tikhoff-Linberg procedure," *Yonsei Medical Journal*, vol. 31, no. 2, pp. 110–122, 1990.

[110] I. Kofránek and Z. Matejovský, "The Tikhoff-Linberg procedure," *Acta Chirurgiae Orthopaedicae et Traumatologiae Cechoslovaca*, vol. 66, pp. 76–81, 1999.

[111] B. E. Linberg, "Interscapulo-thoracic resection for malignant tumors of the shoulder girdle region," *Journal of Bone and Joint Surgery*, vol. 10, p. 344, 1928.

[112] N. J. Machson, "Modification of the interscapulo-thoracic resection (Tichow-Linberg's operation)," *Beiträge zur Orthopädie und Traumatologie*, vol. 15, pp. 212–215, 1968.

[113] G. Bos, F. Sim, D. Pritchard et al., "Prosthetic replacement of the proximal humerus," *Clinical Orthopaedics and Related Research*, vol. 289, no. 224, pp. 178-191, 1987.
[114] R. B. Bourne, "Prophylactic use of antibiotic bone cement: an emerg- ing standard—in the affirmative," *Journal of Arthroplasty*, vol. 19, no. 1, pp. 69–72, 2004.
[115] S. Cannon, "Massive prostheses for malignant bone tumours of the limbs," *The Journal of Bone and Joint Surgery. British Volume*, vol. 79-B, no. 3, pp. 497–506, 1997.
[116] H.-C. Chin, F. J. Frassica, M. D. Markel, D. A. Frassica, F. H. Sim, and E. Y. S. Chao, "The effects of therapeutic doses of irradiation on experimental bone graft incorporation over a porous-coated segmental defect endoprosthesis," *Clinical Orthopaedics and Related Research*, vol. 289, no. 289, pp. 254–266, 1993.
[117] I. Ilyas, R. Pant, A. Kurar, P. Moreau, and D. Younge, "Modular megaprosthesis for proximal femoral tumors," *International Orthopaedics*, vol. 26, no. 3, pp. 170–173, 2002.
[118] E. Mascard, P. Anract, A. Touchene, P. Pouillart, and B. Tomeno, "Com- plications from the hinged GUEPAR prosthesis after resection of knee tumor. 102 cases," *Revue de Chirurgie Orthopedique et Reparatrice de l'Appareil Moteur*, vol. 84, pp. 628–637, 1998.
[119] W. Plotz, H. Rechl, R. Burgkart et al., "Limb salvage with tumor endoprostheses for malig- nant tumors of the knee," *Clinical Orthopaedics and Related Research*, vol. 405, pp. 207–215, 2002.
[120] K. M. Postel, J. Evrard, and J. P. Courpied, *Arthroplastie Totale de Hanche*, Springer-Verlag, Berlin, Germany, 1985.
[121] P. S. Unwin, S. R. Cannon, R. J. Grimer, H. B. S. Kemp, R. S. Sneath, and P. S. Walker, "Aseptic loosening in cemented custom-made prosthetic replacements for bone tumours of the lower limb," *The Journal of Bone and Joint Surgery. British Volume*, vol. 78-B, no. 1, pp. 5–13, 1996.
[122] P. Z. Wirganowicz, J. J. Eckardt, F. J. Dorey, F. R. Eilber, and J. M. Kabo, "Etiology and results of tumor endoprosthesis revision surgery in 64 patients," *Clinical Orthopaedics and Related Research*, vol. 358, pp. 64–74, 1999.
[123] S. D'Adamio, A. Ziranu, G. Cazzato et al., "Antifungal properties of silver coating on tumour endoprostheses: an in vitro study," *European Review for Medical and Pharmacological Sciences*, vol. 23, no. 2, pp. 252–257, 2019.
[124] D. C. Ackland, S. Roshan-Zamir, M. Richardson, and M. G. Pandy, "Moment arms of the shoulder musculature after reverse total shoulder arthroplasty," *The Journal of Bone and Joint Surgery-American Volume*, vol. 92, no. 5, pp. 1221–1230, 2010.
[125] P. Boileau, G. Moineau, Y. Roussanne, and K. O'Shea, "Bony increased offset-reversed shoulder arthroplasty (BIO-RSA)," *JBJS Essential Surgical Techniques*, vol. 7, no. 4, p. e37, 2017.
[126] T. Ji, X. Tang, and W. Guo, "Enhancing soft-tissue reattachment in proximal humeral endoprosthetic reconstruction," *Journal of Orthopaedic Surgery*, vol. 22, no. 1, pp. 100–103, 2014.
[127] M. Moran and P. D. Stalley, "Reconstruction of the proximal humerus with a composite of extracorporeally irradiated bone and endoprosthesis following excision of high grade primary bone sarcomas," *Archives of Orthopaedic and Trauma Surgery*, vol. 129, no. 10, pp. 1339–1345, 2009.
[128] S. A. Lozano-Calderón and N. Chen, "Proximal humerus allograft prosthetic composites: technique, outcomes, and pearls and pitfalls," *Current Reviews in Musculoskeletal Medicine*, vol. 8, no. 4, pp. 324–333, 2015.
[129] J. J. King, L. M. Nystrom, N. B. Reimer, C. P. Gibbs Jr., M. T. Scarborough, and T. W. Wright, "Allograft-prosthetic composite reverse total shoulder arthroplasty for reconstruction of proximal humerus tumor resections," *Journal of Shoulder and Elbow Surgery*, vol. 25, no. 1, pp. 45–54, 2016.
[130] M. El Beaino, J. Liu, V. O. Lewis, and P. P. Lin, "Do early results of proximal humeral allograft-prosthetic composite reconstructions persist at 5-year followup?" *Clinical Orthopaedics & Related Research*, vol. 477, no. 4, pp. 758–765, 2019.
[131] C. Lazerges, L. Dagneaux, B. Degeorge, N. Tardy, B. Coulet, and M. Chammas, "Composite reverse shoulder arthroplasty can provide good function and quality of life in cases of malignant tumour of the proximal humerus," *International Orthopaedics*, vol. 41, no. 12, pp. 2619–2625, 2017.
[132] J. Sanchez-Sotelo, E. R. Wagner, and M. T. Houdek, "Allograft-prosthetic composite reconstruction for massive proximal humeral bone loss in reverse shoulder arthroplasty," *JBJS Essential Surgical Techniques*, vol. 8, no. 1, p. e3, 2018.

28

Intra- and Extra-Articular Deformity of Lower Limb: Tibial Condylar Valgus Osteotomy (TCVO) and Distal Tibial Oblique Osteotomy (DTOO) for Reconstruction of Joint Congruency

Y. Watanabe,[1] N. Takenaka,[2] K. Kinugasa,[3] T. Matsushita,[2] and T. Teramoto[2]

[1] *Department of Orthopaedic Surgery, Teikyo University School of Medicine, Tokyo, Japan*
[2] *Department of Traumatology Fukushima Medical University, Trauma and Reconstruction Center, Southern Tohoku General Hospital, Fukushima, Japan*
[3] *Department of Orthopaedic Surgery, Chikamori Hospital, Kochi, Japan*

Correspondence should be addressed to Y. Watanabe; fracture@zad.att.ne.jp

Guest Editor: Nobuyoshi Watanabe

Osteotomies are the established surgical procedure for the deformity of the lower limb induced by osteoarthritis (OA) of the knee and ankle. Closed-wedge (CW) and open-wedge (OW) high tibial osteotomy (HTO) are extra-articular surgery, which aim to shift the mechanical axis from medial to slightly lateral and reduce the overload in the medial compartment of the varus deformed knee by extra-articular correction. However, varus deformity of the knee with the teeter effect, which could be accompanied with subluxation and thrust due to the medial-lateral soft tissue imbalance, is not resolved only by the shift of mechanical axis. The depression of the medial tibia plateau, so-called pagoda deformity, is the intra-articular deformity, which could potentially cause the teeter effect and involves intra-articular incongruency. In such case, the osteotomy with novel concept should be developed to overcome the issues, both the imbalance of soft tissue and intra-articular deformity. Tibial condylar valgus osteotomy (TCVO) is an intra-articular osteotomy, which improves the joint congruency of the medial-compartment knee OA with subluxation and/or intra-articular deformity and also provides better joint stability. A similar argument is raised in the treatment of the ankle OA. Low tibial osteotomy (LTO) is an extra-articular surgery to correct malalignment of lower leg. Distal tibial oblique osteotomy (DTOO) is a novel surgery to improve the bony congruency of the ankle OA. In DTOO, the distal tibia is cut obliquely from the proximal medial to the distal lateral in the coronal plane and towards the center of the tibiofibular joint to improve the bony congruency of the ankle joint. Tibial condylar valgus osteotomy (TCVO) and distal tibial oblique osteotomy (DTOO) can correct intra-articular deformity of knee and ankle, respectively. The rationale and indication of TCVO and DTOO for the treatment of the lower limb by reconstructing the joint congruency are discussed.

1. Introduction

Deformity of the lower limb induced by osteoarthritis of the knee or ankle causes the adverse effect on daily living due to gait disturbance, which could cause abnormal posture, as well as local problem such as pain. Various surgical procedures have been performed such as femoral, tibial osteotomies, and hip and knee arthroplasties to overcome these issues. Osteotomies are the established surgical options for the treatment of lower limb.

Osteoarthritis of the knee is a representative disease, which involves malalignment of the lower limb with the joint degeneration. Arthroplasty of the knee, involving total knee arthroplasty (TKA), unicompartmental knee arthroplasty (UKA), is established as surgical procedures with good clinical results [1–3]. Around knee osteotomies (AKO) have also been performed extensively for the treatment of this disease and have shown the good clinical outcomes by correcting the alignment of lower limb. High tibial osteotomy (HTO) is performed extensively, which aims to correct the varus knee arthrosis. Many studies demonstrated the good results by cutting the proximal tibia as lateral closed-wedge high tibial valgus osteotomy (CWHTO) or dome valgus osteotomy. Medial open-wedge high tibial valgus osteotomy (OWHTO) has also been developed for the correction of the varus deformed knee and extensively spread by the improvement in surgical technique, fixation devices, and patient selection with fewer complications [4–7]. Hybrid closed-wedge osteotomy, combining OWHTO and CWHTO, has currently performed with disadvantages of traditional CWHTO including lateral-offset, loss of the large bone block below the lateral tibial plateau, and discrepancies in the leg length [8]. High tibial valgus osteotomy is an established surgical procedure to correct varus malalignment in patients with medial-compartment OA of the knee; however, the deformity center of the malalignment of lower limb varies in each case. Distal femoral osteotomy (DFO) has also been performed for the patient with osteoarthritis with the deformity in distal femur and increasingly performed alone or combination with HTO with the improvement in such as surgical technique and fixation devices same as development of medial opening wedge HTO.

The concept of traditional HTO has been the extra-articular correction of the alignment, aiming at the reduction of the overload in the medial compartment of the varus deformed knee by shifting the mechanical axis from medial to slightly lateral. On the other hand, deformities of the lower limb are affected by several factors. The bony deformity and soft tissue balance are the different issues relating to the malalignment. Varus deformity in OA of the knee without excessed medial loosening of soft tissue could be corrected by usual HTO, which is the extra-articular correction with transfer of the mechanical axis. However, the varus deformity of the knee with the teeter effect, which is the medial-lateral soft tissue imbalance, is not resolved only by the shift of mechanical axis to lateral. The depression of the medial tibia plateau, so-called pagoda deformity, is the intra-articular deformity, which could cause intra-articular incongruency and the teeter effect. In such case, the osteotomy with novel concept should be developed to overcome the issues, both the imbalance of soft tissue and intra-articular deformity; otherwise the relief of the pain and disability would not be achieved.

For the treatment of osteoarthritis of ankle joint, the same argument exists as the correction of the varus knee. Low tibial osteotomy (LTO) for osteoarthritis of ankle joint has been performed to change the load distribution on the ankle joint by changing the extra-articular alignment [9, 10]. However, if instability of the talotibial joint exists, novel surgical concept should be induced for the treatment of the osteoarthritis of the ankle joint. Distal tibial oblique osteotomy (DTOO) developed is an operation to improve the bony congruency of the ankle joint by the oblique osteotomy from the proximal medial to the distal lateral in the coronal plane and towards the center of the tibiofibular joint to realign the bony congruency of the ankle joint [11–13].

Considering the correction of lower limb alignment, regardless of cause of mal-alignment, such as post-traumatic, degenerative, or congenital, we need to consider two kinds of deformities: extra-articular and intra-articular deformity. Extra-articular deformity can be discussed under static loading condition, and intra-articular deformity should be discussed under dynamic loading condition.

Extra-articular deformity in frontal plane is evaluated by the measurement of the standing long-leg AP view. Theoretically, there are 728 kinds of extra-articular deformity, and these deformities can be accurately corrected by using hexapod system. Evaluation of intra-articular deformity should be evaluated by dynamic motion of the contours of the bone facing in the joint. Tibial condylar valgus osteotomy (TCVO) and distal tibial oblique osteotomy (DTOO) can correct intra-articular deformity of knee and ankle, respectively.

2. Extra-Articular Deformity and Lower Limb Alignment

Traditionally the degree of extra-articular deformity of the frontal plane has been expressed as the degree of deviation from the mechanical axis of the lower extremity [14] (Figure 1). The mechanical axis of the lower extremity is determined by drawing a line from the center of the femoral head to the center of the ankle joint. The distance between the mechanical axis line and the center of the knee in the frontal plane is called as the mechanical axial deviation (MAD) [15, 16] (Figure 2). Normally, the medial MAD is 1 mm to 15 mm.

The frontal plane knee joint orientation line of the distal femur is drawn as a line tangential to the most distal point on the convexity of the two femoral condyles. The frontal plane knee joint line of the proximal tibia is drawn across the subchondral line of the two tibial plateaus. The angle formed between joint orientation lines on opposite sides of the same joint is called the joint line convergence angle (JLCA) [14]. The ankle JLCA is defined as the angle formed between the tibial joint line axis and the talar joint line axis (Figure 3). In the knee and ankle joints, each JLCA is measured as 0°-2° and -1°-1°, respectively.

The deviation from the normal of the lower extremity alignment can be evaluated by the joint orientation angles, such as MPTA, LDFA, LPDA, etc. measured with the full leg standing frontal X-ray image of the lower limb [14] (Figure 1). Malalignment occurs when the center of the joint does not lie close to mechanical axis line. The MAD is described as either medial (varus) or lateral (valgus) MADs (Figure 1).

Angular deformity has four types: varus/valgus deformity at the frontal plane and procurvatum/recurvatum deformity at the sagittal plane. Similarly, there are four kinds of deformities in translation (medial/lateral at the frontal plane, and anterior/posterior at the sagittal plane) and axial (internal/external rotation and shortening/elongation) deformities. Consequently, there are 728 patterns of extra-articular deformities.

The angular deformity correction of lower limb can be achieved using hinges set on center of rotation of angulation (CORA) of the connecting rods by Ilizarov technique [14]. Currently used hexapod external fixator system can correct multi-directional extra-articular deformity accurately within the rage of measurement in units of 1 mm and 1° [17, 18] (Figures 4 and 5).

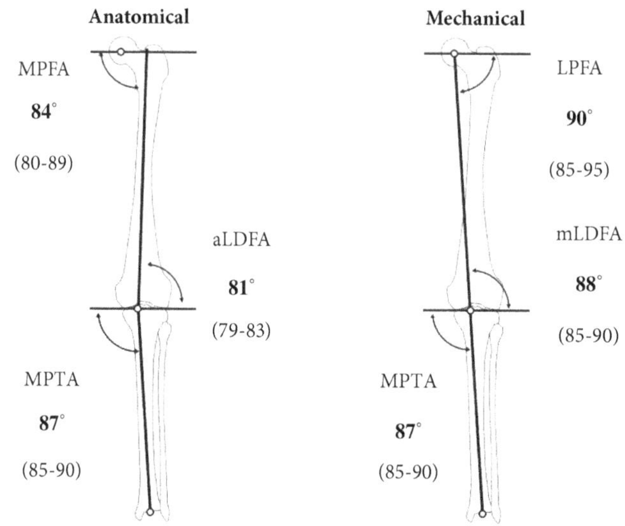

FIGURE 1: Normal lower limb alignment by Paley D.

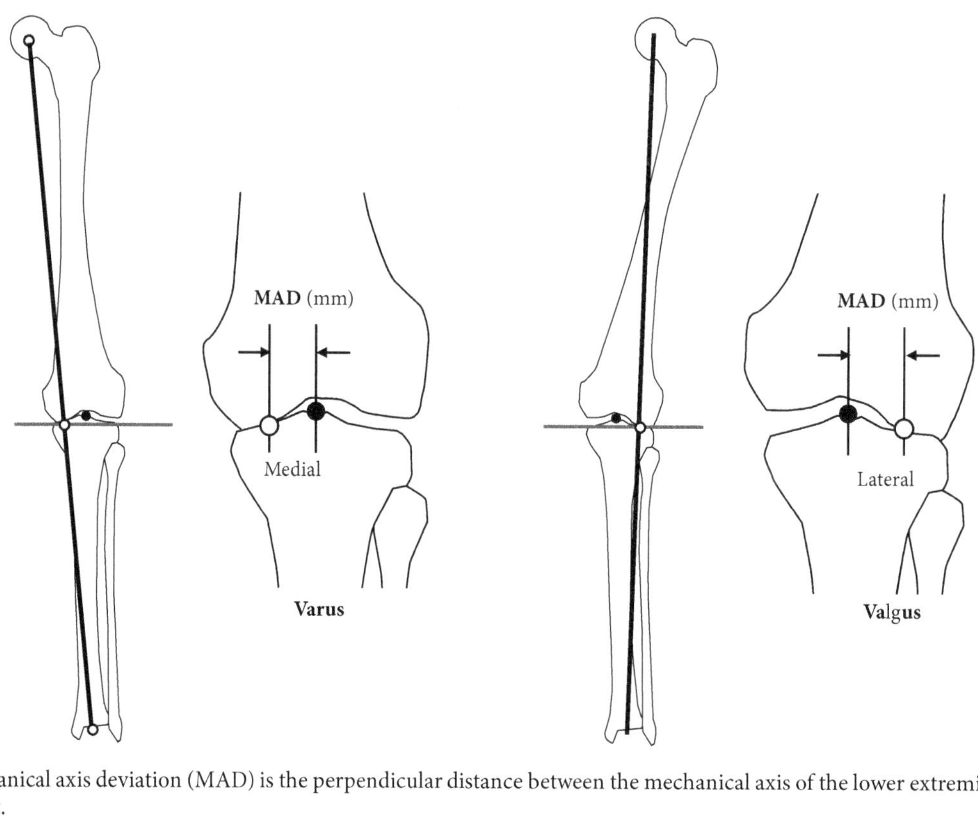

FIGURE 2: Mechanical axis deviation (MAD) is the perpendicular distance between the mechanical axis of the lower extremity and the center of the knee joint.

3. Intra-Articular Deformity and Joint Congruency

Intra-articular deformity means joint congruency. Joint congruency is defined as the fittings of two opposing joint surfaces as they relate to one another considering the spatial contour of each bone at their interface.

In theory, joint congruency can be mainly explained by three factors: contours of bone, functions of ligament, and integrity of articular cartilage and meniscus. Incongruency of the joint immediately causes joint instability or abnormal joint kinematics resulting in the secondary osteoarthritis in the future. For example, mal-union of tibial plateau fracture and/or knee ligament injury such as anterior cruciate

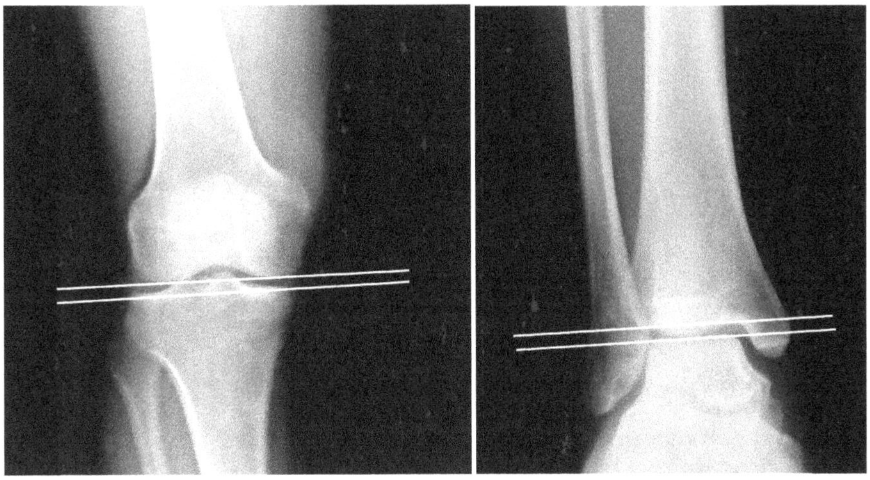

FIGURE 3: Joint line convergence angle (JLCA) for knee and ankle.

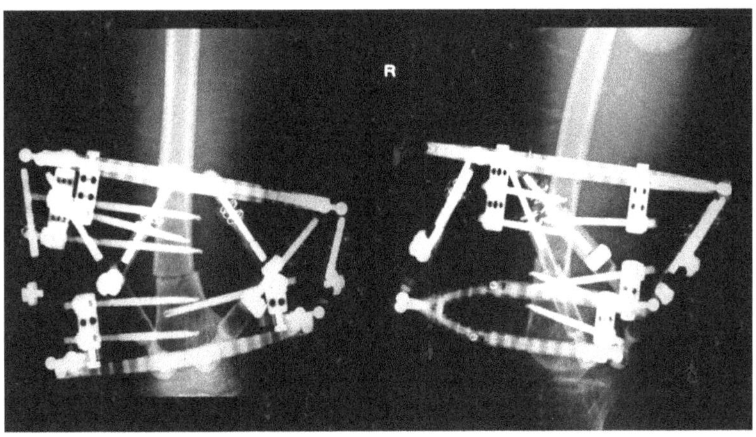

(a)

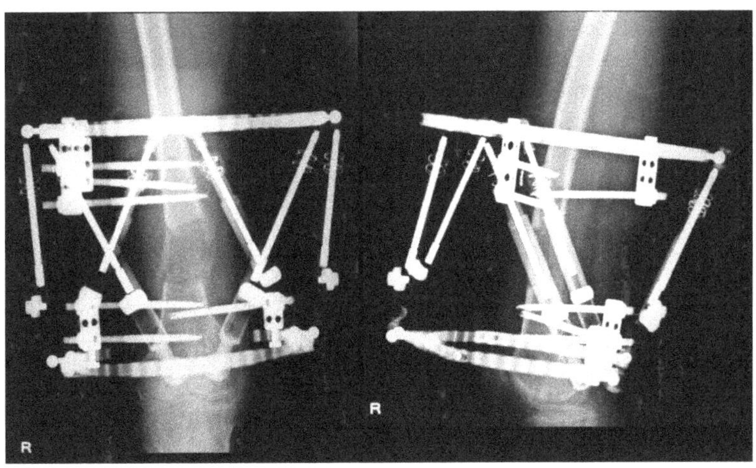

(b)

FIGURE 4: Reconstruction of multidirectional deformity by using the hexapod external fixator system. (a) Application of a hexapod external fixator; (b) completion of the reconstruction program.

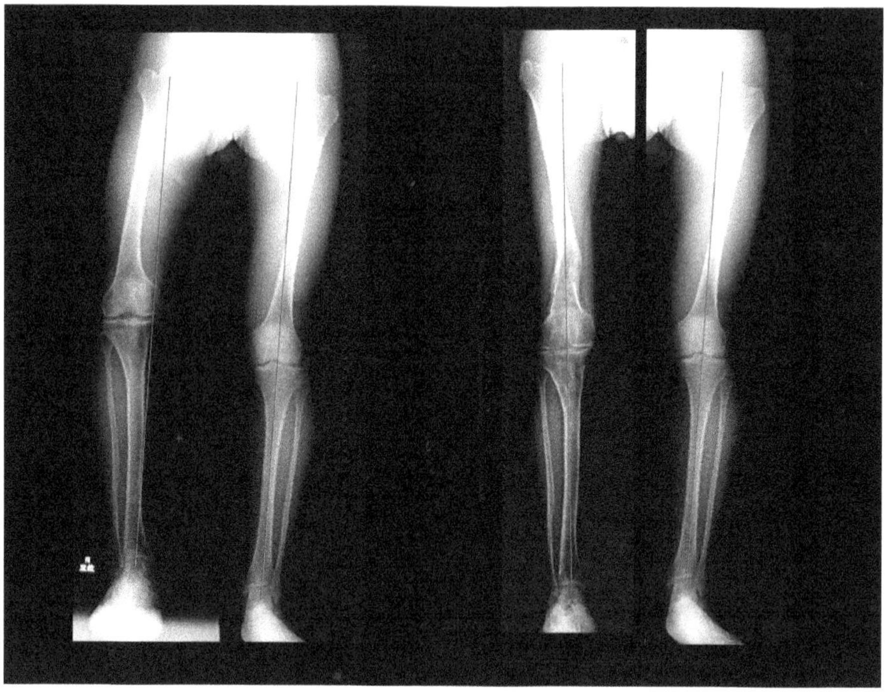

Figure 5: Correction of extra-articular deformity by using hexapod external fixator system. X-ray photos (a) before and (b) after reconstruction.

ligament and/or collateral ligaments causes easily knee instability and secondary osteoarthritis of the involved knee with joint incongruency (Figure 6(a)).

Two primary biomechanical purposes of the articular cartilage are lubrication and shock absorption. The articular cartilage provides a smooth lubricated surface for low friction articulation and acts as a remarkably efficient shock absorber [19, 20].

From the view point of joint congruency, it is considered that the effect of articular cartilage as the shock absorber is not large because the thickness of articular cartilage is thin as 1 - 4 mm. Rather in the cartilaginous element, the menisci may be more important because they have a large effect of filling the gap of the joint [21]. However, cartilage and meniscus do not function enough when the intra-articular bony deformity occurred. Furthermore, ligament function is effective only when the contour of bone is not impaired. Therefore, joint congruency due to the contour of bone plays the most important role.

4. TCVO (Tibial Condylar Valgus Osteotomy) and HTO (High Tibial Osteotomy)

High tibial osteotomy (HTO) is intended to transfer the mechanical axis from medial to slightly lateral to the midline of the knee to decrease the load and subsequently delay osteoarthritis (OA) [22–24]. There are discussions about which alignment is best in HTO but we think that it should be discussed first whether accurate lower extremity alignment can be obtained by the procedures reported [25–31]. If we aim to acquire more accurate lower limb alignment, we should use hexapod external fixator which can theoretically correct extra-articular alignment accurately within the range of measurements in units of 1 mm and 1°.

On the other hand, tibial condylar valgus osteotomy (TCVO) developed by Chiba G et al. in 1989 and published in 1994 is an operation that corrects intra-articular deformity [32, 33] (Figures 6(b) and 7). The main strategy of this surgery is to obtain joint stability and congruency, which is totally different from that of HTO to correct malalignment [32, 33] (Figure 8). TCVO is an operation to acquire the bony joint stability between femur and tibia by the "L" shaped osteotomy of medial tibial condyle and spreading it [32, 33] (Figure 7). It is determined how much the medial tibial condyle is spread by judging joint stability under fluoroscopic dynamic stress test including the rotational stability. However, performing TCVO on a common varus knee improves lower limb alignment (Figure 8). The correction of alignment is an accessory benefit, which is subsequently brought by TCVO. It should not be misunderstood that TCVO is one of HTO subtypes and be aware that the main concept of TCVO is to obtain the joint stability and congruency.

5. Distal Tibial Oblique Osteotomy (DTOO) and Low Tibial Osteotomy (LTO)

The same argument holds for distal tibial oblique osteotomy (DTOO) and low tibial osteotomy (LTO) for osteoarthritis of ankle joint. LTO is an operation of an attempt to change the load distribution on the ankle joint by changing the extra-articular alignment. However, if instability of the talo-tibial

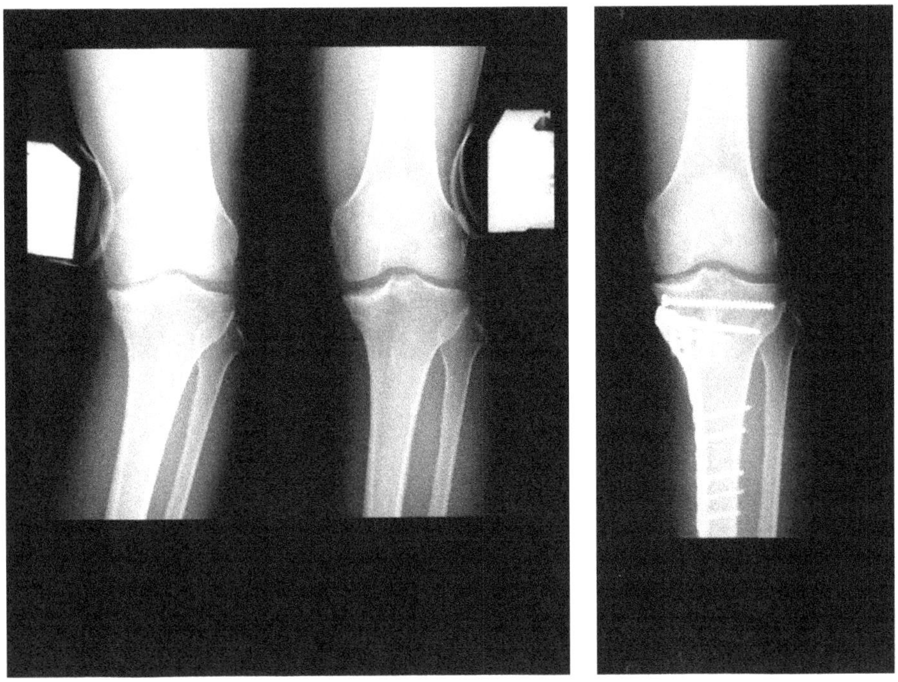

(a) (b)

FIGURE 6: (a) Teeter effect due to intra-articular deformity after medial tibial plateau fracture. (b) After reconstruction by tibial condylar valgus osteotomy (TCVO).

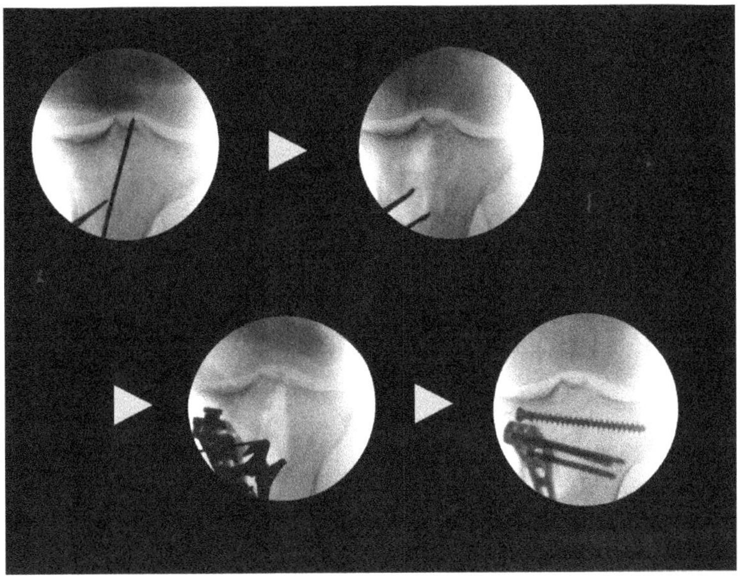

FIGURE 7: Tibial condylar valgus osteotomy (TCVO).

joint exists (Figure 9), improvement of the joint function by LTO depends on luck by self-centering function of the talus.

On the other hand, DTOO developed by Teramoto in 1994 is an operation to improve the bony congruency of the ankle joint [11]. DTOO consists of oblique osteotomy from the proximal medial to the distal lateral in the coronal plane and towards the center of the tibiofibular joint and then widening of the osteotomy site to realign the bony congruency of the ankle joint (Figure 10). DTOO is a surgical technique to realign the ankle joint surface. The shape of the ankle joint surface is changed by cutting and tilting the tibial plafond without osteotomy of the fibula. The inclination of the distal tibial articular surface with respect to the tibial axis is altered, with associated improvement in ankle stability [11–13]. The oblique osteotomy site is spread until the lateral talar articular surface contact with the lateral fibular malleolus.

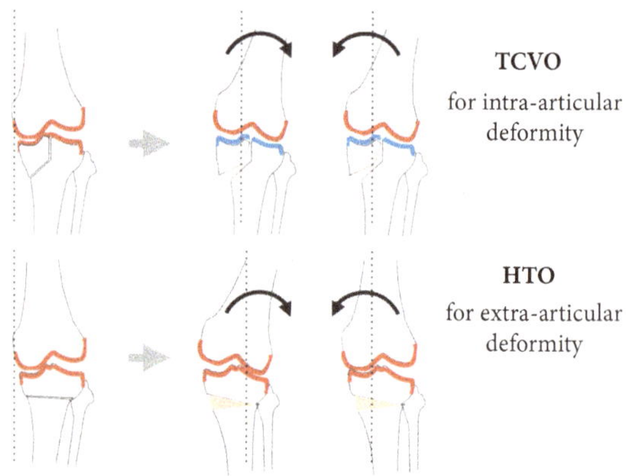

FIGURE 8: TCVO can reconstruct the joint congruency and alignment, however, HTO change only static lower limb alignment. Teeter effect cannot be improved by HTO.

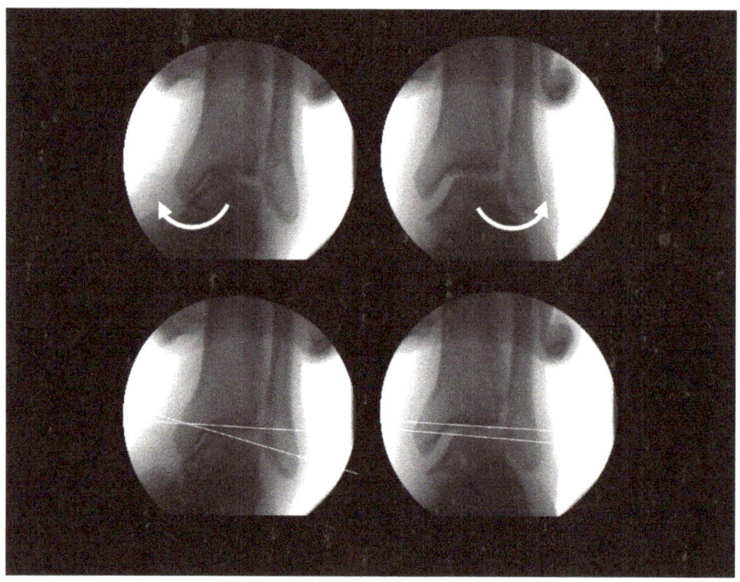

FIGURE 9: Instability of talotibial joint.

The ankle mortise congruency is restored since medial and lateral articular gutters on either side of the talar body are symmetrical which induces the increase of contact area of the talar articular surface with the tibia and fibula. The increased contact area, dispersed load pressure across the ankle joint, and decrease in the load pressure per unit area applied to the ankle joint would improve congruency between the articular surfaces of the talar dome and distal tibial plafond and the medial and lateral gutters of the ankle mortise would improve ankle stability.

6. Discussion

Although osteotomies are effective in managing malalignment of knee and ankle arthrosis, determination regarding the type of osteotomy should be based on the pathology in each patient. The cause of deformity of the knee varies, which involves intra- and extra-articular or the combination of them. Center of the deformity may also vary. Soft tissue balance should be another critical issue for the selection of optimal osteotomy type. Traditional HTO should be an optimal strategy to overcome the malalignment in OA of the knee; however, the excessed medial-lateral soft tissue imbalance and intra-articular deformity are not solved by this surgical procedure. Tibial condylar valgus osteotomy (TCVO) should be an optimal option to overcome these issues that improves intra-articular deformity followed by acquisition of medial-lateral stability of the knee, not lower limb alignment. Although LTO is the good treatment for the deformity in OA of ankle by the extra-articular correction of alignment, treatment for incongruency and instability for OA in ankle is the remaining issue of this surgical technique. Distal tibial oblique osteotomy improves the bony congruency of the ankle joint by the oblique osteotomy.

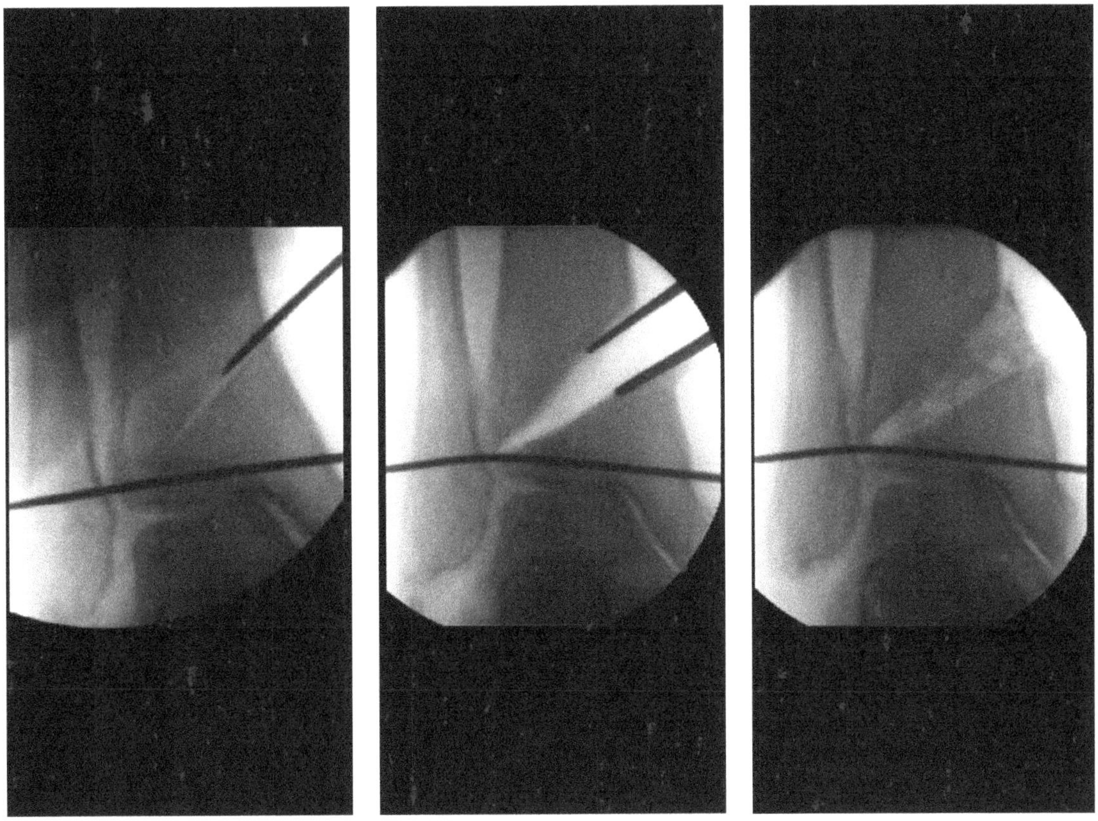

(a) (b) (c)

FIGURE 10: Distal tibial oblique osteotomy (DTOO).

Tibial condylar valgus osteotomy and DTOO that correct intra-articular deformity of knee and ankle are the optimal osteotomies for OA with intra-articular deformity and instability.

References

[1] R. S. Aujla and C. N. Esler, "Total knee arthroplasty for osteoarthritis in patients less than fifty-five years of age: a systematic review," *The Journal of Arthroplasty*, vol. 32, no. 8, pp. 2598–2603, 2017.

[2] H. Siman, A. F. Kamath, N. Carrillo, W. S. Harmsen, M. W. Pagnano, and R. J. Sierra, "Unicompartmental knee arthroplasty vs total knee arthroplasty for medial compartment arthritis in patients older than 75 years: comparable reoperation, revision, and complication rates," *The Journal of Arthroplasty*, vol. 32, no. 6, pp. 1792–1797, 2017.

[3] E. Franceschetti, G. Torre, A. Palumbo et al., "No difference between cemented and cementless total knee arthroplasty in young patients: a review of the evidence," *Knee Surgery, Sports Traumatology, Arthroscopy*, vol. 25, no. 6, pp. 1749–1756, 2017.

[4] T. Duivenvoorden, R. W. Brouwer, A. Baan et al., "Comparison of closing-wedge and opening-wedge high tibial osteotomy for medial compartment osteoarthritis of the knee: a randomized controlled trial with a six-year follow-up," *The Journal of Bone & Joint Surgery—American Volume*, vol. 96, no. 17, pp. 1425–1432, 2014.

[5] S. Floerkemeier, A. E. Staubli, S. Schroeter, S. Goldhahn, and P. Lobenhoffer, "Outcome after high tibial open-wedge osteotomy: A retrospective evaluation of 533 patients," *Knee Surgery, Sports Traumatology, Arthroscopy*, vol. 21, no. 1, pp. 170–180, 2013.

[6] C. Hui, L. J. Salmon, A. Kok et al., "Long-term survival of high tibial osteotomy for medial compartment osteoarthritis of the knee," *The American Journal of Sports Medicine*, vol. 39, no. 1, pp. 64–70, 2011.

[7] I. McNamara, T. B. Birmingham, P. J. Fowler, and J. R. Giffin, "High tibial osteotomy: evolution of research and clinical applications-a canadian experience," *Knee Surgery, Sports Traumatology, Arthroscopy*, vol. 21, no. 1, pp. 23–31, 2013.

[8] R. Takeuchi, H. Ishikawa, Y. Miyasaka, Y. Sasaki, T. Kuniya, and S. Tsukahara, "A novel closed-wedge high tibial osteotomy procedure to treat osteoarthritis of the knee: hybrid technique and rehabilitation measures," *Arthroscopy Techniques*, vol. 3, no. 4, pp. e431–e437, 2014.

[9] Y. Takakura, Y. Tanaka, T. Kumai, and S. Tamai, "Low tibial osteotomy for osteoarthritis of the ankle. Results of a new operation in 18 patients," *The Journal of Bone & Joint Surgery (British Volume)*, vol. 77, no. 1, pp. 50–54, 1995.

[10] Y. Tanaka, Y. Takakura, K. Hayashi, A. Taniguchi, T. Kumai, and K. Sugimoto, "Low tibial osteotomy for varus-type osteoarthritis of the ankle," *The Journal of Bone & Joint Surgery (British Volume)*, vol. 88, no. 7, pp. 909–913, 2006.

[11] T. Teramoto, S. Harada, M. Takaki et al., "The Teramoto distal tibial oblique osteotomy (DTOO): surgical technique and applicability for ankle osteoarthritis with varus deformity," *Strategies in Trauma and Limb Reconstruction*, vol. 13, no. 1, pp. 43–49, 2018.

[12] T. Teramoto, K. Tasiro, K. Ootsuka, M. Takaki, Y. Makino, and T. Asahara, "The changes in the instability of the ankle joint after distal tibial oblique osteotomy performed for the treatment of osteoarthritis of the ankle joint," *Journal of Japanese Association of External Fixation and Limb Lengthening*, vol. 20, pp. 119–126, 2009.

[13] T. Teramoto, S. Harada, M. Takaki et al., "Operative methods of arthroplasty used by intra-articular osteotomy of the knee joint and ankle joint," *Journal of Japanese Association of External Fixation and Limb Lengthening*, vol. 25, pp. 169–176, 2014.

[14] D. Paley, *Principles of Deformity Correction*, Springer, Berlin, Germany, 2002.

[15] R. D. Burghardt, D. Paley, S. C. Specht, and J. E. Herzenberg, "The effect on mechanical axis deviation of femoral lengthening with an intramedullary telescopic nail," *The Journal of Bone & Joint Surgery (British Volume)*, vol. 94, no. 9, pp. 1241–1245, 2012.

[16] J. E. Gordon, R. C. Chen, M. B. Dobbs, S. J. Luhmann, M. M. Rich, and P. L. Schoenecker, "Interobserver and intraobserver reliability in the evaluation of mechanical axis deviation," *Journal of Pediatric Orthopaedics*, vol. 29, no. 3, pp. 281–284, 2009.

[17] J. L. Wilczek and G. A. LaPorta, "The evolution of limb deformity: what has changed over the past ten years?" *Clinics in Podiatric Medicine and Surgery*, vol. 35, no. 1, pp. 123–132, 2018.

[18] J. E. Arvesen, J. Tracy Watson, and H. Israel, "Effectiveness of treatment for distal tibial nonunions with associated complex deformities using a hexapod external fixator," *Journal of Orthopaedic Trauma*, vol. 31, no. 2, pp. e43–e48, 2017.

[19] A. J. Sophia Fox, A. Bedi, and S. A. Rodeo, "The basic science of articular cartilage: structure, composition, and function," *Sports Health*, vol. 1, no. 6, pp. 461–468, 2009.

[20] V. C. Mow, M. H. Holmes, and W. M. Lai, "Fluid transport and mechanical properties of articular cartilage: a review," *Journal of Biomechanics*, vol. 17, no. 5, pp. 377–394, 1984.

[21] Y. Fukuda, S. Takai, N. Yoshino et al., "Impact load transmission of the knee joint-influence of leg alignment and the role of meniscus and articular cartilage," *Clinical Biomechanics*, vol. 15, no. 7, pp. 516–521, 2000.

[22] P. Maquet, "The treatment of choice in osteoarthritis of the knee," *Clinical Orthopaedics and Related Research*, vol. 192, pp. 108–112, 1985.

[23] M. B. Coventry, "Osteotomy about the knee for degenerative and rheumatoid arthritis," *The Journal of Bone & Joint Surgery* vol. 55, no. 1, pp. 23–48, 1973.

[24] Y. Akamatsu, T. Koshino, T. Saito, and J. Wada, "Changes in osteosclerosis of the osteoarthritic knee after high tibial osteotomy," *Clinical Orthopaedics and Related Research*, no. 334, pp. 207–214, 1997.

[25] I. Ivarsson, R. Myrnerts, and J. Gillquist, "High tibial osteotomy for medial osteoarthritis of the knee. A 5 to 7 and an 11 to 13 year follow-up," *The Journal of Bone & Joint Surgery (British Volume)* vol. 72, no. 2, pp. 238–244, 1990.

[26] P. Hernigou, D. Medevielle, J. Debeyre, and D. Goutallier, "Proximal tibial osteotomy for osteoarthritis with varus deformity. A ten to thirteen-year follow-up study," *The Journal of Bone & Joint Surgery*, vol. 69, no. 3, pp. 332–354, 1987.

[27] M. B. Coventry, "Upper tibial osteotomy for osteoarthritis," *The Journal of Bone & Joint Surgery*, vol. 67, no. 7, pp. 1136–1140, 1985.

[28] G. M. Engel and F. G. Lippert 3rd, "Valgus tibial osteotomy: avoiding the pitfalls," *Clinical Orthopaedics and Related Research*, vol. 160, no. 160, pp. 137–143, 1981.

[29] D. B. Kettelkamp and E. Y. Chao, "A method for quantitative analysis of medial and lateral compression forces at the knee during standing," *Clinical Orthopaedics and Related Research*, vol. 83, pp. 202–213, 1972.

[30] T. Koshino, T. Morii, J. Wada, H. Saito, N. Ozawa, and K. Noyori, "High tibial osteotomy with fixation by a blade plate for medial compartment osteoarthritis of the knee," *Orthopedic Clinics of North America*, vol. 20, no. 2, pp. 227–243, 1989.

[31] R. Myrnerts, "Optimal correction in high tibial osteotomy for varus deformity," *Acta Orthopaedica*, vol. 51, no. 4, pp. 689–693, 1980.

[32] G. Chiba, "Tibial condylar valgus osteotomy for osteoarthritis of knee," *OS Now*, vol. 13, pp. 159–166, 1994 (Japanese).

[33] T. Teramoto, "Controversy of high tibial osteotomy," *Journal of Limb Lengthening & Reconstruction*, vol. 1, no. 1, pp. 38–41, 2015.

29

Shoulder Arthrodesis versus Upper Trapezius Transfer for Traumatic Brachial Plexus Injury

Dafang Zhang,[1,2] Rohit Garg,[2,3] Brandon E. Earp,[1,2] Philip Blazar,[1,2] and George S. M. Dyer[1,2]

[1]*Department of Orthopaedic Surgery, Brigham and Women's Hospital, 15 Francis St, Boston, MA 02115, USA*
[2]*Department of Orthopaedic Surgery, Massachusetts General Hospital, 55 Fruit St, Boston, MA 02114, USA*
[3]*Harvard Medical School, 25 Shattuck St, Boston, MA 02115, USA*

Correspondence should be addressed to Dafang Zhang; dizzhang@gmail.com

Academic Editor: Andreas K. Demetriades

Shoulder arthrodesis and upper trapezius transfer are two surgical options for secondary shoulder reconstruction for traumatic brachial plexus injury (BPI). There is a lack of comparative evidence to guide the choice for one procedure over the other. The objectives of this study were to compare (1) rates of complications and reoperation and (2) shoulder range of motion and functional outcome scores following shoulder arthrodesis versus upper trapezius transfer for traumatic BPI. A systematic review and meta-analysis were conducted by a search of four databases of studies assessing shoulder arthrodesis and/or upper trapezius transfer for shoulder reconstruction following adult traumatic BPI. A proportional meta-analysis was performed using a random effects model in anticipation of unobserved heterogeneity. The final meta-analysis included 374 patients from 17 studies, including 232 patients from 11 studies on shoulder arthrodesis and 142 patients from 6 studies on upper trapezius transfer. Shoulder arthrodesis had higher rates of complications and reoperations than upper trapezius transfer for traumatic BPI, but these differences did not reach a statistical significance. Due to the limited sample size, variations in reporting, and study heterogeneity in the published literature, we were not able to draw conclusions regarding shoulder range of motion and functional outcome scores between these two procedures. Shoulder arthrodesis and upper trapezius transfer are both viable options for secondary shoulder reconstruction for traumatic BPI, but with different complications and reoperation profiles. Patients should be counseled on the risk of nonunion and humerus fracture following shoulder arthrodesis.

1. Introduction

Adult traumatic brachial plexus injuries (BPI) are uncommon but devastating injuries to the upper extremity [1]. The primary reconstruction of traumatic BPI generally consists of nerve grafting, nerve transfer, or tendon transfer. Lack of shoulder function is a common problem after traumatic BPI due to paralysis of the deltoid, supraspinatus, and infraspinatus. Such a flail shoulder can arise due to the severity of the initial injury, failure of spontaneous recovery, paucity of viable donor nerves for primary nerve reconstruction, or failure of primary nerve reconstruction [2]. A flail shoulder can cause pain due to inferior instability of the glenohumeral joint, and an unstable glenohumeral joint can adversely affect function by the unwanted dissipation of elbow flexion power [3].

Secondary reconstruction options for the flail shoulder in the setting of traumatic BPI include shoulder arthrodesis [3] and upper trapezius transfer [2, 4]. Intact motor function in the periscapular muscles, including the trapezius, levator scapulae, serratus anterior, and rhomboids, is preferred for an optimal functional result after shoulder arthrodesis, but not required [3]. The prerequisites for upper trapezius transfer include at least M4 strength in the trapezius muscle, passive glenohumeral joint motion to at least 80°, and no advanced degeneration of the glenohumeral joint [5–8]. There is a lack of comparative evidence of shoulder arthrodesis versus upper trapezius transfer for the secondary reconstruction of traumatic BPI to provide patients and surgeons guidance in choosing between these two surgical options.

The objectives of this study were to perform a systematic review and proportional meta-analysis of the available published data to determine whether there are any differences in (1) postoperative complications and reoperations and (2) shoulder range of motion and functional outcome scores after shoulder arthrodesis versus upper trapezius transfer for the secondary reconstruction of traumatic BPI. Our null hypotheses were that no differences in the rate of complication, the rate of reoperation, final range of motion, and functional outcome scores exist between these two procedures.

2. Materials and Methods

A systematic review and meta-analysis were conducted according to the Cochrane Handbook for Systematic Reviews of Interventions guideline and reported according to the Preferred Reporting Items for Systematic Reviews and Meta-Analyses (PRISMA) guideline.

2.1. Types of Studies. Randomized and nonrandomized comparative studies and observational studies were considered for inclusion. Editorials, letters, commentaries, protocols, practice guidelines, systematic reviews, and animal studies were not included. There were no language or publication date criteria for inclusion.

2.2. Types of Interventions. Studies assessing clinical outcomes of shoulder arthrodesis and/or upper trapezius transfer for shoulder reconstruction following adult traumatic BPI were considered for inclusion. We excluded studies of interventions pertaining to brachial plexus birth palsy, iatrogenic BPI, nontraumatic BPI, radiation-induced BPI, isolated axillary nerve palsy, and other pathologies for which shoulder arthrodesis and/or upper trapezius transfer may be performed, such as poliomyelitis. Studies of combined indications were excluded if greater than 10% of patients underwent shoulder arthrodesis and/or upper trapezius transfer for an indication other than traumatic BPI.

2.3. Search Strategy. A comprehensive search of the earliest available publications to September 20, 2020, was conducted of four databases: MEDLINE, EMBASE, CENTRAL, and the U.S. National Institutes of Health registry of clinical trials (https://www.ClinicalTrials.gov). MeSH headings and subheadings were used in various combinations and supplemented with free text to optimize sensitivity. Keywords related to the pathology (e.g., "brachial plexus") were combined with keywords related to the study interventions (e.g., "shoulder arthrodesis" and "trapezius transfer"). The bibliographies of pertinent studies were reviewed for additional studies meeting inclusion criteria.

2.4. Outcome Measures. The main outcome measures of this meta-analysis were (1) postoperative complications and reoperations and (2) shoulder range of motion and functional outcome scores at the time of final follow-up.

2.5. Data Extraction. Titles and abstracts of candidate studies were screened according to inclusion and exclusion criteria, and studies were excluded if they did not pertain to the topic under review. Subsequently, the full-text articles of the remaining potentially eligible studies were retrieved and reviewed for data extraction versus exclusion. Data extraction was performed using a standardized data extraction form, which included study demographics, study interventions, follow-up duration, and outcomes.

2.6. Risk of Bias. All 17 included studies in this systematic review were observational studies (level IV therapeutic evidence). The Methodological Index for Nonrandomized Studies (MINORS) score was used to assess the quality of each study and the potential for bias [9].

2.7. Statistical Analysis. Since the systematic review yielded observational studies of shoulder arthrodesis and/or upper trapezius transfer, not comparative studies, a proportional meta-analysis was performed [10]. A meta-analysis was performed for the prevalence of postoperative complications and reoperations using a random effects model in anticipation of unobserved heterogeneity. Similarly, a meta-analysis of range of motion was performed using a random effects model. Since the observational studies in the meta-analysis are heterogeneous (e.g., age, BPI pattern, surgical technique, and rehabilitation), a random effects model was chosen and assumes that the true effect varies between studies. The combined effect in a random effects model estimates the mean effect in a distribution of effects assumed to be a random sample. Weights are assigned to studies in a random effects model by the inverse of the variance of the effect, taking into account within-study and between-study variances. Compared with a fixed effects model, weights assigned in a random effects model are generally more balanced, such that larger studies are not overly dominant and small studies are not ignored. Heterogeneity was measured using the I^2 statistic. The standard significance criteria of $p < 0.05$ was used. Meta-analysis was performed using MetaXL version 5.3 for Windows (Brisbane, Queensland, Australia).

2.8. Study Characteristics and Quality. Four hundred sixty-three articles were identified by the initial query, including 315 articles by querying shoulder arthrodesis and 148 articles by querying trapezius transfer. After exclusion of duplicate articles, 318 articles remained; these articles were screened according to our inclusion and exclusion criteria. Twenty-eight full-text articles were reviewed, and after application of inclusion and exclusion criteria, 17 articles were included in the final meta-analysis, including 11 articles on shoulder arthrodesis and 6 articles on upper trapezius transfer (Figure 1) [5, 8, 11–23].

The meta-analysis included 374 patients, with a mean age of 29 years, 92% of whom were male. The mean duration of time from injury to surgery was 46 months. The mean duration of postoperative follow-up was 38 months, and minimum postoperative follow-up was 6 months (Table 1). The majority of shoulder arthrodeses was performed for complete BPI, whereas the plurality of upper trapezius transfers was performed for upper trunk BPI (Table 2).

The meta-analysis included 232 patients who underwent shoulder arthrodesis at a mean age of 28 years, 94% of whom were male. The mean duration of time from injury to shoulder arthrodesis was 37 months, and the mean duration of postoperative follow-up was 48 months. The meta-analysis included 142 patients who underwent upper trapezius transfer at a mean age of 29 years, 88% of whom were male. The mean duration of time from injury to upper trapezius transfer was 54 months, and the mean duration of postoperative follow-up was 22 months.

All 17 studies included in this meta-analysis were retrospective observational studies, with a mean MINORS score of 9.8 (range 9-10). As the global ideal MINORS score is 16 for noncomparative studies, this is indicative of a moderate risk of bias in the included studies [25]. All included studies had a minimum of 6 months postoperative follow-up, and 16 out of 17 had a minimum of 1 year postoperative follow-up. Only 9 out of 17 studies specified the pattern of brachial plexus injury. No study reported an adequate discussion of power.

3. Results

3.1. Complications and Reoperations. Eighty-nine complications occurred in 374 procedures (24%) in this meta-analysis. Sixty-seven complications occurred in 232 shoulder arthrodesis procedures (29%), and 22 complications occurred in 142 upper trapezius transfer procedures (15%) (Table 3). The overall weighted prevalence of complication was 0.22 (95% CI 0.15–0.30). The weighted prevalence of complications in the shoulder arthrodesis group was 0.29 (95% CI 0.23–0.36). The weighted prevalence of complications in the upper trapezius transfer group was 0.10 (95% CI 0.01–0.24). The difference in the complication rate between the two procedures was not statistically significant (Figure 2).

Forty-five reoperations (12%) were performed in this meta-analysis. Thirty-seven reoperations were performed in the shoulder arthrodesis group (16%), and 8 reoperations were performed in the upper trapezius transfer group (6%) (Table 4). The overall weighted prevalence of reoperation was 0.11 (95% CI 0.06–0.17). The weighted prevalence of reoperations in the shoulder arthrodesis group was 0.15 (95% CI 0.08–0.23). The weighted prevalence of reoperations in the upper trapezius transfer group was 0.05 (95% CI 0.01–0.11). The difference in the complication rate between the two procedures was not statistically significant (Figure 3).

There was substantial heterogeneity among studies in the proportional meta-analysis of complications ($I^2 = 62\%$) and reoperations ($I^2 = 60\%$). [26] Funnel plots of the proportional meta-analysis of data on complications and reoperations do not demonstrate asymmetry to suggest publication bias (Figure 4).

3.2. Range of Motion and Functional Outcome Scores. Three studies in the shoulder arthrodesis group [11, 20, 21] and one study in the upper trapezius transfer group [15] reported final postoperative active shoulder forward flexion. The pooled final postoperative active shoulder forward flexion was 62° (95% CI 51–72°) in the shoulder arthrodesis group and 78° (95% CI 60–95°) in the upper trapezius transfer group, not a statistically significant difference (Figure 5). Three studies in the shoulder arthrodesis group [16, 21, 22] and three studies in the upper trapezius transfer group [5, 6, 17] reported final postoperative active shoulder abduction. The pooled final postoperative active shoulder abduction was 62° (95% CI 57–67°) in the shoulder arthrodesis group and 76° (95% CI 39–114°) in the upper trapezius transfer group, not a statistically significant difference (Figure 6). There was considerable heterogeneity among studies in the meta-analysis of forward flexion ($I^2 = 89\%$) and abduction ($I^2 = 99\%$) [26].

Three studies in the shoulder arthrodesis group [11, 16, 23] and one study in the upper trapezius transfer group [17] reported functional outcome scores. Atlan et al. reported a mean Disabilities of the Arm, Shoulder, and Hand (DASH) Score of 35.6 and American Shoulder and Elbow Surgeons (ASES) Shoulder Score of 69 in 54 patients who underwent shoulder arthrodesis with mean 37-month follow-up [11]. Esenyel et al. reported on a mean Oxford Shoulder Score (OSS) of 35 in 5 patients who underwent shoulder arthrodesis with mean 58-month follow-up [16]. Thangarajah et al. reported a mean OSS of 27 and subjective shoulder value (SSV) of 45 in 7 patients who underwent shoulder arthrodesis with mean 98-month follow-up [23]. Karki et al. reported a mean DASH score of 38 in 12 patients who underwent upper trapezius transfer with mean 24-month follow-up [17].

4. Discussion

Secondary shoulder reconstruction is commonly required in the treatment of adult traumatic BPI. The need for secondary shoulder reconstruction can arise in a variety of clinical scenarios, ranging from complete BPI with a paucity of donor options for shoulder reanimation to the failure of primary nerve reconstruction. Shoulder arthrodesis and upper trapezius transfer are two surgical options for secondary shoulder reconstruction for traumatic BPI. While there are differences in the indications for these two procedures [3, 5, 7, 8], most traumatic BPI patients are candidates for both, and there is no comparative evidence to guide the choice for one procedure over the other. The goal of the present study was to synthesize the available literature on these procedures and assess for

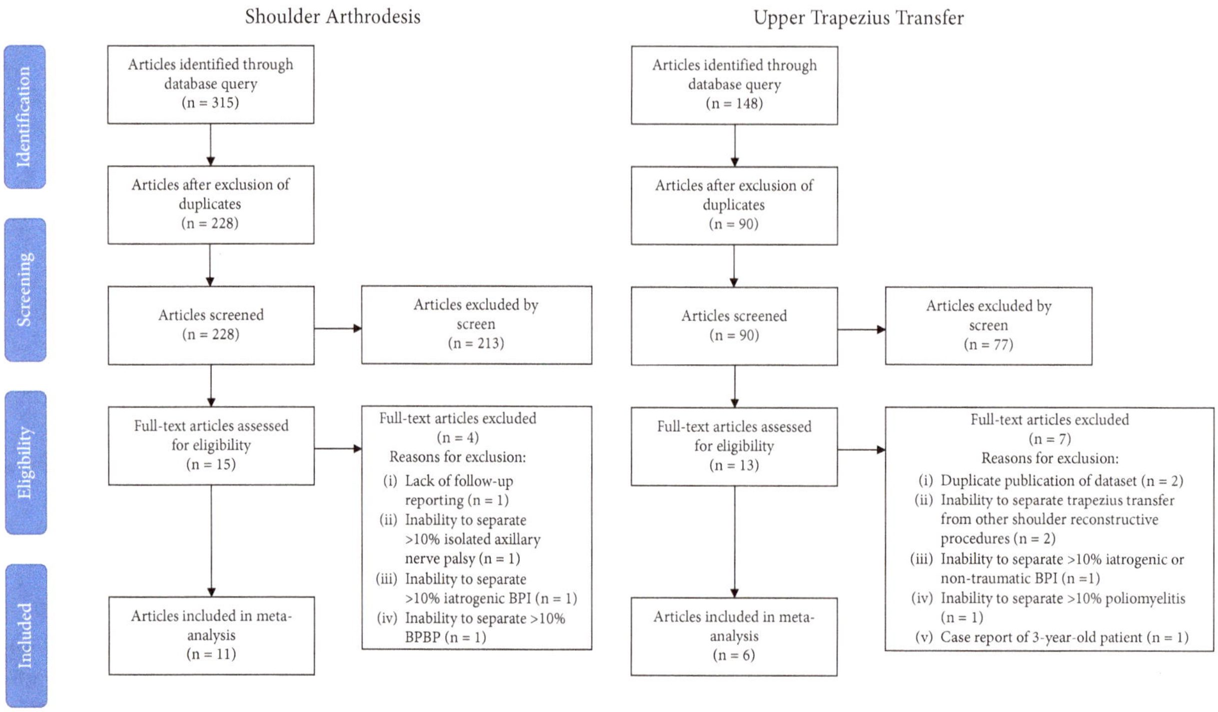

FIGURE 1: Flowchart illustrating the article selection and exclusion process for the systematic review and meta-analysis.

TABLE 1: Baseline study and patient characteristics*.

Study	n	Male (n)	Mean age (years)	Delay to surgery (months)	Follow-up (months)
Shoulder arthrodesis					
Richards et al. [21]	9	8	27	56	25
Rouholamin et al. [22]	12	11	29	NR	34
Richards et al. [20]	46	44	30	NR	44
Emmelot et al. [15]	12	10	19	32	84
Rühmann et al. [8]	14	12	34	47	14
Chammas et al. [13]	27	25	25	33	71
Esenyel et al. [16]	5	5	40	NR	58
Atlan et al. [11]	54	54	24	31	37
Lenior et al. [18]	8	8	33	46	28
Thangarajah et al. [23]	7	6	48	60	98
Degeorge et al. [14]	38	NR	30	NR	58
Upper trapezius transfer					
Aziz et al. [12]	27	23	31	31	15
Mir-Bullo et al. [6]	6	6	28	30	19
Rühmann et al. [24]	80	69	31	73	29
Monreal et al. [7]	10	8	28	37	18
Bertelli et al. [5]	7	7	28	21	12
Karki et al. [17]	12	12	27	24	6

*NR, not reported.

TABLE 2: Patterns of brachial plexus injury for the study cohort.

	C5	C5-C6	C5–C7	C5–C8	C8–T1	C5–T1	Total
Shoulder arthrodesis	1 (1%)	36 (24%)	28 (19%)	0 (0%)	2 (1%)	81 (55%)	148
Upper trapezius transfer	0 (0%)	26 (46%)	15 (27%)	4 (7%)	0 (0%)	11 (20%)	56
Total	1 (0.5%)	62 (30.4%)	43 (21.1%)	4 (2.0%)	2 (1.0%)	92 (45.0%)	204*

*Patterns of brachial plexus injury was available for 204 out of 374 patients in this meta-analysis.

Table 3: Complications following shoulder arthrodesis and upper trapezius transfer.

n	Complication
Shoulder arthrodesis	
22	Nonunion
15	Humerus fracture
11	Symptomatic hardware
5	Deep infection
5	Pin tract infection
2	Skin breakdown
1	Fixation failure
1	Hardware loosening
1	Hematoma
1	Intraarticular screw in acromioclavicular joint
1	Malunion
1	Scapular neck fracture
1	Superficial infection
Upper trapezius transfer	
7	Hardware loosening
4	Deep infection
2	Humerus fracture
2	Persistent glenohumeral joint instability
2	Skin breakdown
2	Transient musculocutaneous nerve palsy
1	Contralateral ulnar neuropathy
1	Silk suture extrusion
1	Superficial infection

differences in complication rates, reoperation rates, shoulder range of motion, and functional outcome scores in patients with traumatic BPI. Due to the heterogeneity of the studies in our meta-analysis, a random effects model was used, which assigned study weights accounting for within-study and between-study variances. With the current available evidence, we found higher rates of complication and reoperation after shoulder arthrodesis compared with upper trapezius transfer for traumatic BPI, but this effect did not reach the statistical significance. Due to the limited sample size, variations in reporting, and study heterogeneity in the published literature, we were not able to draw conclusions regarding differences in shoulder range of motion and functional outcome scores between these two procedures.

This study has several limitations. First, the findings of our meta-analysis are limited by the available literature and the quality of the included studies. Since no comparative studies between shoulder arthrodesis and upper trapezius transfer were identified, a proportional meta-analysis was performed [10]. The included studies had a moderate risk of bias according to the MINORS score [26]. Second, there was substantial heterogeneity in the included studies, in terms of injury severity and pattern, surgical technique and postoperative care, and outcomes reporting. There was a substantial to considerable amount of heterogeneity in the results of our meta-analysis according to the Cochrane Handbook for Systematic Reviews of Interventions guidelines [12]. The large amount of study heterogeneity limited the conclusions that we were able to draw from this study. Third, since this meta-analysis included all adult traumatic BPI, we were unable to substratify our analyses to assess each BPI pattern, such as upper trunk BPI, extended upper trunk BPI, or global BPI. It is possible that some BPI patterns benefit more from one shoulder reconstructive option than another. Finally, there is the potential for publication bias, especially due to the inclusion of smaller case series. If favorable outcomes of surgical interventions were preferentially published in the literature, then our meta-analysis may underestimate the true rates of complications and reoperations and overestimate the true expected shoulder motion and functional outcomes after these procedures.

Shoulder arthrodesis demonstrated higher rates of complications and reoperations compared with upper trapezius transfer for traumatic BPI. It is possible that with greater power, these differences in operative complications and the need for future surgery may have reached a statistical significance. While the difference in these dichotomous outcomes was not statistically significant in our analysis, it is important to note that the reported complications following shoulder arthrodesis tended to be more severe and more frequently require reoperation than those following upper trapezius transfer. Surgeons should be aware of the complications and reoperation profiles of each procedure. Common complications unique to shoulder arthrodesis are nonunion of the arthrodesis and fracture of the humeral shaft distal to arthrodesis. The rate of nonunion of shoulder arthrodesis was 9% in our meta-analysis, but 100% of these required reoperations. Humeral shaft fractures following shoulder arthrodesis arise from stress risers in the bone distal to a stiff construct; in the reported literature, these have been treated successfully both operatively and non-operatively [11, 13, 16, 20]. Upper trapezius transfers are largely successful for improving painful inferior instability from a previously flail shoulder; only 1% of upper trapezius transfer cases in our meta-analysis underwent subsequent shoulder arthrodesis for persistent glenohumeral instability [24].

We were not able to draw conclusions regarding differences in shoulder range of motion and functional outcome scores between shoulder arthrodesis and upper trapezius transfer for traumatic BPI. Functional outcome scores were usually not reported, and when they were, an array of difference scoring systems was used, including DASH, OSS, ASES, and SSV, making direct comparisons challenging. Similarly, postoperative shoulder range of motion was inconsistently reported among the studies in this meta-analysis. There was no consensus about reporting forward flexion, abduction, external rotation, or a combination thereof. Some studies reported only postoperative motion, while others also reported preoperative motion, and still, others reported change in motion. Some studies reported abduction as the angle measured between the trunk and the arm [5, 7], while others utilized preset hand excursion parameters, such as the ability to reach the mouth, the forehead, and the buttock [18]. It is important to note that intact scapulothoracic motion portends a better prognosis for motion after both shoulder arthrodesis and upper trapezius transfer [3]. In our meta-analysis, there was

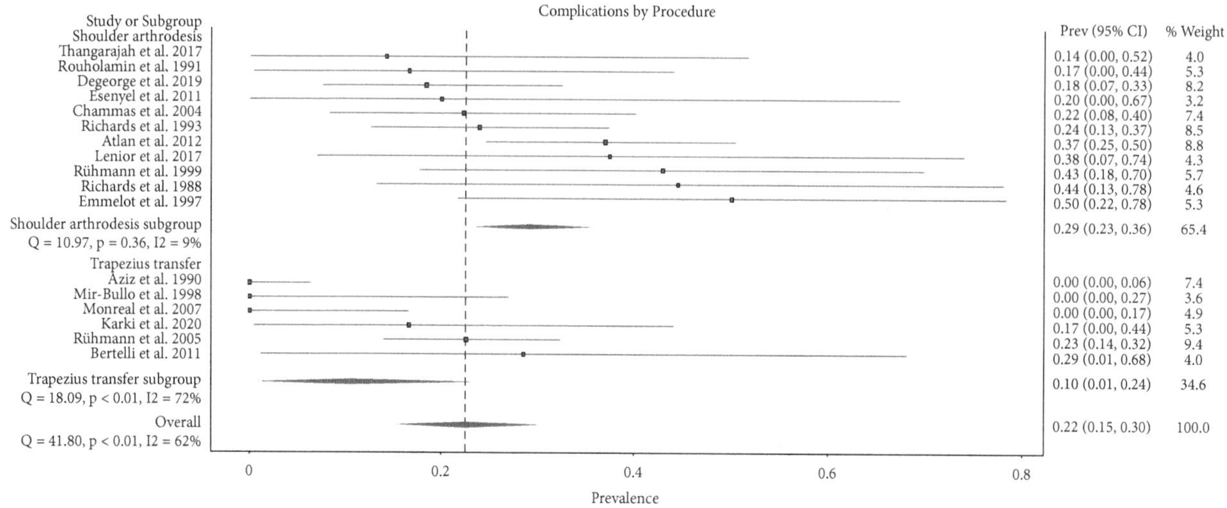

FIGURE 2: Forest plot illustrating the proportions of complications for shoulder arthrodesis versus upper trapezius transfer.

TABLE 4: Reoperations following shoulder arthrodesis and upper trapezius transfer.

n	Reoperation
Shoulder arthrodesis	
23	Revision arthrodesis ± bone grafting for nonunion
7	Humeral shaft open reduction internal fixation
3	Irrigation, debridement, and hardware removal
2	Irrigation and debridement
1	Hematoma evacuation
1	Symptomatic hardware removal
Upper trapezius transfer	
4	Irrigation, debridement, and hardware removal
2	Shoulder arthrodesis
2	Symptomatic hardware removal

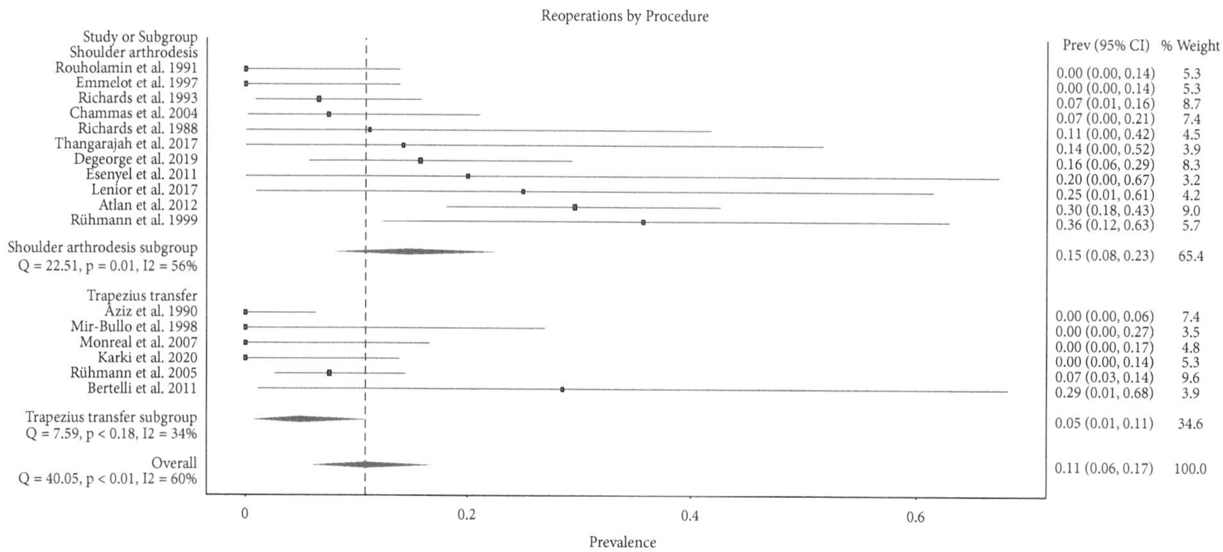

FIGURE 3: Forest plot illustrating the proportions of reoperations for shoulder arthrodesis versus upper trapezius transfer.

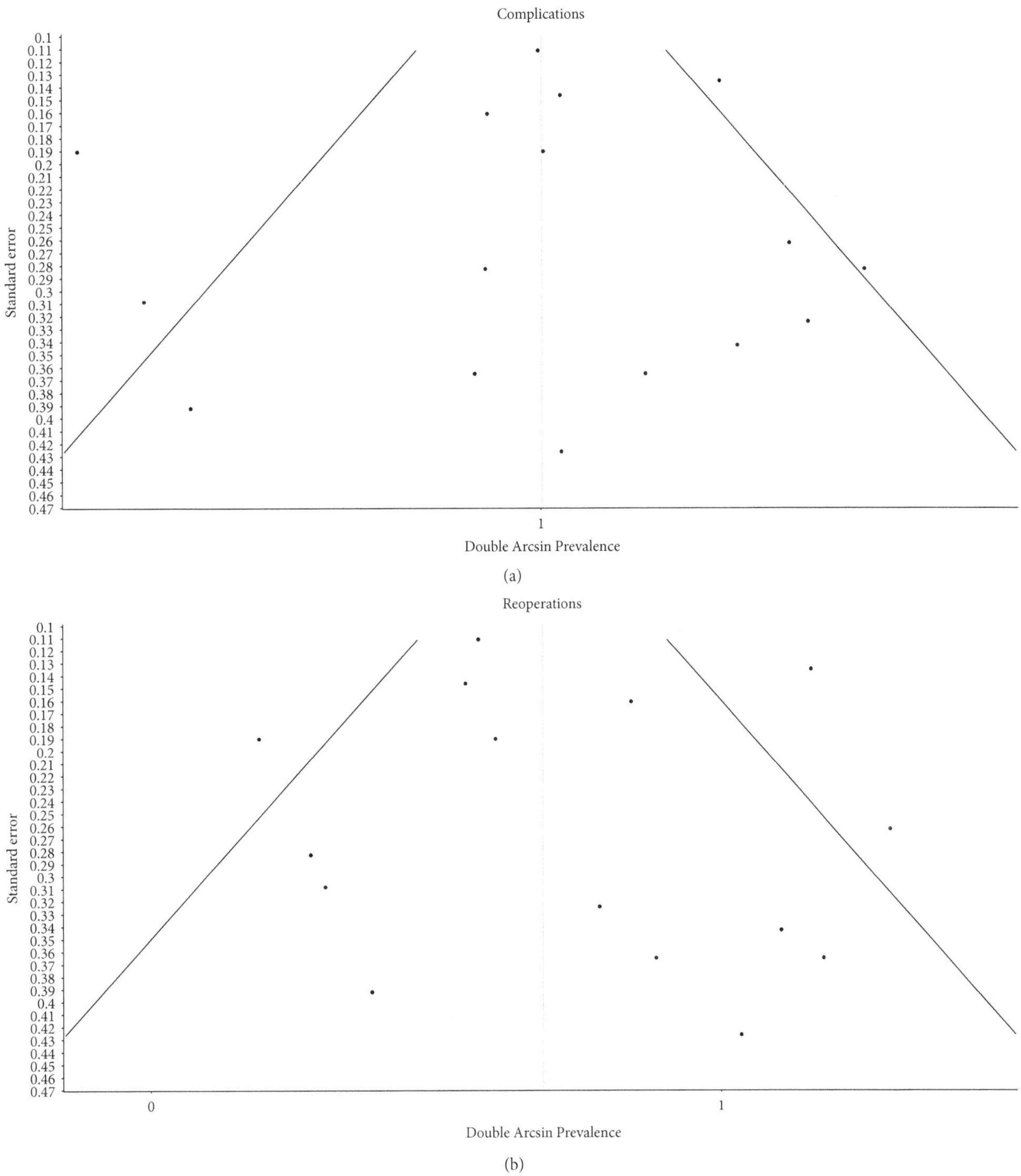

FIGURE 4: Funnel plots of the meta-analysis of data on (a) complications and (b) reoperations after shoulder arthrodesis and upper trapezius transfer for traumatic BPI, illustrating low publication bias. The area within the funnel represents where 95% of data points would be expected in the absence of publication bias.

a higher proportion of complete BPI in the shoulder arthrodesis group; worse scapulothoracic motion in this group may have biased our findings against shoulder arthrodesis. Prospective and comparative studies are needed to evaluate for differences in motion and functional outcomes after these two procedures in traumatic BPI.

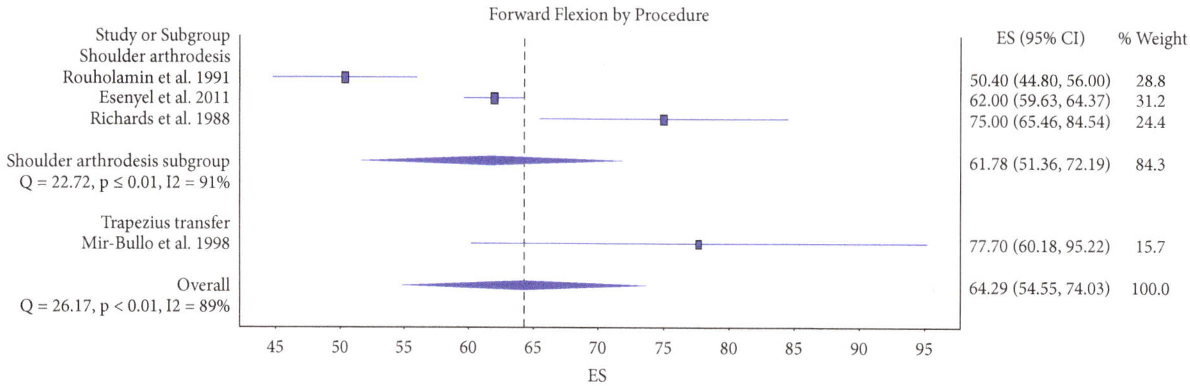

FIGURE 5: Forest plot illustrating active shoulder forward flexion for shoulder arthrodesis versus upper trapezius transfer.

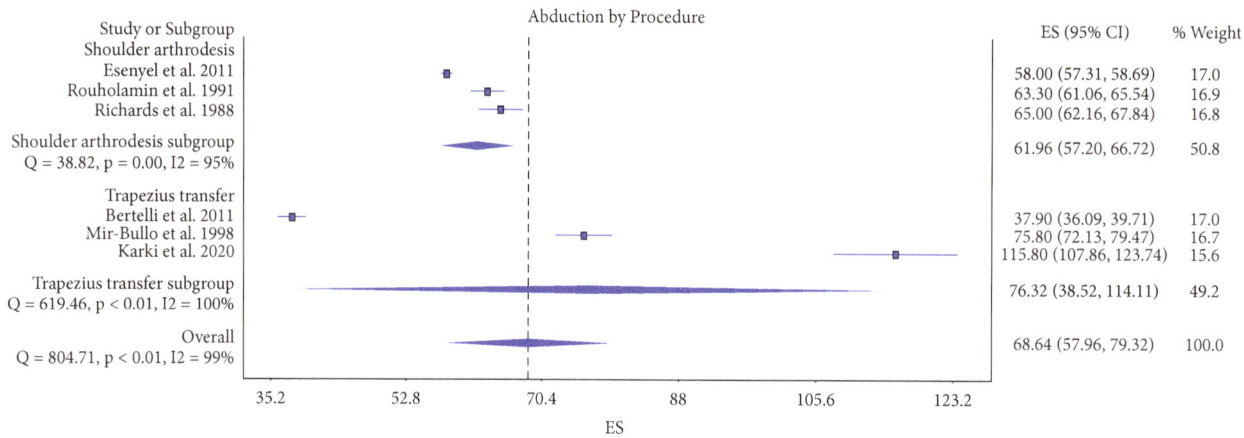

FIGURE 6: Forest plot illustrating active shoulder abduction for shoulder arthrodesis versus upper trapezius transfer.

5. Conclusions

Shoulder arthrodesis and upper trapezius transfer are both viable options for secondary shoulder reconstruction in adult traumatic BPI. Shoulder arthrodesis carries higher rates of complications and reoperations compared with upper trapezius transfer, but the differences are not statistically significant. Patients and surgeons should be aware of different complications and reoperation profiles of these two procedures. In particular, patients should be counseled on the risk of nonunion and humerus fracture with shoulder arthrodesis. Future comparative studies are necessary to clarify the difference in expected functional outcomes and shoulder motion after these two procedures in traumatic BPI.

Additional Points

Location of the study: the work for the study was carried out at Brigham and Women's Hospital.

References

[1] S. S. Noland, A. T. Bishop, R. J. Spinner, and A. Y. Shin, "Adult traumatic brachial plexus injuries," *Journal of the American Academy of Orthopaedic Surgeons*, vol. 27, no. 19, pp. 705–716, 2019.

[2] B. Elhassan, A. T. Bishop, R. U. Hartzler, A. Y. Shin, and R. J. Spinner, "Tendon transfer options about the shoulder in patients with brachial plexus injury," *Journal of Bone and Joint Surgery*, vol. 94, no. 15, pp. 1391–1398, 2012.

[3] D. J. Clare, M. A. Wirth, G. I. Groh, and C. A. Rockwood Jr, "Shoulder arthrodesis," *Journal of Bone and Joint Surgery American Volume*, vol. 83, no. 4, pp. 593–600, 2001.

[4] B. Elhassan, A. Bishop, A. Shin, and R. Spinner, "Shoulder tendon transfer options for adult patients with brachial plexus injury," *The Journal of Hand Surgery*, vol. 35, no. 7, pp. 1211–1219, 2010.

[5] J. A. Bertelli, "Upper and lower trapezius muscle transfer to restore shoulder abduction and external rotation in long-standing upper type palsies of the brachial plexus in adults," *Microsurgery*, vol. 31, no. 4, pp. 263–267, 2011.

[6] X. Mir-Bullo, P. Hinarejos, P. Mir-Batlle, R. Busquets, L. Carrera, and A. Navarro, "Trapezius transfer for shoulder paralysis: 6 patients with brachial plexus injuries followed for 1 year," *Acta Orthopaedica Scandinavica*, vol. 69, no. 1, pp. 69–72, 1998.

[7] R. Monreal, L. Paredes, and H. Diaz, "Leon P Trapezius transfer to treat flail shoulder after brachial plexus palsy," *Journal of Brachial Plexus and Peripheral Nerve Injury*, vol. 2, p. 2, 2007.

[8] O. Rühmann, F. Gossé, C. J. Wirth, and S. Schmolke, "Reconstructive operations for the paralyzed shoulder in brachial

plexus palsy: concept of treatment," *Injury*, vol. 30, no. 9, pp. 609–618, 1999.

[9] K. Slim, E. Nini, D. Forestier, F. Kwiatkowski, Y. Panis, and J. Chipponi, "Methodological index for non-randomized studies (MINORS): development and validation of a new instrument," *ANZ Journal of Surgery*, vol. 73, no. 9, pp. 712–716, 2003.

[10] R. El Dib, P. Nascimento Junior, and A. Kapoor, "An alternative approach to deal with the absence of clinical trials: a proportional meta-analysis of case series studies," *Acta Cirurgica Brasileira*, vol. 28, no. 12, pp. 870–876, 2013 Dec.

[11] F. Atlan, S. Durand, M. Fox, P. Levy, Z. Belkheyar, and C. Oberlin, "Functional outcome of glenohumeral fusion in brachial plexus palsy: a report of 54 cases," *The Journal of Hand Surgery*, vol. 37, no. 4, pp. 683–688, 2012.

[12] W. Aziz, R. Singer, and T. Wolff, "Transfer of the trapezius for flail shoulder after brachial plexus injury," *Journal of Bone and Joint Surgery British Volume*, vol. 72-B, no. 4, pp. 701–704, 1990.

[13] M. Chammas, J. N. Goubier, B. Coulet, G. M. Z. Reckendorf, M. C. Picot, and Y. Allieu, "Glenohumeral arthrodesis in upper and total brachial plexus palsy," *Journal of Bone and Joint Surgery British Volume*, vol. 86, no. 5, pp. 692–695, 2004.

[14] B. Degeorge, C. Lazerges, P. E. Chammas, B. Coulet, F. Lacombe, and M. Chammas, "Comparison of spinal accessory nerve transfer to supra-scapular nerve vs. shoulder arthrodesis in adults with brachial plexus injury," *Orthopaedics and Traumatology: Surgery & Research*, vol. 105, no. 8, pp. 1555–1561, 2019.

[15] C. H. Emmelot, H. K. L. Nielsen, and W. H. Eisma, "Shoulder fusion for paralyzed upper limb," *Clinical Orthopaedics and Related Research*, vol. 340, no. 340, pp. 95–101, 1997.

[16] C. Z. Esenyel, K. Oztürk, Y. Imren, and S. Ayanoğlu, "Shoulder arthrodesis with plate fixation," *Acta Orthopaedica et Traumatologica Turcica*, vol. 45, no. 6, pp. 412–420, 2011.

[17] D. Karki, V. Muthukumar, S. Dash, and A. K. Singh, "Trapezius transfer to restore shoulder function in traumatic brachial plexus injury: revisited and modified," *The journal of hand surgery Asian-Pacific volume*, vol. 25, no. 2, pp. 143–152, 2020.

[18] H. Lenoir, T. Williams, A. Griffart et al., "Arthroscopic arthrodesis of the shoulder in brachial plexus palsy," *Journal of Shoulder and Elbow Surgery*, vol. 26, no. 5, pp. e115–e121, 2017.

[19] A. Nagano, S. Okinaga, N. Ochiai, and T. Kurokawa, "Shoulder arthrodesis by external fixation," *Clinical Orthopaedics and Related Research*, vol. 247, pp. 97–100, 1989.

[20] R. R. Richards, D. Beaton, and A. R. Hudson, "Shoulder arthrodesis with plate fixation: functional outcome analysis," *Journal of Shoulder and Elbow Surgery*, vol. 2, no. 5, pp. 225–239, 1993.

[21] R. R. Richards, R. M. Sherman, A. R. Hudson, and J. P. Waddell, "Shoulder arthrodesis using a pelvic-reconstruction plate. A report of eleven cases," *The Journal of Bone and Joint Surgery*, vol. 70, no. 3, pp. 416–421, 1988.

[22] E. Rouholamin, J. R. Wootton, and A. M. Jamieson, "Arthrodesis of the shoulder following brachial plexus injury," *Injury*, vol. 22, no. 4, pp. 271–274, 1991.

[23] T. Thangarajah and S. M. Lambert, "Glenohumeral arthrodesis for late reconstruction of flail shoulder in patients with traumatic supraclavicular brachial plexus palsy," *Shoulder & Elbow*, vol. 9, no. 4, pp. 266–271, 2017.

[24] O. Rühmann, S. Schmolke, M. Bohnsack, J. Carls, and C. J. Wirth, "Trapezius transfer in brachial plexus palsy," *Journal of Bone and Joint Surgery British Volume*, vol. 87, no. 2, pp. 184–190, 2005.

[25] O. R. Olaiya, A. M. Alagabi, L. Mbuagbaw, and M. H. McRae, "Carpal tunnel release without a tourniquet: a systematic review and meta-analysis," *Plastic and Reconstructive Surgery*, vol. 145, no. 3, pp. 737–744, 2020.

[26] J. P. T. Higgins, J. Thomas, J. Chandler, M. Cumpston, T. Li, and M. J. Page, *Cochrane Handbook For Systematic Reviews Of Interventions*, John Wiley & Sons, Chichester, UK, 2nd edition, 2019.

30

Predicting Success of Two-Stage Exchange for Prosthetic Joint Infection Using C-Reactive Protein/Albumin Ratio

Cierra S. Hong,[1] Sean P. Ryan,[1] Jonathan A. Gabor,[2] Michael A. Bergen,[1] Ran Schwarzkopf,[2] and Thorsten M. Seyler[1]

[1] *Duke University Medical Center, Durham, NC, USA*
[2] *NYU Langone Health, New York City, NY, USA*

Correspondence should be addressed to Cierra S. Hong; cierra.hong@duke.edu

Academic Editor: Benjamin Blondel

Two-stage exchange is most commonly used for treatment of prosthetic joint infections (PJI) but, this may fail to eradicate infections. C-reactive protein/albumin ratio (CAR) has been used to predict survival and operative success in other surgical subspecialties and so, we assess the association between CAR and reimplantation success during two-stage revision for PJI defined by the Musculoskeletal Infection Society following a primary total hip (THA) or knee (TKA) arthroplasty. From January, 2005 to December, 2015, two institutional databases were queried and patient demographics, antibiotic duration, C-reactive protein, and albumin were collected prior to reimplantation. Two-stage revisions were considered successful if patients were off of antibiotics and did not require a repeat surgery. CAR was available for 79 patients (34 hips and 46 knees) with 61 successful two-stage revisions and 18 failures. The average CAR for patients with successful reimplantation was 1.2 (0.2, 3.0) compared to 1.0 (0.4, 3.2) for treatment failure. However, this was not statistically significant (p=0.766). Therefore, CAR is not applicable in predicting the prognosis of two-stage revisions for PJI in total arthroplasty but other preoperative inflammatory-based prognostic scores should be explored.

1. Introduction

In the United States, total hip arthroplasty (THA) and total knee arthroplasty (TKA) are two of the most commonly performed surgeries that treat arthritic pain and improve a patient's functional status. The number of procedures is projected to grow to about half a million and 1.5 million by 2020, respectively [1]. However, this also increases the risk for postoperative complications, including prosthetic joint infections (PJIs), an uncommon but expensive and debilitating complication. From 2001 to 2009, the incidence of PJIs annually in THA and TKA increased from about 2% to 2.18%, almost a twofold increase in the number of infected cases, which led to an additional $200 million in inpatient care costs in the United States [2].

There are multiple strategies to treat and minimize PJI and its associated morbidity and mortality. They include the following medical and surgical managements: debridement, antibiotic, and implant retention (DAIR); one-stage arthroplasty exchange (resection prosthesis followed by reimplantation at the time of explant); two-stage arthroplasty exchange (resection prosthesis followed by reimplantation at a later time point from the explant); and resection arthroplasty [3, 4]. Arthrodesis, amputation, and/or antimicrobial suppression are reserved for chronic or resistant infections [5–7]. In the United States, two-stage exchange is the preferred procedure for eradicating PJIs due to the strong literature support which shows successful outcomes in THA [8] and TKA [9, 10]. However, despite at least a 70% infection-free survival over 10 years [9, 11], those who are not successfully treated with a two-stage revision arthroplasty experience severe complications that can result in soft tissue deficiencies, arthrodesis, amputations, or death [12]. This led to studies investigating risk factors, such as polymicrobial infections and multiple revision surgeries prior to explant of the primary arthroplasty, that predict two-stage revision failures in THA

TABLE 1: Demographic and laboratory data of successful and failed two-stage revision cohorts.

	Successful Two-Stage Revision N = 61	Failed Two-Stage Revision N = 18	p-value
Age (years at primary surgery)	61.0 (56.0, 68.0)	61.0 (54.0, 66.0)	0.578
Gender (female)	28 (45.9)	11 (61.1)	0.257
C-reactive Protein (mg/L)	4.4 (0.8, 9.1)	4.3 (1.8, 10.0)	0.713
Albumin (g/dL)	3.7 (3.1, 4.0)	3.8 (3.5, 4.2)	0.263
CRP/Albumin Ratio (CAR)	1.2 (0.2, 3.0)	1.0 (0.4, 3.2)	0.766

and TKA in order to optimize surgical and medical management of these patients [13, 14].

In other surgical specialties, novel preoperative systemic-inflammation based prognostic scores evaluating C-reactive protein (CRP) and albumin have been shown to predict surgical and overall survival outcomes in addition to risk for disease recurrence after oncologic resections [15–17]. Specifically, the CRP albumin ratio (CAR) has been shown to successfully predict prognosis in many types of cancers most likely because it combines a hallmark of tumorigenesis, inflammation, and preoperative nutritional status [18–21]. However, to our knowledge, CAR has not been investigated in assessing two-stage reimplantation outcomes for PJI in total arthroplasty. In this study, we aim to [1] report the preoperative CAR from patients undergoing a two-stage reimplantation for PJI from two different institutions and [2] assess the correlation with successful postoperative outcomes. We hypothesized that patients who had a successful treatment of their PJI after a two-stage revision for THA or TKA will have elevated preoperative CAR values.

2. Materials and Methods

From January 2005 to December 2015, two institutional databases at tertiary referral centers were retrospectively queried for patients who had a two-stage exchange for PJI after a primary THA or TKA. Patients were included for analysis only if they (1) met either one of the two major or four of the six minor criteria for PJI as defined by the Musculoskeletal Infection Society (MSIS) [22]; (2) completed an explant of their primary THA or TKA and reimplantation at a different surgery date; and (3) had a serum CRP and serum albumin value that were collected within one month of each other and were completed no later than one year before their explant. A total of 79 patients met these inclusion criteria and were retrospectively enrolled in the study. One patient had a two-stage revision for both a primary THA and TKA.

In addition to laboratory data including serum CRP and albumin, clinical demographics, such as age and gender, and antibiotic management were collected. A two-stage exchange arthroplasty was classified successful based off an international multidisciplinary consensus defining successful PJI eradication published by Diaz-Ledezma et al. known as the Delphi consensus criteria [23]. The consensus included the following: (1) no additional surgery to the affected joint after reimplantation; (2) complete PJI eradication which includes no life-long antibiotics for antimicrobial suppression or reinfection by the same organism; and (3) no causes of death related to PJI (i.e., sepsis).

Statistical analysis was performed using Wizard Pro for Mac (E. Miller, Chicago, IL). A univariable logistic regression analysis was performed to assess the primary endpoint, which was whether the two-stage exchange was successfully treating PJI at the two institutions included in the study. Continuous data are presented as median (lower quartile; upper quartile) and were analyzed with a Mann Whitney test between the two cohorts (successful versus unsuccessful two-stage revision) while categorical data are presented as count (percent) and were analyzed with chi-squared test. The results were considered statistically significant when $p<0.05$.

3. Results

From two institutional databases, a total of 79 patients (34 primary THA; 46 primary TKA) developed a PJI as defined by the MSIS and completed a two-stage exchange from 2005 to 2015. Sixty-one of these revisions successfully treated the patient's PJI whereas 18 total joint arthroplasty (5 THA; 13 TKA) required additional surgeries and/or chronic antimicrobial suppression (Figure 1). Demographic data, such as age and gender, in addition to laboratory values of interest are listed in Table 1 for these patients.

Between the two cohorts treated with two-stage exchange for PJI, the median CRP (p=0.713) and albumin (p=0.263) were not significantly different. Additionally, the preoperative CAR was not statistically significant between the cohort with a successful two-stage reimplantation compared to those with a failed reimplantation (successful CAR 1.2 (0.2, 3.0) versus failed CAR 1.0 (0.4, 3.2); p=0.766). In the univariable logistic regression analysis, when considered in isolation, neither CRP (OR 1.00, 95% CI 0.97-1.02; p=0.671) nor albumin (OR 0.99, 95% CI 0.09-1.05; p=0.946) adequately predicted failure of revision. Similarly, CAR did not predict failure (OR 0.975, 95% CI 0.90-1.06; p=0.561).

Forty-two patients (53.2%) had CAR obtained within 30 days of surgery. Thirty of these patients had successful reimplantation and 12 had two-stage exchange revision failures with a CAR median of 1.20 (0.19, 3.43) and 1.03 (0.45, 2.38), respectively. There was no significant difference in preoperative CAR between these two groups (p=0.945) (Table 2).

4. Discussion

PJI, also known as periprosthetic joint infection, can compromise the prosthesis and surrounding bone and soft tissue

Table 2: CAR of successful and failed two-stage revision cohorts within 30-day postoperative period.

	Successful Two-Stage Revision N = 30	Failed Two-Stage Revision N = 12	p-value
CRP/Albumin Ratio (CAR)	1.20 (0.19, 3.43)	1.03 (0.45, 2.38)	0.945

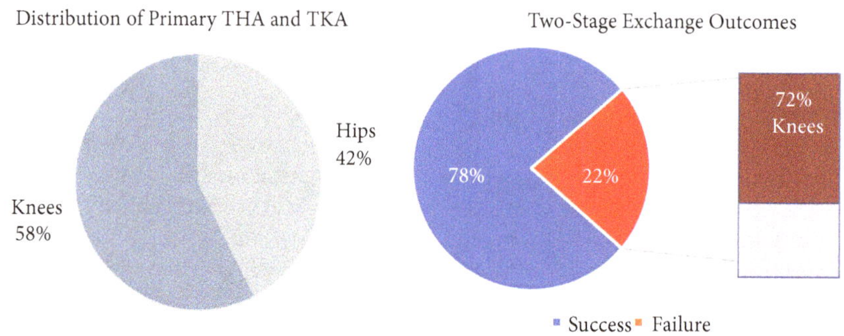

Figure 1: *Left:* distribution of patients included in study cohort. *Right,* distribution of two-stage exchange outcomes after primary THA and TKA.

structures, which significantly increases a patient's morbidity and can lead to patient mortality [4, 24]. In 2011, the MSIS created the major and minor criteria in order to standardize the definition of PJI. It consists of periprosthetic cultures, elevated lab values including C-reactive protein (CRP) and erythrocyte sedimentation rate (ESR), and the presence of a sinus tract into the affected joint [22]. As previously mentioned, in the United States, in addition to antibiotic management, PJI is commonly managed with two-stage exchange arthroplasty due to its success with infection eradication and postoperative survival. However, the outcomes are variable with a reported failure rate up to a third of two-stage knee reimplantations [25] and a tenth of two-stage hip reimplantations [3]. Risk factors including the type of organism causing the PJI [26, 27] and preoperative synovial fluid characteristics [28] have been investigated and shown to predict two-stage exchange failures (Table 3). Another factor that has been studied is the timing of reimplantation after the first-stage explant is completed. Currently, the results remain inconclusive due to the lack of consistency between past studies in regard to the definition of PJI diagnosis and two-stage exchange failure and perioperative surgical and antibiotic treatment protocols between different institutions. For example, Sabry et al. [12] showed that, in patients with primary TKA PJIs, a longer time between explant and reimplantation was associated with infection recurrence. The reported median duration between the two stages associated with the latter was 103 days (range 2-470 days) whereas Rezaie et al. [29] showed the opposite result. Their analysis determined that the time between the two stages in THA and TKA PJI did not have an impact in predicting two-stage exchange failure.

The literature demonstrates multiple risk factors that lead to two-stage revision failures for THA and TKA including obesity, diabetes mellitus, and immunosuppression [39]. However, not only are these risk factors common for different surgical procedures [40, 41] but they also provide no prognostic value for two-stage revisions for PJI. On the other hand, many oncologic surgical specialties have shown that the novel preoperative scores involving systemic-inflammatory markers are valuable for prognosis [42, 43]. This is likely due to the stimulation of inflammatory and acute-phase proteins in addition to the chemokines, cytokines, and immune cells, all of which contribute to tumor progression and dissemination [44]. In a similar manner, PJI stimulates the inflammatory response and systemic markers and can cause many of the classic clinical symptoms associated with this process such as fevers, erythematous warm joints, and pain [4].

Systemic-inflammatory markers were initially investigated individually as prognostic factors as seen with septic patients. Sepsis, which develops from a local infection that becomes systemic, is an inflammatory process that causes acute organ dysfunction and involves many of the factors mentioned above such as acute-phase proteins, chemokines and cytokines [45]. Simple prognostic factors including interleukin-6 (IL-6) [32] and D-dimer (Table 4) were shown to predict mortality in these patients. Eventually, this led to the development of novel systemic prognostic scores, which encompass a multifactorial presentation of the patient, to predict sepsis mortality [35, 38]. The preoperative systemic-inflammatory based prognosis score, CAR, which predicts 180-day mortality in patients with sepsis [38], was of particular interest because it has successfully predicted prognosis in patients undergoing surgery for soft tissue sarcomas [18], esophageal [19], colorectal [20], and pancreatic cancers [21] and has outperformed other scores including neutrophil/lymphocyte ratio, platelet/lymphocyte ratio, and modified Glasgow Prognostic Score in gastric cancer [46]. Individually, elevated CRP [47] and hypoalbuminemia [39] have been associated with failed two-stage exchange outcomes but the present study showed that the preoperative

TABLE 3: Risk factors for two-stage exchange failure and recurrent infections.

Study Authors	Risk Factors
Mortazavi SM, Vegari D, Ho A et al. [26].	Culture-negative PJI; methicillin-resistant PJI; increased reimplantation operative time
Triantafyllopoulos GK, Memtsoudis SG, Zhang W et al. [30].	Female gender, heart and psychiatric diseases
Dwyer MK, Damsgaard C, Wadibia J et al. [28].	Preoperative synovial fluid WBC >60,000 cells/uL, synovial fluid WBC neutrophil >92%, serum ESR >99 mm/hr
Tan TL, Gomez MM, Manrique J et al. [31].	Positive intraoperative culture during reimplantation
Rezaie AA, Goswami K, Shohat N et al. [29].	Charlson comorbidity index
Pelt CE, Grijalva R, Anderson L et al. [14].	(TKA) polymicrobial infection, 4+ surgeries to site of primary TKA before explant
Jhan SW, Lu YD, Lee MS et al. [27].	(THA) BMI 30 kg/m^2, liver cirrhosis, gram-negative organism, presence of sinus tract
Schwarzkopf R, Mikhael B, Wright E et al. [3].	(THA) Previous history of other prosthetic joint infections

Table 4: Prognostic factors for predicting sepsis mortality after two-stage exchange.

Study Authors	Prognostic Factors
Srisangthong P, Wongsa A, Kittiworawitkul P and Wattanathum A [32].	Plasma IL-6 100 pg/mL (28-day mortality)
Parlato M, Cavaillon JM [33].	Lactate, pentraxin 3 (PTX3), pancreatic stone protein, IL-8; microRNA markers 15a/16/193/483-5p, CD14 and CD64 (28-day mortality)
Rodelo JR, De la Rosa G, Valencia ML et al. [34].	D-dimer (28-day mortality)
Artero A, Zaragoza R, Zamarena JJ et al. [35].	Hypoalbuminemia
Chen Y, Chunsheng L [36].	Plasma brain natriuretic peptide >113 pg/mL (28-day mortality)
Ranzani OT, Zampieri FG, Forte DN et al. [37]; Kim MH, Ahn JY, Song JE et al. [38].	CAR (90-day [37] and 180-day [38] mortality)

ratio, which encompasses the inflammatory and nutritional status of a patient, is not a significant indicator of the outcomes of two-stage exchanges after PJI. This is in contrast to the value of CAR as shown in cancer patients.

There were several limitations to this retrospective study. First, the number of patients that met the inclusion criteria was small despite using two different institutional databases. The lack of significant difference of CAR between the successful and failed two-stage exchange was possibly limited by this factor. Secondly, lab values collected up to a year prior to a patient's explant were used to analyze CAR which could not accurately represent the patient's physical state prior to receiving surgery. Finally, patients who had revisions prior to their explant for their two-stage exchange were included, which could also negatively impact the outcomes.

Despite these pitfalls, this study contributes to the literature by applying a successful prognostic model into a field that needs more tools to improve its outcomes. It evaluated the outcomes of two-stage exchanges for THA and TKA in patients from two different institutions who were diagnosed with PJI per the MSIS definition using a novel preoperative systemic-inflammatory prognostic score, CAR. Based on our knowledge of the inflammatory process in PJI and in tumor progression, we hypothesized a correlation, but no significant difference was found with the numbers available. It also highlights the need to prospectively study CAR or other preoperative systemic-inflammation prognostic scores in the setting of PJI as it may provide value in helping to identify the correct timing of reimplantation.

5. Conclusion

This study aims to analyze the predictability of two-stage exchange outcomes to treat PJI defined by the MSIS criteria using a novel preoperative systemic-inflammatory score, CAR. Patient data was collected from two institutional databases and CAR did not predict success or failure after a two-stage exchange in the setting of a PJI. Despite the limitations and conclusion, this study provides insight and explores the prognostic possibilities of preoperative inflammatory scores in the setting of PJIs as they have been previously shown to be successful in other surgical field managing diseases driven by inflammation. Further research is needed to explore the application of other scores, such as neutrophil/lymphocyte, in order to better predict a patient's outcome after a two-stage exchange and to alleviate the financial and emotional burden of PJI.

Disclosure

An earlier version of this work has been presented at the MSIS Annual Meeting 2018.

References

[1] S. M. Kurtz, K. L. Ong, E. Lau, and K. J. Bozic, "Impact of the economic downturn on total joint replacement demand in the United States," *The Journal of Bone and Joint Surgery*, vol. 96, no. 8, pp. 624–630, 2014.

[2] S. M. Kurtz, E. Lau, H. Watson, J. K. Schmier, and J. Parvizi, "Economic burden of periprosthetic joint infection in the United States," *The Journal of Arthroplasty*, vol. 27, no. 8, supplement 1, pp. 61.e1–65.e1, 2012.

[3] R. Schwarzkopf, B. Mikhael, E. Wright, D. M. Estok II, and J. N. Katz, "Treatment failure among infected periprosthetic total hip arthroplasty patients," *The Open Orthopaedics Journal* , vol. 8, no. 1, pp. 118–124, 2014.

[4] A. J. Tande and R. Patel, "Prosthetic joint infection," *Clinical Microbiology Reviews*, vol. 27, no. 2, pp. 302–345, 2014.

[5] H. Sharma, J. De Leeuw, and D. I. Rowley, "Girdlestone resection arthroplasty following failed surgical procedures," *International Orthopaedics*, vol. 29, no. 2, pp. 92–95, 2005.

[6] V. Khanna, D. M. Tushinski, L. J. Soever, A. D. Vincent, and D. J. Backstein, "Above knee amputation following total knee arthroplasty: when enough is enough," *The Journal of Arthroplasty*, vol. 30, no. 4, pp. 658–662, 2015.

[7] M. Wouthuyzen-Bakker, J. M. Nijman, G. A. Kampinga, S. van Assen, and P. C. Jutte, "Efficacy of antibiotic suppressive therapy in patients with a prosthetic joint infection," *Journal of Bone and Joint Infection*, vol. 2, no. 2, pp. 77–83, 2017.

[8] H. J. Cooper and C. J. Della Valle, "The two-stage standard in revision total hip replacement," *The Bone & Joint Journal*, vol. 95-B, no. 11_Supple_A, pp. 84–87, 2013.

[9] T. Mahmud, M. C. Lyons, D. D. Naudie, S. J. MacDonald, and R. W. McCalden, "Assessing the gold standard: a review of 253 two-stage revisions for infected TKA," *Clinical Orthopaedics and Related Research*, vol. 470, no. 10, pp. 2730–2736, 2012.

[10] J. Petrie, A. Sassoon, and G. Haidukewych, "Two-stage revision for the infected total knee arthroplasty: the gold standard,"

Seminars in Arthroplasty, vol. 24, no. 3, pp. 149–151, 2013.

[11] A. N. Ford, A. M. Holzmeister, H. W. Rees, and P. D. Belich, "Characterization of outcomes of 2-stage exchange arthroplasty in the treatment of prosthetic joint infections," *The Journal of Arthroplasty*, vol. 33, no. 7, pp. S224–S227, 2018.

[12] F. Y. Sabry, L. Buller, S. Ahmed, A. K. Klika, and W. K. Barsoum, "Preoperative prediction of failure following two-stage revision for knee prosthetic joint infections," *The Journal of Arthroplasty*, vol. 29, no. 1, pp. 115–121, 2014.

[13] S. Bozhkova, R. Tikhilov, D. Labutin et al., "Failure of the first step of two-stage revision due to polymicrobial prosthetic joint infection of the hip," *Journal of Orthopaedics and Traumatology*, vol. 17, no. 4, pp. 369–376, 2016.

[14] C. E. Pelt, R. Grijalva, L. Anderson et al., "Two-stage revision TKA is associated with high complication and failure rates," *Advances in Orthopedics*, vol. 2014, Article ID 659047, 7 pages, 2014.

[15] M. Shibutani, K. Maeda, H. Nagahara et al., "Prognostic significance of the preoperative ratio of c-reactive protein to albumin in patients with colorectal cancer," *Anticancer Research*, vol. 36, pp. 995–1001, 2016.

[16] M. M. Elahi, D. C. McMillan, C. S. McArdle, W. J. Angerson, and N. Sattar, "Score based on hypoalbuminemia and elevated c-reactive protein predicts survival in patients with advanced gastrointestinal cancer," *Nutrition and Cancer*, vol. 48, no. 2, pp. 171–173, 2004.

[17] Y. Oshiro, R. Sasaki, K. Fukunaga et al., "Inflammation-based prognostic score is a useful predictor of postoperative outcome in patients with extrahepatic cholangiocarcinoma," *Journal of Hepato-Biliary-Pancreatic Sciences*, vol. 20, no. 3, pp. 389–395, 2013.

[18] Y. Liang, W. Xiao, Y. Guan et al., "Prognostic value of the C-reactive protein/Albumin Ratio (CAR) in patients with operable soft tissue sarcoma," *OncoTargets and Therapy*, vol. 10, pp. 98135–98147, 2017.

[19] X. Xu, H. Yu, W. Hu, Q. Song, and W. Mao, "A novel inflammation-based prognostic score, the C-reactive protein/albumin ratio predicts the prognosis of patients with operable esophageal squamous cell carcinoma," *PLoS ONE*, vol. 10, no. 9, 2015.

[20] M. Ishizuka, H. Nagata, K. Takagi, Y. Iwasaki, N. Shibuya, and K. Kubota, "Clinical significance of the C-reactive protein to albumin ratio for survival after surgery for colorectal cancer," *Annals of Surgical Oncology*, vol. 23, pp. 900–907, 2015.

[21] K. Haruki, H. Shiba, Y. Shirai et al., "The C-reactive protein to albumin ratio predicts long-term outcomes in patients with pancreatic cancer after pancreatic resection," *World Journal of Surgery*, vol. 40, pp. 2254–2260, 2016.

[22] J. Parvizi and T. Gehrke, "Definition of periprosthetic joint infection," *The Journal of Arthroplasty*, vol. 29, no. 7, p. 1331, 2014.

[23] C. Diaz-Ledezma, C. A. Higuera, and J. Parvizi, "Success after treatment of periprosthetic joint infection: a delphi-based international multidisciplinary consensus," *Clinical Orthopaedics and Related Research*, vol. 471, no. 7, pp. 2374–2382, 2013.

[24] B. Zmistowski, J. A. Karam, J. B. Durinka, D. S. Casper, and J. Parvizi, "Periprosthetic joint infection increases the risk of one-year mortality," *The Journal of Bone and Joint Surgery-American Volume*, vol. 95, no. 24, pp. 2177–2184, 2013.

[25] Y. S. Lee and A. F. Chen, "Two-stage reimplantation in infected total knee arthroplasty," *Knee Surgery and Related Research*, vol. 30, no. 2, pp. 107–114, 2018.

[26] S. M. J. Mortazavi, D. Vegari, A. Ho, B. Zmistowski, and J. Parvizi, "Two-stage exchange arthroplasty for infected total knee arthroplasty: predictors of failure," *Clinical Orthopaedics and Related Research*, vol. 469, no. 11, pp. 3049–3054, 2011.

[27] S. Jhan, Y. Lu, M. S. Lee, C. Lee, J. Wang, and F. Kuo, "The risk factors of failed reimplantation arthroplasty for periprosthetic hip infection," *BMC Musculoskeletal Disorders*, vol. 18, no. 1, 2017.

[28] M. K. Dwyer, C. Damsgaard, J. Wadibia et al., "Laboratory tests for diagnosis of chronic periprosthetic joint infection can help predict outcomes of two-stage exchange," *The Journal of Bone and Joint Surgery*, vol. 100, no. 12, pp. 1009–1015, 2018.

[29] A. Aali Rezaie, K. Goswami, N. Shohat, A. T. Tokarski, A. E. White, and J. Parvizi, "Time to reimplantation: waiting longer confers no added benefit," *The Journal of Arthroplasty*, vol. 33, no. 6, pp. 1850–1854, 2018.

[30] G. K. Triantafyllopoulos, S. G. Memtsoudis, W. Zhang, Y. Ma, T. P. Sculco, and L. A. Poultsides, "Periprosthetic infection recurrence after 2-stage exchange arthroplasty: failure or fate?" *The Journal of Arthroplasty*, vol. 32, no. 2, pp. 526–531, 2017.

[31] T. L. Tan, M. M. Gomez, J. Manrique, J. Parvizi, and A. F. Chen, "Positive culture during reimplantation increases the risk of subsequent failure in two-stage exchange arthroplasty," *The Journal of Bone and Joint Surgery*, vol. 98, no. 15, pp. 1313–1319, 2016.

[32] P. Srisangthong, A. Wongsa, P. Kittiworawitkul, and A. Wattanathum, "Early IL-6 response in sepsis is correlated with mortality and severity score," *Critical Care*, vol. 17, no. Suppl 2, p. P34, 2013.

[33] M. Parlato and J. Cavaillon, "Host response biomarkers in the diagnosis of sepsis: a general overview," *Journal of Molecular Biology and Methods*, vol. 1237, pp. 149–211, 2015.

[34] J. R. Rodelo, G. De la Rosa, M. L. Valencia et al., "D-dimer is a significant prognostic factor in patients with suspected infection and sepsis," *The American Journal of Emergency Medicine*, vol. 30, no. 9, pp. 1991–1999, 2012.

[35] A. Artero, R. Zaragoza, J. J. Camarena, S. Sancho, R. González, and J. M. Nogueira, "Prognostic factors of mortality in patients with community-acquired bloodstream infection with severe sepsis and septic shock," *Journal of Critical Care*, vol. 25, no. 2, pp. 276–281, 2010.

[36] Y. Chen and C. Li, "Prognostic significance of brain natriuretic peptide obtained in the ED in patients with SIRS or sepsis," *The American Journal of Emergency Medicine*, vol. 27, no. 6, pp. 701–706, 2009.

[37] O. T. Ranzani, F. G. Zampieri, D. N. Forte, L. C. P. Azevedo, and M. Park, "C-reactive protein/albumin ratio predicts 90-day mortality of septic patients," *PLoS ONE*, vol. 8, no. 3, Article ID e59321, 2013.

[38] M. H. Kim, J. Y. Ahn, J. E. Song et al., "The C-reactive protein/albumin ratio as an independent predictor of mortality in patients with severe sepsis or septic shock treated with early goal-directed therapy," *PLoS ONE*, vol. 10, no. 7, Article ID e0132109, 2015.

[39] L. Fagotti, J. Tatka, M. J. Salles, and M. C. Queiroz, "Risk factors and treatment options for failure of a two-stage exchange," *Current Reviews in Musculoskeletal Medicine*, vol. 11, no. 3, pp. 420–427, 2018.

[40] D. C. Sing, T. F. Luan, B. T. Feeley, and A. L. Zhang, "Is obesity a risk factor for adverse events after knee arthroscopy?" *Arthroscopy: The Journal of Arthroscopic and Related Surgery*

vol. 32, no. 7, pp. 1346–1353.el, 2016.

[41] K. L. Hackman, M. J. Bailey, G. I. Snell, and L. A. Bach, "Diabetes is a major risk factor for mortality after lung transplantation," *American Journal of Transplantation*, vol. 14, no. 2, pp. 438–445, 2014.

[42] Y. Liu, X. He, J. Pan, S. Chen, and L. Wang, "Prognostic role of Glasgow prognostic score in patients with colorectal cancer: evidence from population studies," *Scientific Reports*, vol. 7, no. 1, 2017.

[43] Y. Yu, L. Qian, and J. Cui, "Value of neutrophil-to-lymphocyte ratio for predicting lung cancer prognosis: a meta-analysis of 7,219 patients," *Molecular and Clinical Oncology*, vol. 7, no. 3, pp. 498–506, 2017.

[44] C. I. Diakos, K. A. Charles, D. C. McMillan, and S. J. Clarke, "Cancer-related inflammation and treatment effectiveness," *The Lancet Oncology*, vol. 15, no. 11, pp. e493–e503, 2014.

[45] D. C. Angus and T. van der Poll, "Severe sepsis and septic shock," *The New England Journal of Medicine*, vol. 369, no. 9, pp. 840–851, 2013.

[46] X. Liu, X. Sun, J. Liu et al., "Preoperative C-reactive protein/albumin ratio predicts prognosis of patients after curative resection for gastric cancer," *Translational Oncology*, vol. 8, no. 4, pp. 339–345, 2015.

[47] M. S. Cha, S. H. Cho, D. H. Kim et al., "Two-stage total knee arthroplasty for prosthetic joint infection," *Knee Surgery and Related Research*, vol. 27, no. 2, pp. 82–89, 2015.

31

Prosthetic Joint Infection Trends at a Dedicated Orthopaedics Specialty Hospital

Robert P. Runner,[1] Amanda Mener,[2] James R. Roberson,[1] Thomas L. Bradbury,[1] George N. Guild,[1] Scott D. Boden,[1] and Greg A. Erens[1]

[1]*Emory University Department of Orthopaedics, Atlanta, GA, USA*
[2]*Emory University School of Medicine, Atlanta, GA, USA*

Correspondence should be addressed to Robert P. Runner; rrunner@emory.edu

Academic Editor: Thorsten M. Seyler

Introduction. Historically, a majority of prosthetic joint infections (PJIs) grew Gram-positive bacteria. While previous studies stratified PJI risk with specific organisms by patient comorbidities, we compared infection rates and microbiologic characteristics of PJIs by hospital setting: a dedicated orthopaedic hospital versus a general hospital serving multiple surgical specialties. *Methods.* A retrospective review of prospectively collected data on 11,842 consecutive primary hip and knee arthroplasty patients was performed. Arthroplasty cases performed between April 2006 and August 2008 at the general university hospital serving multiple surgical specialties were compared to cases at a single orthopaedic specialty hospital from September 2008 to August 2016. *Results.* The general university hospital PJI incidence rate was 1.43%, with 5.3% of infections from Gram-negative species. In comparison, at the dedicated orthopaedic hospital, the overall PJI incidence rate was substantially reduced to 0.75% over the 8-year timeframe. Comparing the final two years of practice at the general university facility to the most recent two years at the dedicated orthopaedics hospital, the PJI incidence was significantly reduced (1.43% vs 0.61%). Though the overall number of infections was reduced, there was a significantly higher proportion of Gram-negative infections over the 8-year timeframe at 25.3%. *Conclusion.* In transitioning from a multispecialty university hospital to a dedicated orthopaedic hospital, the PJI incidence has been significantly reduced despite a greater Gram-negative proportion (25.3% versus 5.3%). These results suggest a change in the microbiologic profile of PJI when transitioning to a dedicated orthopaedic facility and that greater Gram-negative antibiotic coverage could be considered.

1. Introduction

In the last decade, the demand for hip and knee arthroplasty has grown more than 150% and is expected to continue to grow, with a projected 673% increase in demand for primary total knee arthroplasty by 2030 [1]. With this increase in hip and knee arthroplasty, there will likely be a corresponding increase in postoperative infections. The current infection rate for joint arthroplasty ranges from 0.6% to 2.4% [2]. Furthermore, within two years of knee arthroplasty, the rate of infection is estimated at 1.55% [3]. These postoperative infections can have debilitating consequences for patients, often necessitating extensive antibiotic use with potential side effects and repeat operations. The purpose of this study was to identify and compare the incidence of prosthetic joint infection (PJI) and characterize the microbiologic profile of these infections that occurred between two hospital settings: a general university hospital and a dedicated orthopaedic specialty hospital.

Gram-positive bacteria have been most commonly implicated in PJIs [4–6]. To combat surgical site infections, routine use of prophylactic antibiotics has been implemented; however previous studies have shown that there is a lack of consensus regarding the optimal protocol for prophylactic antibiotic use. According to the Surgical Care Improvement Project Advisory Committee and the American Academy of Orthopaedic Surgeons, the preferred antibiotic prophylaxis for patients undergoing hip or knee replacements is cefazolin or cefuroxime [7, 8]. Cephalosporins are commonly used as antibiotic prophylaxis given their bactericidal activity against Gram-positive and Gram-negative organisms [9]. Previously, it has been shown that the timing of prophylactic antibiotics was critical with the lowest infection rate occurring if antibiotics were administered within one hour before surgery [10, 11]. Furthermore, in addition to the timing of antibiotics, other indications for antibiotic use must be considered, such as the prevalence of resistant strains in the surrounding population. Because of the increased incidence of methicillin-resistant *Staphylococcus aureus* [12, 13], the use of vancomycin has increased. However, the routine use of vancomycin to potentially prevent surgical site infections is a controversial topic. It has previously been shown that diabetes, chronic steroid use, and obesity are risk factors of PJI [14–24] but the root cause of PJI is multifactorial. Additionally, infection season and month has been correlated to an increased risk of PJIs, with summer months accounting for more PJIs compared to winter months [25, 26]. Overall, there is not a clear understanding of the specific factors that contribute to postoperative infections, nor a defined method for preventing these infections from occurring.

Historically, at large academic settings, orthopaedic procedures have been performed alongside other surgical specialties in the same operating rooms. However, recently, there has been a shift towards more dedicated orthopaedics units within general hospitals and even dedicated orthopaedics hospitals. Dedicated orthopaedic units have been associated with decreased complication rates [27, 28]. Even the establishment of a dedicated orthopaedic trauma room at general university hospitals has resulted in a reduction in after-hours surgery and complications [29, 30], improving efficiency and morbidity and mortality. However, less is established in the literature regarding the impact of transitioning to a dedicated orthopaedic hospital in potentially reducing PJIs, improving efficiency, and minimizing complications. The purpose of this study was to compare the infection rates and microbiologic characteristics between a general university and a dedicated orthopaedic specialty hospital in primary arthroplasty patients. The null hypothesis was that the infection rate and microbiologic profile between the institutions would be similar.

2. Materials and Methods

Institutional Review Board approval was obtained for this retrospective review of prospectively collected data on 11,842 consecutive primary hip at knee arthroplasty patients performed at a single academic residency program. Arthroplasty cases performed between April 2006 and August 2008 at the general university hospital serving multiple surgical specialties were compared to cases at a single dedicated orthopaedics specialty hospital from September 2008 through August 2016. As the surveillance program at the general university hospital only started in 2006, arthroplasty cases before this date were excluded.

As the original start of data collection was prior to current definitions of PJI [31–33], the definition of infection was kept consistent throughout data collection for both hospitals as all primary arthroplasty patients required return to the operative room for debridement of deep infection within one year of index procedure.

Table 1: *Overall incidence rates decreased at dedicated orthopaedics hospital.* Overall incidence rate of PJIs between the general university hospital and dedicated orthopaedics hospital. p = .0224 by X^2 analysis.

	Infected	Overall	Incidence
General university hospital	19	1325	1.43%
Dedicated orthopaedics hospital	68	9055	0.75%

Table 2: *2-year incidence rates decreased at dedicated orthopaedics hospital.* Incidence rate of PJIs over a 2-year timeframe between the general university hospital and dedicated orthopaedics hospital. p = .0087 by X^2 analysis.

	Infected	Overall	Incidence
General university hospital	19	1325	1.43%
Dedicated orthopaedics hospital	17	2787	0.61%

Operative variables examined were as follows: procedure date, whether a resident or fellow was scrubbed on the case, and surgery time. Surgery time was defined in minutes from incision start to surgery end time. Demographic variables collected were as follows: age, gender, smoking history, diabetes status, and history of steroid use. Infection variables on the cultured organism identified (if any), bacterial species, and Gram-negative or Gram-positive status were obtained.

2.1. Statistical Analysis. To evaluate differences between the general university hospital and dedicated orthopaedics specialty hospital categorical variables were analyzed with X^2 analysis. For continuous variables of age and BMI, Mann–Whitney U nonparametric analysis was utilized. $p<0.05$ was the cutoff for significance. All statistical analysis was performed in GraphPad Prism (San Diego, CA),

3. Results

To begin comparing the infection rates and microbiologic characteristics between the general university hospital and dedicated orthopaedics specialty hospital, the incidence rate of infections in each hospital setting was calculated. The general university hospital PJI incidence rate was 1.43%. In comparison, at the dedicated orthopaedics specialty hospital, the overall PJI incidence rate was substantially reduced to 0.75% (p=.0224) (Table 1). When comparing the final two years of practice at the general university facility to the most recent two years at the dedicated orthopaedics specialty hospital, the PJI incidence was significantly reduced from the 1.43% incidence at the general university hospital to 0.61% infection rate at the dedicated orthopaedics specialty hospital (p=.0087) (Table 2), with a decrease in the length of surgery for infected cases occurring at the dedicated orthopaedics specialty hospital compared to the general university hospital (Table 3).

To identify differences in infection rates between the general university hospital and dedicated orthopaedics specialty

TABLE 3: In cases that developed an infection, there was a reduced surgery time for cases performed at the dedicated orthopaedics hospital compared to the general university hospital.

	Surgery time (minutes)
General university hospital	146.08
Dedicated orthopaedics hospital	131.31

hospital, demographic variables for all PJIs (hip and knee combined) were analyzed, as obesity, history of steroid use, and diabetes have all been previously identified as risk factors to PJIs [15–24]. Table 4 identifies demographic variables between patients with PJIs at both the academic general and dedicated orthopaedics specialty hospital. There was no significant difference in the average age (64.4 versus 61.6 years, p =0.13) or BMI (30.5 versus 31.5, p =0.52) between the groups. Additionally, there were no statistically significant differences in the proportion of males and females with all PJIs at the academic general and dedicated orthopaedics specialty hospital (p=.043), nor were there differences in the proportion of diabetic patients (p =.40), proportion of procedures with a resident/fellow scrubbed (p=0.67), positive history of steroid use (p=0.31), nor smoking history (p =0.37) between these two populations. In subgroup analysis of TKA patients based on hospital location, there was no difference in the proportion of males and females (p=0.90), diabetic patients (p=0.13), nor history of steroid use (p=0.09) in knee PJIs at the general university hospital nor dedicated orthopaedics specialty hospital (Table 5). Although there was an observed difference in the proportion of cases with a resident/fellow scrubbed (p=0.02) and smoking status (p=0.04), we interpret these findings to be reflective of the small number of knee PJIs at the general university hospital (n=8) compared to the dedicated orthopaedics specialty hospital (n=35), as well as the significant proportion of nonreported smoking statuses at the general university hospital (12.5%) (Table 5). Additionally, there was no difference in the proportion of males and females (p=0.30), diabetic patients (p=0.83), whether a resident or fellow was scrubbed (p=0.15), history of steroid use (p=0.56) nor smoking status (p=0.24) in THA PJI (Table 6). These results indicate that, despite the decreased incidence of infections at the dedicated orthopaedics specialty hospitals, the overall baseline characteristics of the patient populations were mostly similar.

Next, the characteristics of the bacterial organisms cultured from patients with PJIs at the general university were compared to those at the dedicated orthopaedics specialty hospital, as Gram-positive bacteria have been most commonly implicated in PJIs [4–6]. At the general university hospital only 5.3% of cultured organisms were Gram-negative (Figure 1(a)). Interestingly, while 69.0% of cultured organisms from the PJI patients at the dedicated orthopaedics specialty hospital were Gram-positive, 25.3% of cultured organisms were Gram-negative (Figure 2(a)). Importantly, while the majority of cultured organisms from PJIs at both the dedicated orthopaedics specialty hospital and general university hospital were *Staphylococcus* species (Figures 1 and 2) with no statistically significant difference in the diversity of bacterial organisms in either setting (p=0.92), and there was a noticeable contrast in the variety of bacterial organisms isolated from the general university hospital compared to the dedicated orthopaedics specialty hospital. In particular, there were 3 bacterial organisms isolated from PJIs at the general university hospital (Figure 1(b)), compared to 17 different bacterial organisms isolated from PJIs at the dedicated orthopaedics specialty hospital (Figure 2(b)). More specifically, from PJIs at the dedicated orthopaedics specialty hospital, there were a variety of Gram-negative species isolated, such as *Klebsiella*, *Proteus*, *Pseudomonas*, *Serratia*, *E. coli*, *Bacteroides*, *Eikenella*, *Morganella*, and *Veilllonella*, among others (Figure 2(b)). These results suggest that while the overall incidence of PJIs at a dedicated orthopaedics specialty hospital is reduced compared to a general university hospital, there was a nonstatistically significant trend towards an increased percentage of Gram-negative infections (p=0.15), with a greater variety of bacterial organisms isolated from PJIs.

Finally, infection season and month have been correlated to an increased risk of PJIs, with summer months accounting for more PJIs compared to winter months [25, 26]. When examining procedure season and month at the general university hospital, there was a trend towards more infections occurring from procedures performed in the spring compared to other seasons (Figure 3(a)), with the most infections occurring in October and April (Figure 3(b)). However, at dedicated orthopaedics specialty hospital, there was a trend towards an increase in PJIs from procedures that occurred during the fall (Figure 4(a)) and during October (Figure 4(b)). When the procedure month and season between the general university and specialty orthopaedic hospital were directly compared by X^2 analysis, neither were significantly different (p=0.72 and p=0.22 for the procedure month and season, resp.).

4. Discussion

4.1. The Transition from General University to Dedicated Orthopaedics Hospital. Although the transition from general hospitals to specialized hospitals has existed for over 100 years with the 1857 opening of a dedicated cardiac hospital in London [34], over the recent years in the United States, there has been a growing interest in physician-owned hospitals offering specialty care. While only 100 specialty hospitals existed in 1990, that number more than tripled by 2005 [35]. In particular, there has been an increase in specialty cardiac and orthopaedic hospitals. Studies of these specialty hospitals have shown that specialty hospitals generally have better outcomes than general hospitals. A 2005 study showed patients who underwent percutaneous coronary intervention and coronary artery bypass grafting (CABG) at cardiac specialty hospitals were less likely to have associated complications of myocardial infarction and had lower odds ratio for death after CABG and lower readmission rates when compared to general hospitals [36]. Furthermore, Heinemann et al. demonstrated that spinal cord injury (SCI) patients treated at a specialized SCI center had greater daily functional gain compared to a general hospital [37]. Patients at one specialty cardiac specialty hospital had a 12.1% decrease in in-hospital

TABLE 4: *Demographic variables at general university versus dedicated orthopaedic hospital.* Demographic variables, such as BMI, sex, diabetes, whether a resident/fellow was scrubbed, positive history of steroid use, and smoking status were examined at the general university versus dedicated orthopaedics specialty hospitals. NR = not reported. For comparisons of age and BMI, Mann–Whitney *U* nonparametric analysis utilized. For all other variables, X^2 analysis utilized.

	General	Specialty	*p*-value
Age			
Mean	64.4	61.6	0.13
BMI	30.5	31.5	0.52
Sex			0.43
Male	12 (63.2%)	36 (52.9%)	
Female	7 (36.8%)	32 (47.1%)	
Diabetes	5 (26.3%)	12 (17.6%)	0.40
Resident/fellow scrubbed	11 (57.9%)	43 (63.2%)	0.67
Positive history of steroid use	2 (10.5%)	3 (8.3%)	0.31
Smoker			0.37
Never	11 (57.9%)	44 (64.7%)	
Former	2 (10.5%)	13 (19.1%)	
Current	4 (21.1%)	9 (13.2%)	
NR	2 (10.5%)	2 (2.9%)	

TABLE 5: *Demographic variables at general university versus dedicated orthopaedic hospital for TKA PJIs.* Demographic variables, such as BMI, sex, diabetes, whether a resident/fellow was scrubbed, positive history of steroid use, and smoking status were examined at the general university versus dedicated orthopaedics specialty hospitals. NR = not reported. *p* value was calculated by X^2 analysis.

	General	Specialty	*p* value
Sex			0.90
Male	5 (62.5%)	21 (60%)	
Female	3 (37.5%)	14 (40%)	
Diabetes	3 (37.5%)	5 (14.3%)	0.13
Resident/fellow scrubbed	2 (25.0%)	24 (68.6%)	0.02
Positive history of steroid use	2 (25.0%)	2 (5.7%)	0.09
Smoker			0.04
Never	6 (75.0%)	20 (57.1%)	
Former	0 (0.0%)	9 (25.7%)	
Current	1 (12.5%)	6 (17.1%)	
NR	1 (12.5%)	0 (0.0%)	

TABLE 6: *Demographic variables at general university versus dedicated orthopaedic hospital for THA PJIs.* Demographic variables, such as BMI, sex, diabetes, whether a resident/fellow was scrubbed, positive history of steroid use, and smoking status were examined at the general university versus dedicated orthopaedics specialty hospitals. NR = not reported. *p* value was calculated by X^2 analysis.

	General	Specialty	*p* value
Sex			0.30
Male	7 (63.6%)	15 (45.5%)	
Female	4 (36.4%)	18 (54.5%)	
Diabetes	2 (18.2%)	7 (21.2%)	0.83
Resident/fellow scrubbed	9 (81.8%)	19 (57.6%)	0.15
Positive history of steroid use	0 (0.0%)	1 (3.0%)	0.56
Smoker			0.24
Never	5 (45.4%)	24 (72.7%)	
Former	2 (18.2%)	4 (12.1%)	
Current	3 (27.3%)	3 (9.0%)	
NR	1 (9.1%)	2 (6.0%)	

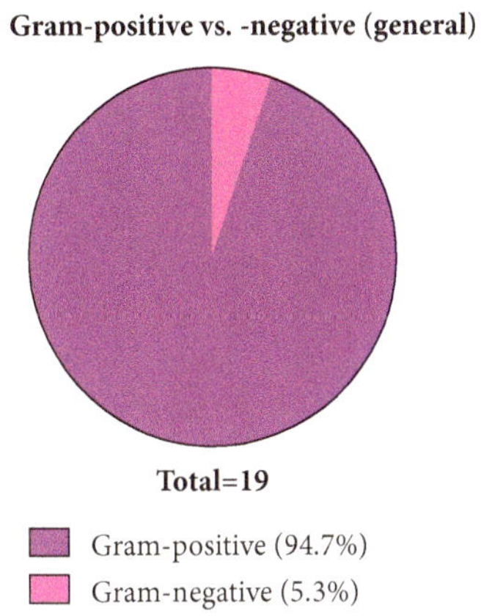

(a)

General Hospital			
Organism	Hip	Knee	Total
Staphylococcus	8 (80.0%)	4 (44.4%)	12 (63.2%)
Streptococcus	0	2 (22.2%)	2 (10.5%)
Enterococcus	0	1 (11.1%)	1 (5.3%)
E. coli	1 (10.0%)	0	1 (5.3%)
No growth	1 (10.0%)	2 (22.2%)	3 (15.8%)

(b)

FIGURE 1: *At general university hospital, a majority of infections are caused by Gram-positive organisms.* (a) The percentages of isolated organisms that were Gram-negative, Gram-positive, or neither or experienced no growth were examined at the general university hospital. (b) The bacterial organisms in hip and knee PJIs at the general university hospital were characterized.

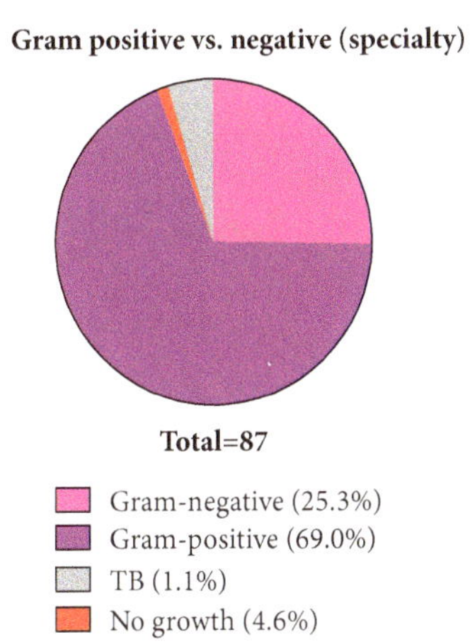

(a)

Specialty Hospital			
Organism	Hip	Knee	Total
Staphylococcus	19 (46.3%)	26 (56.5%)	45 (51.7%)
Klebsiella	1 (2.1%)	1 (2.2%)	2 (2.3%)
Proteus	2 (4.9%)	0	2 (2.3%)
Enterobacter	1 (2.1%)	1 (2.2%)	2 (2.3%)
Pseudomonas	2 (4.9%)	3 (6.5%)	5 (5.7%)
Serratia	1 (2.1%)	0	1 (1.1%)
E. coli	2 (4.9%)	1 (2.2%)	3 (3.4%)
Mycobacterium tuberulosis	0	1 (2.2%)	1 (1.1%)
Streptococcus	4 (9.8%)	1 (2.2%)	5 (5.7%)
Veillonella	0	1 (2.2%)	1 (1.1%)
Prevotella	0	2 (4.3%)	2 (2.3%)
Citrobacter	0	1 (2.2%)	1 (1.1%)
Eikenella	0	1 (2.2%)	1 (1.1%)
Enterococcus	2 (4.9%)	3 (6.5%)	5 (5.7%)
Coryneform	2 (4.9%)	3 (6.5%)	5 (5.7%)
Morganella morganii	1 (2.1%)	0	1 (1.1%)
Bacteroides	1 (2.1%)	0	1 (1.1%)
No growth	3 (7.3%)	1 (2.2%)	4 (4.6%)

(b)

FIGURE 2: *Increased proportion of Gram-negative PJIs at dedicated orthopaedics hospital.* (a) The percentages of isolated organisms that were Gram-negative, Gram-positive, or neither or experienced no growth were examined at the dedicated orthopaedics specialty hospital. (b) The bacterial organisms in hip and knee PJIs at the dedicated orthopaedics specialty hospital were characterized.

mortality rate compared to patients in a general community and teaching hospitals, indicating that specialized care may provide a wide range of benefits to patients to patients in terms of morbidity and mortality. In orthopaedics specifically, Greenwald et al. found lower overall mortality and readmission rates at the orthopaedic specialty hospitals they examined [38]. However, few studies exist to examine the specific differences among care in orthopaedics specifically at a specialty versus general hospital. Additionally, there is little understanding of how the transition to a dedicated orthopaedics hospital may impact infection rates. Therefore, our study addresses a critical gap in understanding how the infection rates and microbiologic characteristics may differ between a general university hospital and dedicated

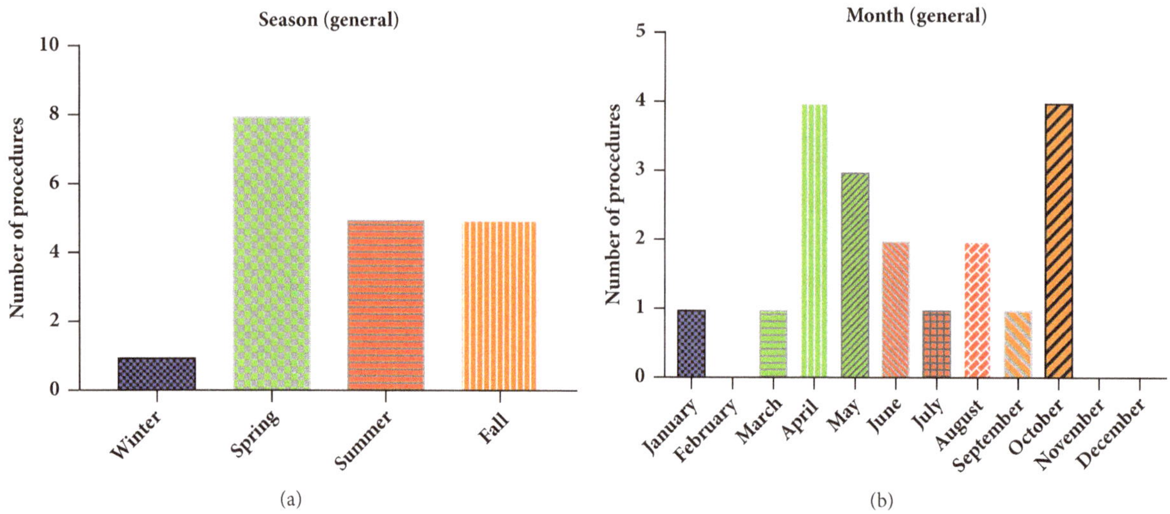

FIGURE 3: *No trends in seasonality nor procedure month at general university hospital.* (a) The season during which procedures resulting in PJIs at the general university hospital were performed is shown. (b) The particular month during which procedures resulting in PJIs at the general university hospital were performed is shown, with the months color-coded corresponding to the season.

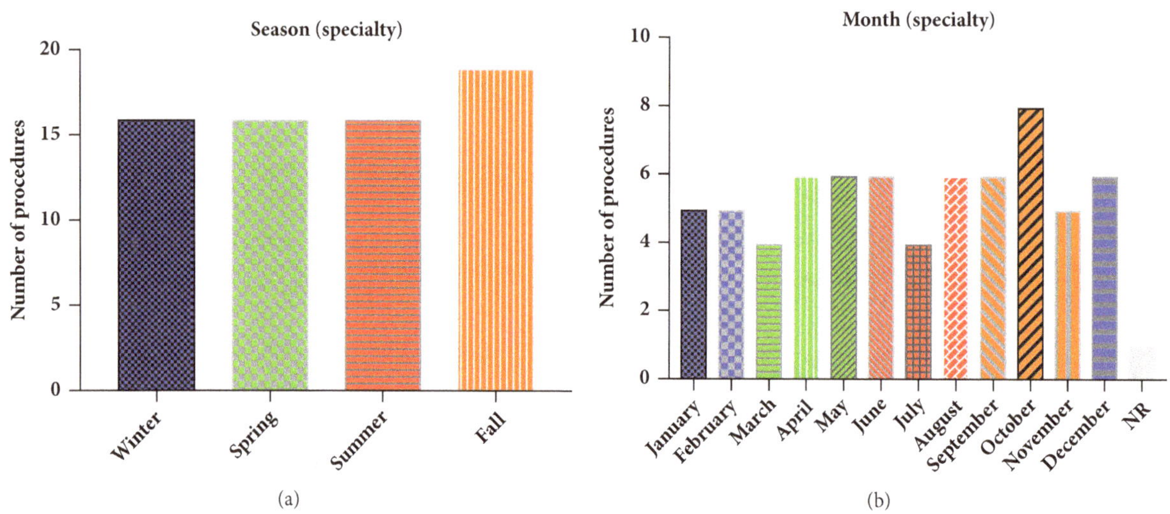

FIGURE 4: *No trends in seasonality nor procedure month at dedicated orthopaedics hospital.* (a) The season during which procedures resulting in PJIs at the dedicated orthopaedics specialty hospital were performed is shown. (b) The particular month during which procedures resulting in PJIs at the dedicated orthopaedics specialty hospital were performed is shown, with the months color-coded corresponding to the season.

orthopaedic specialty hospital. In particular, we found an overall lower infection rate at the dedicated orthopaedics specialty hospital with a greater bacterial diversity and higher rate of Gram-negative infections.

While seasonality could certainly impact the increased incidence of Gram-negative PJIs at the dedicated orthopaedics specialty hospital, given that prior studies showed an increased incidence of Gram-negative infections in the summer months [25, 26], we do not interpret our results to indicate that seasonality impacts the incidence of Gram-negative infections observed at the dedicated orthopaedics specialty hospital compared to the general university hospital. While it is interesting to note the seasonal differences in our two cohorts, given the small sample sizes and minor differences, we cannot reasonably conclude that seasonality impacts the variety of Gram-negative infections observed at the dedicated orthopaedic specialty hospital.

4.2. Gram-Negative Infections and PJIs. Although a lower overall infection rate at the dedicated orthopaedics specialty hospital was observed compared to the general university hospital, there was a greater variety of Gram-negative bacteria among the PJIs at the specialty hospital. While much remains to be determined regarding Gram-negative PJIs in the orthopaedic literature, as the most common organisms implicated in PJIs are *Staphylococcus* species [39], some studies have detailed approaches for combatting Gram-negative PJIs in particular settings. Zmitowski et al. reported 31/277 (11.2%)

of PJIs as colonized with Gram-negative bacteria, with *E. coli* being the most common pathogen; other colonizers included *Proteus, Serratia,* and *Klebsiella* [40]—similar pathogens were observed in this series, but at a higher proportion of Gram-negative infections. Furthermore, given that Zmitowski et al. described Gram-negative organisms resistant to third-generation cephalosporins, ciprofloxacin, or gentamicin, when applied to this study, those findings potentially suggest that the Gram-negative bacteria reported in our study may have been resistant to current prophylactic regimens consisting primarily of cephalosporins. Antimicrobial resistance is a particular issue in Gram-negative infections, and, in 2009, Martinez-Pastor et al. reported 47 cases of PJIs due to Gram-negative bacteria, with the most frequent pathogens being members of the *Enterobacteriaceae* family and *Pseudomonas* species, with some resistance occurring to ciprofloxacin in the *Enterobacteriaceae* family [41]. One case report of PJI following total hip arthroplasty found *Clostridium perfingens,* despite receiving intravenous cefuroxime [42], again indicating that prophylactic administration of cephalosporins may not prevent the development of Gram-negative PJIs. In another retrospective observational study, 242 cases of Gram-negative PJIs were reported over a 7-year timespan with *Enterobacteriaceae* (78%) and *Pseuduomonas* species (20%) as the most common isolates, with 19% of isolates being ciprofloxacin-resistant [43]. Together, these previous reports of Gram-negative PJIs, while limited in scope, indicate that even prophylactic administration of cephalosporins may not provide sufficient coverage for all PJI-causing pathogens, particularly in the case of some Gram-negative bacteria. Further studies will be necessary to characterize the prevalence of Gram-negative infections in other hospital settings, and specifically in the rising number of orthopaedic specialty hospitals.

Furthermore, over the time period in which our study was conducted from 2008 to 2016, several new techniques for identifying clinical bacterial isolates have become more widely utilized in clinical laboratories. Standard protocols involve obtaining culture specimes intraoperatively through swabs and tissue samples, followed by sterile transport to a clinical microbiology laboratory for processing and culture. Newer methods include amplifying bacterial genomes of interest through polymerase chain reactions (PCR) or sequencing of bacterial genomes, known as 16S rRNA sequencing for targeting prokaryote rather than eukaryote genome, or alternatively mass spectrometry and 16S rRNA quantitative PCR to estimate bacterial load [44–46]. Although these advances in isolating clinical bacterial species could theoretically contribute to differences of bacterial species identified over the same timeframe if these newer sensitive tests were utilized in the specialty hospital and not the general hospital, given that our study relied on culture results in both settings, differences in these methods are not applicable to the results presented here.

4.3. Strengths and Limitations. This study provided a unique opportunity to examine one university system in its transition from orthopaedics practice at a general university hospital to a dedicated orthopaedic specialty hospital. By studying one university system, rather than comparing a community hospital to a separate specialty hospital, we attempted to control for many factors. Although the operative venue changed in 2008, there was no change in the surgeons, residents, patient population served, or discrete changes in surgical technique or irrigation solution, including betadine washes, thus minimizing confounding variables. Despite this strength, given the rare occurrence of infection it is difficult to perform in-depth statistical analysis to elucidate risk factors for infection within this sample. Additionally, as there has been other infection control measures to reduce infection over the past decade it would be speculative to presume that the transition to a dedicated specialty hospital is the sole reason for the reduced infection rate. Additional benefits to reduce infection at a dedicated orthopaedic hospital can include streamlined anesthesia teams and sterile supply processing with dedicated OR staff resulting in shorter OR times, as shown in Table 3, and consistent attention to sterility needed for arthroplasty cases. Additionally, although we are unable to quantify measures of stricter adherence to Surgical Care Improvement Project guidelines or reduction in OR traffic, the consistent attention to sterility is paramount for total joint replacements. Finally, as this study examined the transition from a general hospital to a specialty hospital within an academic setting that has a large catchment area with a diverse patient population, we acknowledge that these results may not be translatable to other practice settings.

4.4. Conclusions and Future Directions. In this study, the infection rates and demographic and microbiologic characteristics between patients with PJIs at a general university hospital, were compared to the PJIs after the same university system transitioned to a dedicated orthopaedic specialty hospital. There was a decreased overall infection rate; however, a greater proportion of infections were from Gram-negative organisms with a variety of Gram-negative organisms isolated. These results indicate a potential nuance in dedicated orthopaedic specialty hospital care and need to further study infection prevention and treatment strategies to continue to minimize PJI.

Disclosure

This manuscript was presented at the Southern Orthopaedic Association 34th Annual Meeting.

References

[1] S. Kurtz, K. Ong, E. Lau, F. Mowat, and M. Halpern, "Projections of primary and revision hip and knee arthroplasty in the United States from 2005 to 2030," *The Journal of Bone & Joint Surgery* vol. 89, no. 4, pp. 780–785, 2007.

[2] H.-Y. Chiang, L. A. Herwaldt, A. E. Blevins, E. Cho, and M. L. Schweizer, "Effectiveness of local vancomycin powder to decrease surgical site infections: A meta-analysis," *The Spine Journal*, vol. 14, no. 3, pp. 397–407, 2014.

[3] K. L. Garvin and B. S. Konigsberg, "Infection Following Total Knee Arthroplasty," *The Journal of Bone & Joint Surgery*, vol. 93, no. 12, pp. 1167–1175, 2011.

[4] L. Pulido, E. Ghanem, A. Joshi, J. J. Purtill, and J. Parvizi, "Periprosthetic joint infection: the incidence, timing, and predisposing factors," *Clinical Orthopaedics and Related Research*, vol. 466, no. 7, pp. 1710–1715, 2008.

[5] E. S. R. Darley and A. P. MacGowan, "Antibiotic treatment of Gram-positive bone and joint infections," *Journal of Antimicrobial Chemotherapy*, vol. 53, no. 6, pp. 928–935, 2004.

[6] E. Moran, S. Masters, A. R. Berendt, P. McLardy-Smith, I. Byren, and B. L. Atkins, "Guiding empirical antibiotic therapy in orthopaedics: the microbiology of prosthetic joint infection managed by debridement, irrigation and prosthesis retention," *Infection*, vol. 55, no. 1, pp. 1–7, 2007.

[7] C. S. Oishi, W. V. Carrion, and F. T. Hoaglund, "Use of parenteral prophylactic antibiotics in clean orthopaedic surgery. A review of the literature," *Clinical Orthopaedics and Related Research*, vol. 296, no. 249, 1993.

[8] D. J. Schurman, H. P. Hirshman, G. Kajiyama, K. Moser, and D. S. Burton, "Cefazolin concentrations in bone and synovial fluid," *The Journal of Bone & Joint Surgery*, vol. 60, no. 3, pp. 359–362, 1978.

[9] H. C. Neu, "Cephalosporin Antibiotics as Applied in Surgery of Bones and Joints," *Clinical Orthopaedics and Related Research*, vol. 190, no. 50, 1984.

[10] D. C. Classen, R. S. Evans, S. L. Pestotnik, S. D. Horn, R. L. Menlove, and J. P. Burke, "The timing of prophylactic administration of antibiotics and the risk of surgical-wound infection," *The New England Journal of Medicine*, vol. 326, no. 5, pp. 281–286, 1992.

[11] J. Commission, *Specifications Manual for Joint Commission National Quality Core Measures*, The Joint Commission, Oakbrook Terrace, IL, USA, 2014.

[12] S. K. Fridkin, J. C. Hageman, M. Morrison et al., "Methicillin-resistant Staphylococcus aureus disease in three communities," *The New England Journal of Medicine*, vol. 352, no. 14, pp. 1436–1505, 2005.

[13] B. Hota, C. Ellenbogen, M. K. Hayden, A. Aroutcheva, T. W. Rice, and R. A. Weinstein, "Community-associated methicillin-resistant Staphylococcus aureus skin and soft tissue infections at a public hospital: Do public housing and incarceration amplify transmission?" *JAMA Internal Medicine*, vol. 167, no. 10, pp. 1026–1033, 2007.

[14] M. A. Olsen, J. J. Nepple, K. D. Riew et al., "Risk factors for surgical site infection following orthopaedic spinal operations," *The Journal of Bone & Joint Surgery*, vol. 90, no. 1, pp. 62–69, 2008.

[15] P. O'Toole, M. G. Maltenfort, A. F. Chen, and J. Parvizi, "Projected Increase in Periprosthetic Joint Infections Secondary to Rise in Diabetes and Obesity," *The Journal of Arthroplasty*, vol. 31, no. 1, pp. 7–10, 2016.

[16] Z. Ma, F. Guo, J. Qi, W. Xiang, and J. Zhang, "Meta-analysis shows that obesity may be a significant risk factor for prosthetic joint infections," *International Orthopaedics*, vol. 40, no. 4, pp. 659–667, 2016.

[17] M. H. A. Nocon, C. Russell, G. Westrich, B. Brause, and A. Miller, "The Influence of Obesity on the Infection Risk of Prosthetic Joint Infection in the Geriatric Orthopedic Population," in *Open Forum Infectious Diseases*, p. S98, Oxford University Press, 2017.

[18] L. Font-Vizcarra, E. Tornero, G. Bori, J. Bosch, J. Mensa, and A. Soriano, "Relationship between intraoperative cultures during hip arthroplasty, obesity, and the risk of early prosthetic joint infection: A prospective study of 428 patients," *The International Journal of Artificial Organs*, vol. 34, no. 9, pp. 870–875, 2011.

[19] K. J. Bozic, D. T. Ward, E. C. Lau et al., "Risk factors for periprosthetic joint infection following primary total hip arthroplasty: a case control study," *The Journal of Arthroplasty*, vol. 29, no. 1, pp. 154–156, 2014.

[20] C. D. Watts, M. T. Houdek, E. R. Wagner, M. P. Abdel, and M. J. Taunton, "Insulin Dependence Increases the Risk of Failure After Total Knee Arthroplasty in Morbidly Obese Patients," *The Journal of Arthroplasty*, vol. 31, no. 1, pp. 256–259, 2016.

[21] A. W. Chambers, K. W. Lacy, M. H. L. Liow, J. P. M. Manalo, A. A. Freiberg, and Y.-M. Kwon, "Multiple hip intra-articular steroid injections increase risk of periprosthetic joint infection compared with single injections," *The Journal of Arthroplasty*, vol. 32, no. 6, pp. 1980–1983, 2017.

[22] E. F. Berbari, A. D. Hanssen, and M. C. Duffy, "Risk factors for prosthetic joint infection: case-control study," *Clinical Infectious Diseases*, vol. 27, no. 5, pp. 1247–1254, 1998.

[23] S. Kaspar and J. de V de Beer, "Infection in hip arthroplasty after previous injection of steroid," *The Bone & Joint Journal*, vol. 87, no. 4, p. 454, 2005.

[24] A. L. McIntosh, A. D. Hanssen, D. E. Wenger, and D. R. Osmon, "Recent intraarticular steroid injection may increase infection rates in primary THA," *Clinical Orthopaedics and Related Research*, no. 451, pp. 50–54, 2006.

[25] P. Kane, C. Chen, Z. Post, K. Radcliff, F. Orozco, and A. Ong, "Seasonality of infection rates after total joint arthroplasty," *Orthopedics*, vol. 37, no. 2, pp. e182–e186, 2014.

[26] M. J. Durkin, K. V. Dicks, A. W. Baker et al., "Seasonal variation of common surgical site infections: Does season matter?" *Infection Control and Hospital Epidemiology*, vol. 36, no. 9, pp. 1011–1016, 2015.

[27] C. Doro, J. Dimick, R. Wainess, G. Upchurch, and A. Urquhart, "Hospital Volume and Inpatient Mortality Outcomes of Total Hip Arthroplasty in the United States," *The Journal of Arthroplasty*, vol. 21, no. 6, pp. 10–16, 2006.

[28] D. H. Solomon, E. Losina, J. A. Baron et al., "Contribution of hospital characteristics to the volume-outcome relationship: Dislocation and infection following total hip replacement surgery," *Arthritis & Rheumatology*, vol. 46, no. 9, pp. 2436–2444, 2002.

[29] T. Bhattacharyya, M. S. Vrahas, S. M. Morrison et al., "The value of the dedicated orthopaedic trauma operating room," *Journal of Trauma - Injury Infection and Critical Care*, vol. 60, no. 6, pp. 1336–1340, 2006.

[30] D. Lemos, E. Nilssen, B. Khatiwada et al., "Dedicated orthopedic trauma theatres: effect on morbidity and mortality in a single trauma centre," *Canadian Journal of Surgery*, vol. 52, no. 2, pp. 87–91, 2009.

[31] D. R. Osmon, E. F. Berbari, A. R. Berendt et al., "Diagnosis and management of prosthetic joint infection: clinical practice guidelines by the infectious diseases Society of America," *Clinical Infectious Diseases*, vol. 56, no. 1, pp. e1–e25, 2013.

[32] J. Parvizi, T. L. Tan, K. Goswami et al., "The 2018 definition of periprosthetic hip and knee infection: an evidence-based and validated criteria," *The Journal of Arthroplasty*, vol. 33, no. 5, p. 1309, 2018.

[33] J. Parvizi, B. Zmistowski, E. F. Berbari et al., "New definition

for periprosthetic joint infection: from the workgroup of the musculoskeletal infection society," *Clinical Orthopaedics and Related Research*, vol. 469, no. 11, pp. 2992–2994, 2011.

[34] R. Voelker, "Specialty hospitals generate revenue and controversy," *Journal of the American Medical Association*, vol. 289, no. 4, pp. 409-410, 2003.

[35] J. K. Iglehart, "The emergence of physician-owned specialty hospitals," *The New England Journal of Medicine*, vol. 352, no. 1, pp. 78–84, 2005.

[36] P. Cram, G. E. Rosenthal, and M. S. Vaughan-Sarrazin, "Cardiac revascularization in specialty and general hospitals," *The New England Journal of Medicine*, vol. 352, no. 14, pp. 1454–1507, 2005.

[37] A. W. Heinemann, G. M. Yarkony, E. J. Roth et al., "Functional outcome following spinal cord injury: A comparison of specialized spinal cord injury center vs general hospital short-term care," *JAMA Neurology*, vol. 46, no. 10, pp. 1098–1102, 1989.

[38] L. Greenwald, J. Cromwell, W. Adamache et al., "Specialty versus community hospitals: Referrals, quality, and community benefits," *Health Affairs*, vol. 25, no. 1, pp. 106–118, 2006.

[39] J. Parvizi, E. Ghanem, S. Menashe, R. L. Barrack, and T. W. Bauer, "Periprosthetic infection: What are the diagnostic challenges?" *The Journal of Bone & Joint Surgery*, vol. 88, Suppl 4, pp. 138–147, 2006.

[40] B. Zmistowski, C. J. Fedorka, E. Sheehan, G. Deirmengian, M. S. Austin, and J. Parvizi, "Prosthetic joint infection caused by gram-negative organisms," *The Journal of Arthroplasty*, vol. 26, no. 6, pp. 104–108, 2011.

[41] J. C. Martínez-Pastor, E. Muñoz-Mahamud, F. Vilchez et al., "Outcome of acute prosthetic joint infections due to gram-negative bacilli treated with open debridement and retention of the prosthesis," *Antimicrobial Agents and Chemotherapy*, vol. 53, no. 11, pp. 4772–4777, 2009.

[42] J. F. Baker, M. H. Vioreanu, and J. A. Harty, "Clostridium perfringens infection complicating periprosthetic fracture fixation about the hip: Successful treatment with early aggressive debridement," *Hip International*, vol. 22, no. 1, pp. 122–125, 2012.

[43] D. Rodríguez-Pardo, C. Pigrau, J. Lora-Tamayo et al., "Gram-negative prosthetic joint infection: outcome of a debridement, antibiotics and implant retention approach. A large multicentre study," *Clinical Microbiology and Infection*, vol. 20, no. 11, pp. O911–O919, 2014.

[44] R. Patel, "MALDI-TOF MS for the diagnosis of infectious diseases," *Clinical Chemistry*, vol. 61, no. 1, pp. 100–111, 2015.

[45] L. Váradi, J. L. Luo, D. E. Hibbs et al., "Methods for the detection and identification of pathogenic bacteria: Past, present, and future," *Chemical Society Reviews*, vol. 46, no. 16, pp. 4818–4832, 2017.

[46] A. Spichler, B. L. Hurwitz, D. G. Armstrong, and B. A. Lipsky, "Microbiology of diabetic foot infections: from Louis Pasteur to 'crime scene investigation'," *BMC Medicine*, vol. 13, no. 1, article 2, 2015.

32

Efficacy of the Combined Administration of Systemic and Intra-Articular Tranexamic Acid in Total Hip Arthroplasty Secondary to Femoral Neck Fracture

Joseph Maalouly,[1] Antonios Tawk,[2] Rami Ayoubi,[1] Georges Katoul Al Rahbani,[2] Aida Metri,[2] Elias Saidy,[1] Gerard El-Hajj,[3] and Alexandre Nehme[1]

[1]*Department of Orthopedic Surgery and Traumatology, Saint George Hospital University Medical Center, Balamand University, P.O. Box 166378, Achrafieh, Beirut 1100 2807, Lebanon*
[2]*Faculty of Medicine and Medical Sciences, University of Balamand, Aschrafieh, Beirut, Lebanon*
[3]*Department of Medical Imaging and Radiology, Saint George Hospital University Medical Center, Balamand University, P.O. Box 166378, Achrafieh, Beirut 1100 2807, Lebanon*

Correspondence should be addressed to Joseph Maalouly; josephmaalouly2@gmail.com

Academic Editor: Allen L. Carl

Background. Total hip arthroplasty (THA) is associated with substantial blood loss in the postoperative course. Tranexamic acid (TXA) is a potent antifibrinolytic agent, routinely administered by intravenous (IV) and topical (intra-articular, IA) route, which can possibly interrupt the cascade of events due to hemostatic irregularities close to the source of bleeding. However, scientific evidence of combined administration of TXA in THA secondary to a femoral neck fracture is still meagre. The present study aims to compare the patients who were administered combined IV and topical TXA with a control group in terms of blood loss, transfusion rate, and incidence of deep vein thrombosis (DVT) and thromboembolism (TE). *Patients and Methods.* 195 patients with femoral neck fracture underwent THA and were placed into two groups: (1) IV and IA TXA group which had 58 patients and (2) no TXA control group which had 137 patients. In the TXA group, 1 g IV TXA was administered 30 minutes before incision, and 1 g IA TXA was administered intraoperatively after fascia closure. No drains were placed, and soft spica was applied to the hip. *Results.* Combined usage of IV and IA TXA showed better results when compared to the control group in terms of blood transfusion rate (31%) and hemoglobin drop (28%). No cases of DVT or TE were noted among the two study groups. *Conclusion* Combined use of IV and IA TXA provided significantly better results compared to no TXA use with respect to all variables related to postoperative blood loss in THA. Moreover, TXA use is safe in terms of incidence of symptomatic DVT and TE.

1. Introduction

Large amounts of perioperative blood loss and large transfusion rates are associated with total joint replacement surgeries. Total hip arthroplasty (THA) patients are transfused at rates of 16–37% [1]. Femoral neck fractures are pathological entities associated with high mortality and morbidity and are projected to reach more than 6 million cases in the next 30 years [2]. When compared to hemiarthroplasty, THA is associated with better functional outcome scores and decreased reported pain throughout the postoperative course. However, there is an increased risk in THA regarding blood loss, surgery time, and risk of dislocation [3]. The perioperative blood loss in THA may lead to hematomas formation and in certain cases to acute anemia, subsequently resulting in blood transfusions with their associated risks (cardiopulmonary events and transfusion reactions) and health care costs [4]. In addition, allogeneic blood transfusions can also raise the patient's risk of adverse immunological reaction, disease transmission, and postoperative infection [5]. Therefore, every operation stimulates the fibrinolytic process transiently [6]. There is no replacement, of course, for effective surgical technique and local hemostasis intraoperatively. Nevertheless, through various means such as hypotensive anesthesia [7], drain clamping [8], preoperative autologous blood donation [9], and the use of antifibrinolytic agents, a surgeon can reduce the risk of blood loss.

Tranexamic acid (TXA) is a potent antifibrinolytic agent, which may interrupt the cascade of events due to hemostatic irregularities close to the bleeding source. Tranexamic acid, a synthetic analogue of amino acid lysine, prevents fibrinolysis by competitively blocking plasminogen lysine-binding sites, resulting in reduced proteolytic activity on fibrin monomers and fibrinogen, resulting in clot stabilization. [10]. It reaches a concentration of 90%–100% in joints compared with its plasma concentration [11]. In addition, TXA concentrations of up to 10 mg/mL of blood do not influence platelet counts, coagulation times, or various coagulation factors in whole blood or citrated blood from healthy subjects [12].

However, isolated case reports of thrombus formation have been reported, leading to concerns about the risk of thromboembolic complications in a patient population that is already at high risk for deep vein thrombosis (DVT) and pulmonary embolism (PE). This prevented widespread acceptance of IV antifibrinolytics in full joint replacement operations [13, 14].

Furthermore, multiple studies [15–17] including a meta-analysis [18] showed the potential of topical (IA) TXA to be equivalent or even better than intravenous (IV) TXA. In addition, a recent study by Lin et al. [19] found that the efficacy of combined TXA administration is higher than topical use alone. Thus, it is imperative to say that a combined administration of TXA may prove to be more effective compared with topical or intravenous TXA use alone.

The present study was therefore conducted to compare the efficacy of the combined use of IV and IA TXA with that of no use of TXA in terms of total blood loss and allogeneic transfusion rate and to assess the safety profile of each regimen in terms of DVT and TE incidence. As the additional use of topical TXA increases the probability of enhanced antifibrinolytic activity, we hypothesized that there will be a significant difference between the group with the combined use of IV and IA TXA and the group without TXA use in terms of blood loss, allogeneic blood transfusion rate, and hemoglobin (Hb) drop.

2. Materials and Methods

For this study, written informed consent was obtained from all the patients recruited.

A retrospective study of a single institution was conducted. All patients aged 50 to 100 diagnosed with femoral neck fracture and scheduled for primary arthroplasty by the senior author were eligible. The study excluded patients with history of renal impairment, cardiovascular disease (previous myocardial infarction, atrial fibrillation), or cerebrovascular disease (previous stroke or peripheral vascular surgery). Patients with history of thromboembolic disease, allergy to TXA, bleeding disorder, or receiving anticoagulant

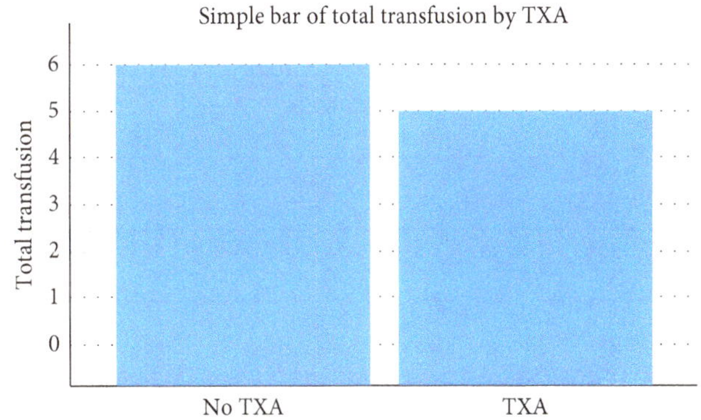

Figure 1: Superiority of the TXA regimen.

drug treatment were also excluded. Preoperative blood transfusions for patient preparation were not taken into account. Between January 2016 and September 2019, 195 patients (75 males and 120 females) were successfully recruited into two groups: (1) IV and IA TXA; and (2) no TXA.

30 minutes prior to incision, 1 g of IV TXA was given. All hip surgeries were operated with the standard posterolateral approach to the hip in order to decrease variability within the study, and noncemented prostheses were used. No drains were placed, and the closure of the wound was performed in a standard fashion in all cases. Soft spica was applied after dressing application. Intra-articular tranexamic acid 1 g in 20 mL NaCl was used after fascia closure in all surgeries. Postoperatively, all patients underwent a standard institution thromboembolic prophylaxis protocol. Pneumatic calf pumps were given immediately postoperatively until the patient started ambulating. As per the National Institute for Health and Care Excellence (NICE) recommendation, subcutaneous lovenox (enoxaparin sodium) 40 mg once daily (Sanofi, Paris, France) was given to all patients on the first postoperative day (POD) and continued until discharge from the hospital around 6 days postoperatively. Anticoagulation therapy was continued at home for a total of 35 days from the operation. All patients underwent inpatient postoperative physiotherapy with the aim of early mobilization. No screening for deep vein thrombosis was done in the postoperative period to detect asymptomatic occurrence. For symptomatic patients, evaluation with ultrasonography of the lower limb deep veins and CT scan of the chest (PE protocol) was done.

The primary outcomes of this study were transfusion incidences, postoperative drop in serum hemoglobin level while the secondary outcomes include duration of surgery, length of hospital stay, wound complications, and thromboembolic events within 30 days of surgery. Outcomes such as total blood loss, intraoperative blood, and hidden blood loss were not taken into account in this study.

At the institution where this study was performed, a serum hemoglobin level of less than 8.0 g/dl was considered the transfusion trigger. For patients presenting with anemic symptoms or any anemia-related organ dysfunctions, the transfusion trigger was less than 10.0 g/dl.

Table 1: The demographics of the studied population in the current study.

Group statistics	Group	N	Mean	Std. deviation	Std. error mean
Pre-op Hgb	No TXA	137	12.133	1.9545	0.1670
	TXA	58	12.224	1.5226	0.1999
D1 PO Hgb	No TXA	137	10.560	1.3907	0.1188
	TXA	58	11.048	1.3806	0.1813
D5 PO Hgb	No TXA	137	10.251	1.0346	0.0884
	TXA	57	10.309	1.0863	0.1439
Total transfusion	No TXA	137	1.58	1.443	0.123
	TXA	58	1.10	1.209	0.159
Age	No TXA	137	70.42	16.478	1.408
	TXA	58	73.76	13.187	1.732
Hb preop-Hb postop1	No TXA	58	1.573	0.56	0.05
Hb preop-Hb postop1	TXA	137	1.176	0.15	0.02

Table 2: Correlation between TXA use and hemoglobin levels and total transfusion.

Correlations		Total transfusion	TXA	D5 PO Hgb	Pre-op Hgb	D1 PO Hgb
Total transfusion	Pearson correlation	1	−0.158*	−0.200**	−0.599**	−0.450**
	Sig. (2-tailed)		0.027	0.005	0.000	0.000
	N	195	195	194	195	195
TXA	Pearson correlation	−0.158*	1	0.025	0.023	0.160*
	Sig. (2-tailed)	0.027		0.726	0.751	0.026
	N	195	195	194	195	195
D5 PO Hgb	Pearson correlation	−0.200**	0.025	1	0.277**	0.436**
	Sig. (2-tailed)	0.005	0.726		0.000	0.000
	N	194	194	194	194	194
Pre-op Hgb	Pearson correlation	−0.599**	0.023	0.277**	1	0.474**
	Sig. (2-tailed)	0.000	0.751	0.000		0.000
	N	195	195	194	195	195
D1 PO Hgb	Pearson correlation	−0.450**	0.160*	0.436**	0.474**	1
	Sig. (2-tailed)	0.000	0.026	0.000	0.000	
	N	195	195	194	195	195

*Correlation is significant at the 0.05 level (2-tailed). **Correlation is significant at the 0.01 level (2-tailed). Pre-op = preoperative, Hgb = hemoglobin, D = day, PO = postoperative.

3. Statistical Analysis

Statistical analysis was carried out in consultation with the in-house biostatistician, using SPSS® 25.0 (IBM, Armonk, New York, United States). Statistical significance was defined as a p value of ≤0.05. Testing for normality was done with the Shapiro-Wilk test. We used Levene's test for equality of variances and Student's t-test for equality of means.

4. Results

Our results show a decrease in the transfusion rate in the TXA group as seen in Figure 1. No statistically significant difference was found between the two studied groups in matter of age (Table 1) and BMI. Table 2 shows that there is a significant negative Pearson correlation between TXA and blood transfusions ($p < 0.05$) and a positive Pearson correlation between TXA and hemoglobin levels on the first postoperative day. This is interpreted as tranexamic acid use decreases blood transfusions and leads to higher first day hemoglobin levels. Furthermore, a negative Pearson correlation is present between hemoglobin levels preoperatively and blood transfusions ($p < 0.01$), and a positive correlation between hemoglobin preoperatively and hemoglobin levels at day 1 and day 5 postoperatively ($p < 0.01$). This suggests that a higher preoperative hemoglobin reduces the need for transfusions and these patients have higher hemoglobin levels postoperatively. Levene's test was used for equality of variances and Student's t-test for equality of means as shown in Table 3. Our findings show no statistically significant difference in terms of preoperative hemoglobin levels and hemoglobin levels at day 5 postoperatively, while statistically significant difference between the two groups was noted in terms of day 1 postoperative hemoglobin levels and total amount of transfusions used intraoperatively and postoperatively. Since $p < 0.05$ is less than our chosen significance level $\alpha = 0.05$, we can reject the null hypothesis and conclude that statistically significant difference is present between the TXA group and the control group in terms of day 1 postoperative hemoglobin levels and total amount of transfusion.

5. Discussion

In the current study, the primary endpoint is the decrease in the hemoglobin drop and the decrease in transfusion rate seen with IV and IA administration of TXA in THA. The

Table 3: *t*-test for the TXA group and the control group.

Independent samples test										
		Levene's test for equality of variances		*t*-test for equality of means						
		F	Sig.	*T*	Df	Sig. (2-tailed)	Mean difference	Std. error difference	95% confidence interval of the difference Lower	Upper
Pre-op Hgb	Equal variances assumed	4.680	0.032	−0.317	193	0.751	−0.0913	0.2879	−0.6591	0.4765
	Equal variances not assumed			−0.350	136.438	0.727	−0.0913	0.2605	−0.6064	0.4238
D1 PO Hgb	Equal variances assumed	0.000	0.988	−2.247	193	0.026	−0.4884	0.2174	−0.9172	−0.0597
	Equal variances not assumed			−2.253	108.127	0.026	−0.4884	0.2167	−0.9180	−0.0588
D5 PO Hgb	Equal variances assumed	0.486	0.487	−0.351	192	0.726	−0.0580	0.1655	−0.3844	0.2684
	Equal variances not assumed			−0.344	100.365	0.732	−0.0580	0.1689	−0.3930	0.2770
Total transfusion	Equal variances assumed	1.450	0.230	2.225	193	0.027	0.480	0.216	0.055	0.906
	Equal variances not assumed			2.390	127.083	0.018	0.480	0.201	0.083	0.878
Age	Equal variances assumed	1.707	0.193	−1.367	193	0.173	−3.335	2.440	−8.149	1.478
	Equal variances not assumed			−1.495	132.919	0.137	−3.335	2.232	−7.749	1.079

Pre-op = preoperative, Hgb = hemoglobin, *D* = day, PO = postoperative.

drop in hemoglobin (Hgb) was 28% lower in THA when TXA was used. This translated into a much lower risk of requiring a blood transfusion in the THA patients in which TXA was used. The patients with TXA required 31% less transfusion on average than the control group. The protocol used in this study consisted of 1 g IV tranexamic acid 30 minutes before incision and 1 g injection after fascia closure without placing any drains and with soft spica application looks to be effective and safe. There was no reported symptomatic thromboembolic event.

Currently, TXA is FDA approved only for tooth extraction in hemophilia patients. TXA distributes widely in the extracellular and intracellular compartments when given IV [20]. It spreads rapidly into the synovial fluid until the TXA concentration in the synovial fluid reaches the serum concentration [21]. Its biological half-life in the joint fluid is three hours, and glomerular filtration eliminates 90% within 24 hours [22, 23]. Compared to IV administration, intra-articular TXA advocates believe that the benefits include easy administration, maximum concentration at the bleeding site, and minimal systemic absorption. The objective of both delivery systems is to achieve a concentration of approximately 10 mg/mL [20].

Antifibrinolytics have been in use since the 1960s as a class of drugs [22]. TXA is an amino acid lysine analogue. It competitively inhibits the activation of plasminogen and the binding of plasmin to fibrin, inhibiting the degradation of fibrin [13]. Since it works by increasing the breakdown of fibrin when created, it is not necessarily a procoagulant but promotes coagulation already in progress. This makes TXA potentially suitable for use in reducing postoperative bleeding, where surgical hemostasis has been achieved and fibrinolytic activity needs to be suppressed to help maintain hemostasis without promoting the formation of venous thrombus.

In a meta-analysis of all operations, tranexamic acid has been shown to reduce the risk of transfusion by a third [23]. It was used successfully through an intravenous route in orthopedic surgery, with several studies showing significant reductions in bleeding and transfusion risk following THA [24]. Nevertheless, the possibility of thromboembolic complications following systemic administration remains a concern [13, 14].

Kagoma et al. [25] studied the impact of antifibrinolytics on blood transfusion reduction, showing a decrease in blood transfusion rate, after total knee and hip arthroplasties.

Rajesparan et al. reported less blood loss in the TXA group in a study of 73 patients undergoing THA [26]. Gill and Rosenstein found that the use of IV TXA in different doses significantly reduced intraoperative and total blood loss during the review of 13 randomized controlled trials [27].

Zhou et al. meta-analysis of 19 randomized control experiments using different doses of IV TXA in THA found marked reductions in total, intraoperative, postoperative, and secret blood loss in the TXA group compared to the control group [28].

No significant difference in safety between the different methods was noted after a comprehensive review of the literature [29]. For THA, Amin et al. suggested administering a dose of 15 mg/kg IV given 10 minutes before incision and 3 g in 100 mL of saline soak as defined intraoperatively by Melvin [30].

Based on the evidence in the literature, Hayes et al. recommend a regimen consisting of a 1 g IV dose of TXA to be administered before incision or tourniquet inflation with an additional 1 g IV dose given at closure [31].

Based on the current evidence-based medicine, clinicians and patients need to know the possible clinical benefits and risks of TXA, when deciding on their therapy management following THA. Regarding efficacy and safety, our study suggests that TXA should be indicated in patients undergoing THA secondary to femoral neck fracture. In view of our data, our protocol of 1 g IV tranexamic acid 30 minutes before incision and 1 g injection after fascia closure seems to be effective and safe. The dosing regimen appears to be one of the lowest reported dose in the literature with a good safety profile and efficiency.

6. Conclusion

After thorough review of the literature and according to our data, it is our recommendation that 1 g of TXA in IV be given 30 minutes prior to incision and 1 g TXA intra-articular after fascia closure without drains and with the application of a soft spica, as this is seen to be beneficial in terms of blood loss, blood transfusions, and postoperative hemoglobin drop. This seems important as it decreases hospital costs and risks to the patient from the transfusion and anemia. Our protocol appears safe and effective and may be the safest effective dosing regimen.

6.1. Limitations. This study has several limitations. First, the participants included in our study excluded high risk patients. These included patients with a history of cardiovascular disease, cerebrovascular disease, thromboembolic events, renal failure, allergy to TXA, bleeding diathesis, and those on anticoagulation therapy. Second, differences in surgical techniques and blood transfusion protocol are likely to have contributed to the differences observed among studies. Third, this is a retrospective study. Few studies reported the type of surgical hemostasis utilized; these techniques are known to reduce bleeding during surgery [31].

References

[1] B. E. Bierbaum, J. J. Callaghan, J. O. Galante, H. E. Rubash, R. E. Tooms, and R. B. Welch, "An analysis of blood management in patients having a total hip or knee arthroplasty," *The Journal of Bone & Joint Surgery*, vol. 81, no. 1, pp. 2–10, 1999.

[2] P. Kannus, H. Haapasalo, M. Sankelo et al., "Possibility to increase women's bone mass by physical activity wanes rapidly after puberty," *Bone*, vol. 18, no. 1, pp. S113–S63, 1996.

[3] M. Maceroli, L. E. Nikkel, B. Mahmood et al., "Total hip arthroplasty for femoral neck fractures," *Journal of Orthopaedic Trauma*, vol. 30, no. 11, pp. 597–604, 2016.

[4] J. E. Ollivier, S. Van Driessche, F. Billuart, J. Beldame, and J. Matsoukis, "Tranexamic acid and total hip arthroplasty: optimizing the administration method," *Annals of Translational Medicine*, vol. 4, no. 24, 2016.

[5] K. Charoencholvanich and P. Siriwattanasakul, "Tranexamic acid reduces blood loss and blood transfusion after TKA: a prospective randomized controlled trial," *Clinical Orthopaedics and Related Research*, vol. 469, no. 10, pp. 2874–2880, 2011.

[6] B. Risberg, "The response of the fibrinolytic system in trauma," *Acta Chirurgica Scandinavica. Supplementum*, vol. 522, pp. 245–271, 1985.

[7] N. E. Sharrock and E. A. Salvati, "Hypotensive epidural anesthesia for total hip arthroplasty: a review," *Acta Orthopaedica Scandinavica*, vol. 67, no. 1, pp. 91–107, 1996.

[8] P. Zan, J. J. Yao, L. Fan et al., "Efficacy of a four-hour drainage clamping technique in the reduction of blood loss following total hip arthroplasty: a prospective cohort study," *Medical Science Monitor*, vol. 23, pp. 2708–2714, 2017.

[9] Z. Haien, J. Yong, M. Baoan, G. Mingjun, and F. Qingyu, "Post-operative auto-transfusion in total hip or knee arthroplasty: a meta-analysis of randomized controlled trials," *PLoS One*, vol. 8, no. 1, Article ID e55073, 2013.

[10] C. J. Dunn and K. L. Goa, "Tranexamic acid," *Drugs*, vol. 57, no. 6, pp. 1005–1032, 1999.

[11] B. Åstedt, "Clinical pharmacology of tranexamic acid," *Scandinavian Journal of Gastroenterology*, vol. 22, no. 137, pp. 22–25, 1987.

[12] Pfizer, product information, cyklokapron (tranexamic acid); 2011.

[13] P. M. Mannucci, "Hemostatic drugs," *New England Journal of Medicine*, vol. 339, no. 4, pp. 245–253, 1998.

[14] R. Raveendran and J. Wong, "Tranexamic acid reduces blood transfusion in surgical patients while its effects on thromboembolic events and mortality are uncertain," *Evidence Based Medicine*, vol. 18, no. 2, pp. 65-66, 2013.

[15] S. Alshryda, J. Mason, M. Vaghela et al., "Topical (intra-articular) tranexamic acid reduces blood loss and transfusion rates following total knee replacement," *The Journal of Bone and Joint Surgery-American Volume*, vol. 95, no. 21, pp. 1961–1968, 2013.

[16] R. N. Maniar, G. Kumar, T. Singhi, R. M. Nayak, and P. R. Maniar, "Most effective regimen of tranexamic acid in knee arthroplasty: a prospective randomized controlled study in 240 patients," *Clinical Orthopaedics and Related Research*, vol. 470, no. 9, pp. 2605–2612, 2012.

[17] J.-G. Seo, Y.-W. Moon, S.-H. Park, S.-M. Kim, and K.-R. Ko, "The comparative efficacies of intra-articular and IV tranexamic acid for reducing blood loss during total knee arthroplasty," *Knee Surgery, Sports Traumatology, Arthroscopy*, vol. 21, no. 8, pp. 1869–1874, 2013.

[18] M. Panteli, C. Papakostidis, Z. Dahabreh, and P. V. Giannoudis, "Topical tranexamic acid in total knee replacement: a systematic review and meta-analysis," *The Knee*, vol. 20, no. 5, pp. 300–309, 2013.

[19] S.-Y. Lin, C.-H. Chen, Y.-C. Fu, P.-J. Huang, J.-K. Chang, and H.-T. Huang, "The efficacy of combined use of intraarticular and intravenous tranexamic acid on reducing blood loss and transfusion rate in total knee arthroplasty," *The Journal of Arthroplasty*, vol. 30, no. 5, pp. 776–780, 2015.

[20] I. M. Nilsson, "Clinical pharmacology of aminocaproic and tranexamic acids," *Journal of Clinical Pathology*, vol. 33, no. 1, pp. 41–47, 1980.

[21] A. Ahlberg, O. Eriksson, and H. Kjellman, "Diffusion of tranexamic acid to the joint," *Acta Orthopaedica Scandinavica*, vol. 47, no. 5, pp. 486–488, 1976.

[22] J. D. Eubanks, "Antifibrinolytics in major orthopaedic surgery," *American Academy of Orthopaedic Surgeon*, vol. 18, no. 3, pp. 132–138, 2010.

[23] K. Ker, P. Edwards, P. Perel, H. Shakur, and I. Roberts, "Effect of tranexamic acid on surgical bleeding: systematic review and cumulative meta-analysis," *BMJ*, vol. 344, Article ID e3054, 2012.

[24] J. J. Callaghan, M. R. O'Rourke, and S. S. Liu, "Blood management," *The Journal of Arthroplasty*, vol. 20, no. 4, pp. 51–54, 2005.

[25] Y. K. Kagoma, M. A. Crowther, J. Douketis, M. Bhandari, J. Eikelboom, and W. Lim, "Use of antifibrinolytic therapy to reduce transfusion in patients undergoing orthopedic surgery: a systematic review of randomized trials," *Thrombosis Research*, vol. 123, no. 5, pp. 687–696, 2009.

[26] K. Rajesparan, L. C. Biant, M. Ahmad, and R. E. Field, "The effect of an intravenous bolus of tranexamic acid on blood loss in total hip replacement," *The Journal of Bone and Joint Surgery. British Volume*, vol. 91-B, no. 6, pp. 776–783, 2009.

[27] J. B. Gill and A. Rosenstein, "The use of antifibrinolytic agents in total hip arthroplasty," *The Journal of Arthroplasty*, vol. 21, no. 6, pp. 869–873, 2006.

[28] X.-D. Zhou, L.-J. Tao, J. Li, and L.-D. Wu, "Do we really need tranexamic acid in total hip arthroplasty? a meta-analysis of nineteen randomized controlled trials," *Archives of Orthopaedic and Trauma Surgery*, vol. 133, no. 7, pp. 1017–1027, 2013.

[29] N. H. Amin, T. S. Scudday, and F. D. Cushner, "Systemic versus topical tranexamic acid," *Techniques in Orthopaedics*, vol. 32, no. 1, pp. 23–27, 2017.

[30] J. S. Melvin, L. S. Stryker, and R. J. Sierra, "Tranexamic acid in hip and knee arthroplasty," *Journal of the American Academy of Orthopaedic Surgeons*, vol. 23, no. 12, pp. 732–740, 2015.

[31] A. Hayes, D. B. Murphy, and M. McCarroll, "The efficacy of single-dose aprotinin 2 million KIU in reducing blood loss and its impact on the incidence of deep venous thrombosis in patients undergoing total hip replacement surgery," *Journal of Clinical Anesthesia*, vol. 8, no. 5, pp. 357–360, 1996.

Permissions

All chapters in this book were first published by Hindawi Publishing Corporation; hereby published with permission under the Creative Commons Attribution License or equivalent. Every chapter published in this book has been scrutinized by our experts. Their significance has been extensively debated. The topics covered herein carry significant findings which will fuel the growth of the discipline. They may even be implemented as practical applications or may be referred to as a beginning point for another development.

The contributors of this book come from diverse backgrounds, making this book a truly international effort. This book will bring forth new frontiers with its revolutionizing research information and detailed analysis of the nascent developments around the world.

We would like to thank all the contributing authors for lending their expertise to make the book truly unique. They have played a crucial role in the development of this book. Without their invaluable contributions this book wouldn't have been possible. They have made vital efforts to compile up to date information on the varied aspects of this subject to make this book a valuable addition to the collection of many professionals and students.

This book was conceptualized with the vision of imparting up-to-date information and advanced data in this field. To ensure the same, a matchless editorial board was set up. Every individual on the board went through rigorous rounds of assessment to prove their worth. After which they invested a large part of their time researching and compiling the most relevant data for our readers.

The editorial board has been involved in producing this book since its inception. They have spent rigorous hours researching and exploring the diverse topics which have resulted in the successful publishing of this book. They have passed on their knowledge of decades through this book. To expedite this challenging task, the publisher supported the team at every step. A small team of assistant editors was also appointed to further simplify the editing procedure and attain best results for the readers.

Apart from the editorial board, the designing team has also invested a significant amount of their time in understanding the subject and creating the most relevant covers. They scrutinized every image to scout for the most suitable representation of the subject and create an appropriate cover for the book.

The publishing team has been an ardent support to the editorial, designing and production team. Their endless efforts to recruit the best for this project, has resulted in the accomplishment of this book. They are a veteran in the field of academics and their pool of knowledge is as vast as their experience in printing. Their expertise and guidance has proved useful at every step. Their uncompromising quality standards have made this book an exceptional effort. Their encouragement from time to time has been an inspiration for everyone.

The publisher and the editorial board hope that this book will prove to be a valuable piece of knowledge for researchers, students, practitioners and scholars across the globe.

List of Contributors

Hargita Dömötör, Ádám L. Varga and Gábor Nardai
Department of Anesthesiology and Intensive Care, Péterfy Hospital and National Institute of Trauma, Budapest, Hungary

Róbert Sződy and Ferenc Tóth
Department of Traumatology, Péterfy Hospital and National Institute of Trauma, 1081, Fiumeiút 17, Budapest, Hungary

Laurence Grüber, Georges Kohut and Théa Voser
Clinique Générale Saint-Anne, Cabinet Kohut. Rue Hans-Geiler 6, Fribourg 1700, Switzerland

Leo M. Nherera
Health Economics and Market Access, Smith & Nephew, 5600 Clearfork Main St, Fort Worth, TX 76107, USA

Sanjay Verma
Health Economics and Market Access, Smith & Nephew, 5 Croxley Green Business Park, Hatters Ln, Watford WD18 8YE, Watford, UK

Paul Trueman
Health Economics and Market Access, Smith & Nephew, 101 Hessle Rd, Hull HU3 2BN, UK

Simon Jennings
London North West University Healthcare NHS Trust, Acton Lane Park Royal, London NW10 7NS, UK

Meredith P. Crizer, Amer Haffar, Andrew Battenberg, Mikayla McGrath, Ryan Sutton and Jess H. Lonner
Rothman Orthopaedic Institute at Thomas Jefferson University, Philadelphia, PA, USA

J. Chin, J. Blackett, D. C. Kieser, C. Frampton and G. Hooper
Department of Orthopaedic Surgery and Musculoskeletal Medicine, University of Otago, Christchurch, New Zealand

Christopher Fang and Eric L. Smith
Department of Orthopedic Surgery, New England Baptist Hospital, 125 Parker Hill Ave, Boston, MA 02120, USA

Kenneth McAlpine, Michael Gustin, Ruijia Niu and David Freccero
Department of Orthopedic Surgery, Boston Medical Center, One Boston Medical Center Pl, Boston, MA 02118, USA

Matthew Gordon
Department of Orthopedic Surgery, Tufts Medical Center, 800 Washington St, Boston, MA 02111, USA

Jakub Szczesiul and Marek Bielecki
Department of Orthopedic, Traumatology and Hand Surgery, Medical University of Białystok, Białystok, Poland
Department of Orthopedic, Traumatology and Hand Surgery, Uniwersytecki Szpital Kliniczny w Białymstoku, Białystok, Poland

Qing Li
School of Aerospace, The University of Sydney, Mechanical and Mechatronic Engineering, Building J07, Sydney, NSW2006, Australia

Yolanda Gu
School of Aerospace, The University of Sydney, Mechanical and Mechatronic Engineering, Building J07, Sydney, NSW2006, Australia
Optimized Ortho, 17 Bridge Street, Pymble, NSW2073, Australia

Jim Pierrepont and Catherine Stambouzou
Optimized Ortho, 17 Bridge Street, Pymble, NSW2073, Australia

Jonathan Baré
Melbourne Orthopaedic Group, 33 The Avenue, Windsor, VIC 3191, Australia

Umaima R. Khairy and Sadiq J. Hamandi
Biomedical Engineering Department, College of Engineering, Al-Nahrain University, Baghdad, Iraq

Ahmed S. Abid Ali
Orthopedics Department, College of Medicine, Al-Nahrain University, Baghdad, Iraq

Atef Mohamed Morsy, Emad Gaber Elbana and Ahmed Gaber Mostafa
The Orthopaedic Department, Beni-Suef University, Beni-Suef, Egypt

Mark Ashraf Edward and Mahmoud A. Hafez
The Orthopaedic Department, Faculty of Medicine, October 6 University, Giza, Egypt

Hunter Warwick, Andrew George, Claire Howell, Cynthia Green and William A. Jiranek
Department of Orthopaedic Surgery, Duke University Hospital, Durham, NC 27710, USA

Thorsten M. Seyler
Department of Orthopaedic Surgery, Duke University Hospital, Durham, NC 27710, USA
Department of Orthopaedic Surgery, Duke University Medical Center, Durham, NC, USA
Duke University Medical Center, Durham, NC, USA

Koichiro Okuyama
Akita Rosai Hospital, Japan

Keiji Kamo
Akita Rosai Hospital, Japan
Akita Hip Research Group, Japan
Akita Hip Research Group (AHRG), Akita, Japan

Yoichi Shimada
Akita Hip Research Group, Japan
Department of Orthopedic Surgery, Akita University Graduate School of Medicine, Japan

Naohisa Miyakoshi
Department of Orthopedic Surgery, Akita University Graduate School of Medicine, Japan
Department of Orthopedic Surgery, Akita University Graduate School of Medicine, Akita, Japan

Yasushi Oshima, Norishige Iizawa, Tokifumi Majima and Shinro Takai
Department of Orthopaedic Surgery, Nippon Medical School, 1-1-5 Sendagi, Bunkyo-ku, Tokyo 113 8603, Japan

Nobuyoshi Watanabe
Department of Orthopaedic Surgery, Kyoto Kujo Hospital, 10 Karahashi Rajomoncho, Minami-ku, Kyoto 601-8453, Japan

Mitsuhiro Kawata
School of Health Sciences, Bukkyo University, 7 Higashitoganoo-cho, Nakagyo-ku, Kyoto 604-8418, Japan

Jacob M. Wilson, Kevin X. Farley and Eric R. Wagner
Department of Orthopaedic Surgery, Emory Orthopaedics & Spine Center, 59 S Executive Park NW, Atlanta, GA 30329, USA

George N. Guild and Thomas L. Bradbury
Department of Orthopaedic Surgery, Emory Orthopaedics & Spine Center, 59 S Executive Park NW, Atlanta, GA 30329, USA
Emory University Department of Orthopaedics, Atlanta, GA, USA

Matthew Aizpuru
Emory School of Medicine, 201 Dowman Dr., Atlanta, GA 30322, USA

Yazan Al Thaher
Faculty of Pharmacy, Philadelphia University, Amman 19392, Jordan

Othman A. Alfuqaha
Scientific Research Office, Jordan University Hospital, #e University of Jordan, Amman 11942, Jordan

Ahmed Dweidari
Department of Special Procedure, Division of Orthopedics, School of Medicine, #e University of Jordan, Amman 11942, Jordan

Tetsuya Kawano, Hiroaki Kijima, Masashi Fujii and Takanori Miura
Department of Orthopedic Surgery, Akita University Graduate School of Medicine, Akita, Japan
Akita Hip Research Group (AHRG), Akita, Japan

Shin Yamada, Natsuo Konishi, Hitoshi Kubota, Hiroshi Tazawa, Takayuki Tani, Norio Suzuki, Yoshihiko Okudera, Ken Sasaki, Yosuke Iwamoto and Itsuki Nagahata
Akita Hip Research Group (AHRG), Akita, Japan

E. Grant Sutter, Samuel S. Wellman and Michael P. Bolognesi
Department of Orthopaedic Surgery, Duke University Medical Center, Durham, NC, USA

Kenta Konno, Shigeo Hagiwara, Junichi Nakamura, Yuya Kawarai, Sumihisa Orita, Yawara Eguchi and Seiji Ohtori
Department of Orthopaedics Surgery, Graduate School of Medicine, Chiba University, 1-8-1 Inohana, Chuo-ku, Chiba 260-8670, Japan

Adam M. Katchky
Department of Orthopedics and Rehabilitation, University of Vermont, Burlington, VT, USA

Mitchell L. Smith
Melbourne Orthopaedic Group, Windsor, VIC, Australia

Andrew J. Shimmin and Jonathan V. Baré
Melbourne Orthopaedic Group, Windsor, VIC, Australia
Department of Surgery, Monash University, Melbourne, VIC, Australia

Stephen J. McMahon
Department of Surgery, Monash University, Melbourne, VIC, Australia
Malabar Orthopaedic Clinic, Windsor, VIC, Australia

Jeremy Latham
Spire Southampton Hospital, Southampton, UK

Shaifuzain Ab Rahman, Amran Ahmed Shokri, Muhammad Rajaie Ahmad and Nur Syahida Termizi
Department of Orthopedic, Hospital Universiti Sains Malaysia, 16150 Kubang Kerian, Kelantan, Malaysia

Ahmad Filza Ismail
Department of Community Medicine, Hospital Universiti Sains Malaysia, 16150 Kubang Kerian, Kelantan, Malaysia

Olcay Guler and Hakan Sofu
Department of Orthopedics and Traumatology, Medical Faculty, Altınbaş University, Istanbul, Turkey

Gürkan Gümüşsuyu and Hüseyin Bahadır Gökçen
Department of Orthopedics and Traumatology, Medical Faculty, Istinye University, Istanbul, Turkey

Abdulrahman D. Algarni
Department of Orthopedic Surgery, King Saud University, Riyadh, Saudi Arabia

Dani M. Gaillard-Campbell and Thomas P. Gross
Midlands Orthopaedics & Neurosurgery, 1910 Blanding Street, Columbia, SC 29201, USA

Michael H. Bourne, Tony L.Miller and E. Marc Mariani
Salt Lake Orthopaedic Clinic, St. Mark's Hospital, Salt Lake City, Utah, USA

Kensei Yoshimoto, Masahiko Noguchi, Akifumi Yamada and Yuki Nasu
Orthopaedic Foot and Ankle Center, Shiseikai Daini Hospital, 5-19-1 Kamisoshigaya, Setagaya-ku, Tokyo, 157-8550, Japan

Joseph F. Fetto
The Brooklyn Hospital Medical Center, Brooklyn, NY 11201, USA

Antonio D'Arienzo, Edoardo Ipponi, Alfio Damiano Ruinato, Silvia De Franco, Simone Colangeli, Lorenzo Andreani and Rodolfo Capanna
Department of Orthopaedic and Trauma Surgery, University of Pisa, Pisa, Italy

Y. Watanabe
Department of Orthopaedic Surgery, Teikyo University School of Medicine, Tokyo, Japan

N. Takenaka, T. Matsushita and T. Teramoto
Department of Traumatology Fukushima Medical University, Trauma and Reconstruction Center, Southern Tohoku General Hospital, Fukushima, Japan

K. Kinugasa
Department of Orthopaedic Surgery, Chikamori Hospital, Kochi, Japan

Dafang Zhang, Brandon E. Earp, Philip Blazar and George S. M. Dyer
Department of Orthopaedic Surgery, Brigham and Women's Hospital, 15 Francis St, Boston, MA 02115, USA
Department of Orthopaedic Surgery, Massachusetts General Hospital, 55 Fruit St, Boston, MA 02114, USA

Rohit Garg
Department of Orthopaedic Surgery, Massachusetts General Hospital, 55 Fruit St, Boston, MA 02114, USA
Harvard Medical School, 25 Shattuck St, Boston, MA 02115, USA

Cierra S. Hong, Sean P. Ryan and Michael A. Bergen
Duke University Medical Center, Durham, NC, USA

Jonathan A. Gabor and Ran Schwarzkopf
NYU Langone Health, New York City, NY, USA

Robert P. Runner, James R. Roberson, Scott D. Boden and Greg A. Erens
Emory University Department of Orthopaedics, Atlanta, GA, USA

Amanda Mener
Emory University School of Medicine, Atlanta, GA, USA

Joseph Maalouly, Rami Ayoubi, Elias Saidy and Alexandre Nehme
Department of Orthopedic Surgery and Traumatology, Saint George Hospital University Medical Center, Balamand University, Achrafieh, Beirut 1100 2807, Lebanon

Antonios Tawk, Georges Katoul Al Rahbani and Aida Metri
Faculty of Medicine and Medical Sciences, University of Balamand, Aschrafieh, Beirut, Lebanon

Gerard El-Hajj
Department of Medical Imaging and Radiology, Saint George Hospital University Medical Center, Balamand University, P.O. Box 166378, Achrafieh, Beirut 1100 2807, Lebanon

Index